CASE REVIEW
Pediatric Imaging

Series Editor
David M. Yousem, MD
Professor, Department of Radiology
Director of Neuroradiology
Johns Hopkins Hospital
Baltimore, Maryland

Other Volumes in the Case Review Series
Brain Imaging
Breast Imaging
Cardiac Imaging
Emergency Radiology
Gastrointestinal Imaging
General and Vascular Ultrasound
Genitourinary Imaging
Head and Neck Imaging
Musculoskeletal Imaging
Nuclear Medicine
OB/GYN Ultrasound
Pediatric Imaging
Spine Imaging
Thoracic Imaging
Vascular and Interventional Imaging

Robert J. Ward, MD
Musculoskeletal Imaging
Department of Radiology
Lahey Clinic
Burlington, Massachusetts

Hans Blickman, MD, PhD, FACR
Professor & Chairman
Department of Radiology
UMC Nijmegen
The Netherlands

WITH 524 ILLUSTRATIONS

CASE REVIEW

Pediatric Imaging

CASE REVIEW SERIES

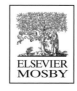

ELSEVIER
MOSBY

ELSEVIER
MOSBY

Mosby, Inc.
An Affiliate of Elsevier Inc.
11830 Westline Industrial Drive
St. Louis, Missouri 63146

PEDIATRIC IMAGING   ISBN: 0-323-00505-5

Notice

Radiology is an ever-changing field. Standard safety precautions must be followed, but as new research and clinical experience broaden our knowledge, changes in treatment and drug therapy may become necessary or appropriate. Readers are advised to check the most current product information provided by the manufacturer of each drug to be administered to verify the recommended dose, the method and duration of administration, and contraindications. It is the responsibility of the licensed prescriber, relying on experience and knowledge of the patient, to determine dosages and the best treatment for each individual patient. Neither the publisher nor the author assumes any liability for any injury and/or damage to persons or property arising from this publication.

The Publisher

Library of Congress Cataloging-in-Publication Data

Ward, Robert J., MD.
   Pediatric imaging : case review / Robert J. Ward, Hans Blickman. – 1st ed.
     p. ; cm.
   Includes bibliographical references.
   ISBN 0-323-00505-5
   1. Pediatric diagnostic imaging—Case studies. 2. Pediatric radiography – Case studies.
3. Children—Diseases—Diagnosis—Case studies. I. Blickman, Hans. II.Title.
   [DNLM: 1. Diagnostic Imaging—Methods—Child—Case Report. 2. Diagnostic
Imaging—methods—Infants—Case Reports. 3. Pediatrics—methods—Case Report. WN 240
W262p 2005]
   RJ51.R3.W37 2005
   618.92'00754—dc22

                                          2003060752

In memory of Dennis J. Kagan

My experience in teaching medical students, residents, fellows, practicing radiologists, and clinicians has been that they love the case conference format more than any other approach. I hope that the reason for this is not a reflection on my lecturing ability, but rather that people stay awake, alert, and on their toes more when they are in the hot seat (or may be the next person to assume the hot seat). In the dozens of continuing medical education courses I have directed, the case review sessions are almost always the most popular parts of the courses.

The idea of this Case Review series grew out of a need for books designed as exam preparation tools for the resident, fellow, or practicing radiologist about to take the boards or the certificate of additional qualification (CAQ) exams. Anxiety runs extremely high concerning the content of these exams, administered as unknown cases. Residents, fellows, and practicing radiologists are very hungry for formats that mimic this exam setting and that cover the types of cases they will encounter and have to accurately describe. In addition, books of this ilk serve as excellent practical reviews of a field and can help a practicing board-certified radiologist keep his or her skills sharpened. Thus heads banged together, and Mosby and I arrived at the format of the volume herein, which is applied consistently to each volume in the series. We believe that these volumes will strengthen the ability of the reader to interpret studies. By formatting the individual cases so that they can "stand alone," these case review books can be read in a leisurely fashion, a case at a time, on the whim of the reader.

The content of each volume is organized into three sections based on difficulty of interpretation and/or the rarity of the lesion presented. There are the Opening Round cases, which graduating radiology residents should have relatively little difficulty mastering. The Fair Game section consists of cases that require more study, but most people should get into the ballpark with their differential diagnoses. Finally, there is the Challenge section. Most fellows or fellowship-trained practicing radiologists will be able to mention entities in the differential diagnoses of these challenging cases, but one shouldn't expect to consistently "hit home runs" a la Mark McGwire. The Challenge cases are really designed to whet one's appetite for further reading on these entities and to test one's wits. Within each of these sections, the selection of cases is entirely random, as one would expect at the boards (in your office or in Louisville).

For many cases in this series, a specific diagnosis may not be what is expected – the quality of the differential diagnosis and the inclusion of appropriate options are most important. Teaching how to distinguish between the diagnostic options (taught in the question and answer and comment sections) will be the goal of the authors of each Case Review volume.

The best way to go through these books is to look at the images, guess the diagnosis, answer the questions, and then turn the page for the answers. If there are two cases on a page, do them two at a time. No peeking!

Mosby (through the strong work of Liz Corra) and I have recruited most of the authors of THE REQUISITES series (editor, James Thrall, MD) to create Case Review books for their subspecialties. To meet the needs of certain subspecialties and to keep each of the volumes to a consistent, practical size, some specialties will have more than one volume (e.g., ultrasound, interventional and vascular radiology, and neuroradiology). Nonetheless, the pleasing tone of THE REQUISITES series and its emphasis on condensing the fields of radiology into its foundations will be inculcated into the Case Review volumes. In many situations, THE REQUISITES authors have enlisted new coauthors to breathe a novel approach and excitement into the cases submitted. I think the fact that so many of THE REQUISITES authors are "on board" for this new series is a testament to their dedication to teaching. I hope that the success of THE REQUISITES is duplicated with the new Case Review series. Just as THE REQUISITES series provides coverage of the essentials in each subspecialty and successfully meets that overwhelming need in the market, I hope that the Case Review series successfully meets the overwhelming need in the market for practical, focused case reviews.

David M. Yousem, MD

Pediatric Radiology is a subspecialty of radiology that has suffered a chronic shortage of fellowship-trained specialists. This has necessitated general radiologists assuming a greater burden in reading pediatric cases, and this has exacerbated the unease with which radiologists must apply lessons learned in adults to children…and then wonder if that is appropriate. Children get different diseases than adults and should be evaluated with different means.

Fortunately, Drs. Rob Ward and Hans Blickman have now provided a stellar case review volume that will appeal to general radiologists, pediatric radiologists in training, and practicing pediatric radiologists and pediatricians. These outstanding authors have addressed the many organ systems and modalities applied to the "age-challenged" component of our society. The pearls of wisdom supplied can be readily applied to the next stack of films/screenful of electronic images you read that contains pediatric studies. I applaud their hard work in readying this volume for press.

The philosophy of the Case Review Series is to review each specialty in a challenging interactive way. Each book in the series has gradations of difficulty so that the reader can assess his or her proficiency and can use this self-evaluation to guide continued education. Since each case in the book is distinct, this is the kind of text that can be picked up and read at any time in your day, in your career.

I am very pleased to welcome the Pediatric Radiology Case Review edition to the growing Case Review Family that includes Vascular and Interventional Imaging Case Review by Suresh Vedantham and Jennifer Gould, Nuclear Medicine Case Review by Harvey A. Zeissman and Patrician Rehm, General and Vascular Ultrasound Case Review by William D. Middleton, Musculoskeletal Case Review by Joseph Yu, Obstetrical and Gynecologic Ultrasound Case Review by Al Kurtz and Pam Johnson, Spine Imaging by Brian Bowen, Thoracic Imaging by Phil Boiselle and Theresa McLoud, Genitourinary Imaging by Ron Zagoria, William Mayo-Smith, and Glenn Tung, Gastrointestinal Imaging by Peter Feczko and Robert Halpert, Brain Imaging by Laurie Loevner, and Head and Neck Imaging by David M. Yousem.

David M. Yousem, M.D.
Case Review Series Editor

Don't let anyone fool you; there are two radiologies. There is the radiology of the boards typified by gamesmanship, Aunt Minnies, and command of the "zebras." There is also the radiology of practice characterized by common sense, good judgment, and a fund of knowledge. A well-equipped radiologist ought to be well acquainted with both.

Whether or not you embrace this duality of radiology, it is likely here to stay. There is, however, an increasing degree of overlap between these two radiologies as practical issues and common scenarios have penetrated the examination. The radiology boards are by no means an exclusive exercise in the esoteric as they strive to assure a basic level of competence with which to assist optimally in practical patient care. We hope to help prepare you for both.

In this author's opinion, the tools needed to succeed in Louisville include motivation, hard work, focus, and time. How you spend your time is vital. From the combined perspective of the only Case Review author (Robert J. Ward) to date to have used the series to successfully navigate the halls of the Executive West (the ABR board exam) and a seasoned ABR examiner (Hans Blickman), we are confident in recommending these books as a primary preparatory resource. In conjunction with attending guided board review, the case based approach is the most effective way to hone skills and expand your knowledge base for the impending exam.

While we had one foot planted in academics, intending this book to be useful for board preparation, the other was planted firmly in the practical world of everyday practice. There is a substantial amount of practical information included in the cases that ought to aid in your future or everyday practice. We are firm believers that good medicine is practiced by people with a deep understanding of pathophysiology. This paradigm appears somewhat less than universal as much of medical education is relegated to multiple choice examinations focused on the mastery of trivia.

Our approach has been to emphasize pathophysiology as a means to understanding diagnostic imaging findings. It is far easier in our opinion to remember the findings of rheumatoid arthritis if you understand the disease process. This approach however, must be balanced by the importance in brevity required in a boards study tool.

An additional note: We have avoided tipping off the diagnosis within the question section of the case as to allow the reader a more honest opportunity at formulating a reasonable differential. Do not be misled by the questions: they are often related only to the organ system of the case and in some instances bear no relation to the diagnosis.

We hope this book aids in your successful certification as well as a resource and review for your practice.

Robert J. Ward, M.D.
Hans Blickman, M.D., PhD.

Feedback is encouraged at RobWardMD@aol.com

A book is neither a solo effort nor a project with a definite starting point. My preparation began with word decoding, reading, writing, science, biology, medicine, and radiology residency to name a few. Careers are built on foundations and without the support of parents, siblings, teachers, college professors, medical school professors, and radiology mentors this book would not have been possible, that is at least one with my name on it.

Firstly, I'd like to thank my parents, notably my mom, who gave up much of her time during my early school years to hammer the importance of education, pride, and finishing what you start. None of this would have been possible without that bedrock foundation. Thanks to my dad and sister Nicole for their unending support.

Of mention are the teachers through my grade school years who rarely get the credit they truly deserve. Nicholas Byrne, Walter Pevny, Wilma Everson, James Strohmeyer, James McGuire, John Logsdon, Rodney Sheratsky, Ph.D., and Grant Simons, M.D.

College and early employment brought much wisdom from Erik J. Antener, Cristobal Alvarez, Chi Y. Kim, Stephen Roth, Ph.D., and Edward McGuire, Ph.D.

Medical School introduced me to the wisdom of Eric Lazaro, M.D., Arthur G. Calise, D.O., Jules Titelbaum, M.D., and Jeremias Murillo, M.D. Graduating would not have been possible if it was not for the fierce and incomparable support and friendship of Grace A. Conley, M.D. Thanks Grace, you are one of a kind. Thanks to Alessio Pigazzi, M.D. for the introduction that launched my radiology career.

I must thank John A. Bardini, M.D. and Evan W. Harris, M.D. for introducing me to radiology. Thank you to George Williams, M.D., Leonard Zawodniak, M.D., Daniel Flynn, M.D. and Maria Melacci, R.N. for bringing sanity to internship.

With respect to radiology, very special thanks go to Victor W. Lee, M.D., Hans Blickman, M.D., Ph.D., and Stephen J. Eustace, M.D. for opening the radiology door, holding it, and kicking me through, respectively. I would also like to thank Carol A. Boles, M.D. and Leon Lenchik, M.D. for their musculoskeletal mentorship.

Very special thanks to Rachel A. Schoenberger whose support, advice, and friendship have been absolutely indispensable over the past five years.

This book would not have been possible without the guidance and input of Carlo Buonomo, M.D., Vinaya K. Reddy, M.D., David Yousem, M.D., Thomas Ptak, M.D., Christine Menias, M.D., Sanjeev Bhalla, M.D., Christopher Roth, M.D., Kartik Boorgu, M.D., Paresh Rijsinghani, M.D., Inna Goldberg, M.D., David Rusch, M.D., Peter Hildebrand, M.D., Carl Geyer, M.D., Karen Reuter, M.D., and Cheryl Keller.

Thanks go to Meghan McAteer for all her production help.

And finally, this project may have never been completed if not for the tireless editorial efforts of Hilarie Surrena.

Robert J. Ward, M.D.

The more senior one gets, the more one realizes that radiology is best practiced as a team on multiple levels. This is never more obvious when one undertakes an endeavor such as this that you hope will benefit the specialty, especially its future: the residents.

In discussions, exchange of material and seeking of advise many have indirectly contributed to this volume. I particularly want to thank Dr. Carlo Buonomo and Dr. Richard Tello (both Boston) who critically reviewed parts of the text.

This effort was also a truly international pediatric radiology collaborative effort with input from Drs. Pat Barnes (Stanford), Lya van Die/Carla Boetes/Albert Lemmens/Jacky de Rooy (UMC Nijmegen, Netherlands), Dr. Simon Robben (UMC Maastricht, Netherlands) as well as the preeminent neuroradiologists of the Netherlands Drs Frederik Barkhof and Mark van Buchem. All deserve our gratitude.

It took us a while to finish this job. My co-author deserves praise for seeing it through, with my returning to my native the Netherlands 4 years ago and undertaking the chairmanship of a major medical center's department of radiology. He will be, and actually is, an outstanding radiologist and colleague. Rob, to paraphrase my grandmother: what you wait for is extra good!

The patience of Mosby/Saunders/Elsevier is also appreciated. As I am preparing the third edition of the pediatric requisites I look forward to continuing our cooperative effort.

Hans Blickman, M.D., PhD.

CONTENTS

Opening Round Cases

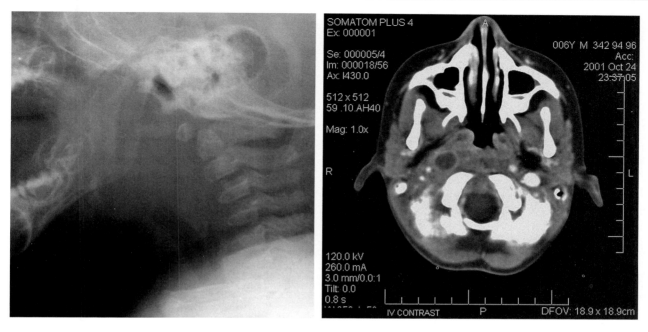

1. What additional plain film test might you order to confirm the findings?
2. What should the soft tissue width be in a child less than 3?
3. What finding suggests pseudosubluxation over subluxation?
4. What is the differential diagnosis of this finding?

Retropharyngeal Abscess

1. Inspiratory film, as expiratory film in children may demonstrate artifactual prevertebral soft tissue swelling.

2. Prevertebral soft tissue width should never exceed one half the width of the accompanying vertebral body.

3. Straightening of the lordotic curve due to spasm may result in pseudosubluxation of C2 on C3. Subluxation in a normal curve is pathologic until proven otherwise.

4. Hemorrhage, infection, lymphadenopathy secondary to lymphoma, neuroblastoma, or retropharyngeal goiter.

References

Gaglani MJ et al.: Neonatal radiology casebook. Retropharyngeal abscess in the neonate. *J Perinatol* 16(3 Pt 1):231–233, 1996. Review.

Castellote A, Vazquez E, Vera J, et al.: Cervicothoracic lesions in infants and children. *Radiographics* 19(3): 583–600, 1999.

Cross-Reference

Pediatric Radiology: THE REQUISITES, 2nd edn, pp 9–10.

Comment

The importance of careful examination of the lateral c-spine cannot be overstated. Strict adherence to a systematic approach is the best way to insure against missed findings and tragic outcomes. A good place to start is an overview of the film. Does the spine "feel" right? Examine *all* (swimmer's view if necessary) of the cervical vertebral bodies for fractures, joint space narrowing, uniform spacing of the spinous processes and preservation of the anterior, posterior, and laminar lines. Inspect the prevertebral soft tissues for widening greater than one half of a vertebral body, or the presence of gas. In the context of trauma, one may only see focal swelling at the level of vertebral injury. Don't ignore this clue, follow up with CT! Further investigation of the soft tissues ought to focus on the oro- and hypopharynx.

The etiology of retropharyngeal abscess is most commonly related to nodal drainage from acute tonsillitis. The most common organism is group B *Streptococcus*. Clinical presentation includes fever, stiff neck, and dysphagia. The presence of gas in the absence of trauma is nearly pathognomonic. A few pitfalls are worthy of mention. Soft tissue fullness may mimic swelling on expiratory films. Inspiratory films or fluoroscopy will aid in the distinction. Don't be fooled by C2 on C3 pseudosubluxation,

a common finding in pediatric neck spasm—a straightened or reversed lordotic curve. Normal lordosis with subluxation is pathologic until proven otherwise.

CT findings demonstrate an ill-defined, enhancing, soft tissue mass located just off the midline in the retropharyngeal space. A retropharyngeal mass will posteriorly displace the longus coli muscles, while a prevertebral mass will displace the muscles anteriorly.

Treatment ranges from antibiotics to radiographic or surgical drainage of discrete collections.

Notes

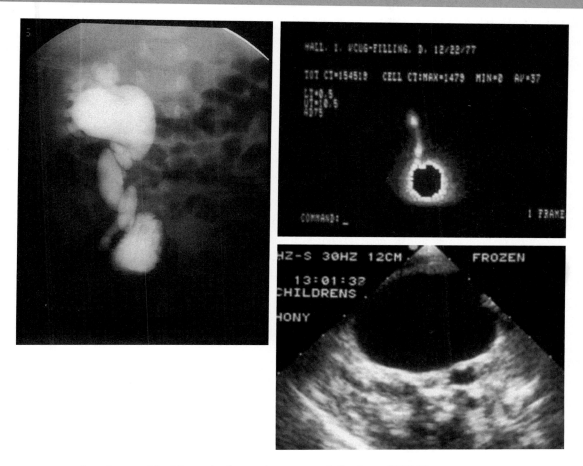

1. What percentage of patients with this entity has urinary tract infections (UTIs)?

2. What are the sequelae of renal scarring?

3. What is the therapy?

4. What are the common presenting symptoms?

Vesicoureteral Reflux

1. 35%.

2. Hypertension, growth retardation, and chronic renal failure.

3. Surgical reimplantation of ureter if antibiotic therapy fails.

4. Urinary tract infections, urgency, dribbling, incontinence, abdominal mass, poor weight gain, and hypertension.

Reference

Fernbach SK, Feinstein FA, Schmidt MB: Pediatric voiding cystourethrography: a pictorial guide. *Radiographics* 20:155–168, 2000.

Cross-Reference

Pediatric Radiology: THE REQUISITES, pp 181–182.

Comment

Vesicoureteral reflux (VUR) is a pathologic condition in which urine flows upstream from the bladder to the kidneys, causing infection in the acute period and eventual scarring and dysfunction over time. VUR is caused by an abnormally wide opening at the ureterovesicular junction (UVJ). Normally the ureter enters the bladder at an acute angle, creating a valve that prevents back flow. If the valve is distorted by either a ureter that inserts perpendicular to the serosal surface or an anatomic bladder abnormality such as a diverticulum, the ostia will remain open and allow retrograde flow of urine. Over time, long-standing reflux will eventually lead to renal infection with subsequent scarring.

Clinically, UTIs rank second behind upper respiratory infections in all childhood infections. The big players in urinary tract infections are those entities that either push urine up from the bladder as in VUR or keep urine from flowing antegrade as in ureteropelvic junction (UPJ), UVJ, ureteroceles, or posterior urethra valves. Evaluation for these entities includes an antegrade (intravenous pyelogram, IVP), an ultrasound, or retrograde (voiding cystourethrogram, VCUG). The VCUG is performed by gravity-dripping water-soluble contrast into the catheterized bladder until the patient voids. Voiding spot films (easier said than done) as well as an abdomen radiograph are taken to evaluate for urethral anatomy as well as the presence of reflux. Reflux severity is graded I—V. The sequelae of pyelonephritis secondary to VUR (scarring) are demonstrated with the use of scintigraphy.

Notes

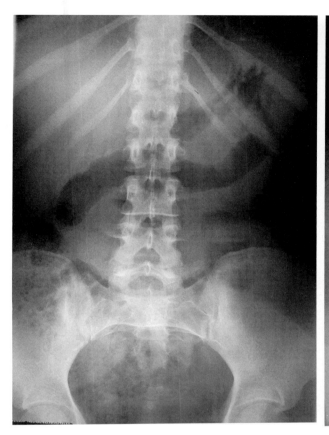 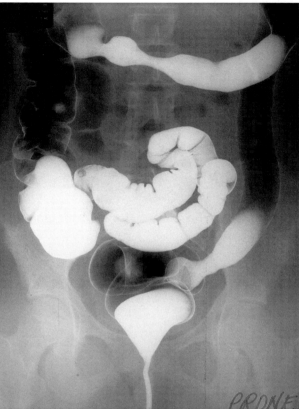

1. What are the associated findings of this entity?

2. Is there an association with polyps?

3. Is the terminal ileum involved?

4. What is the etiologic agent in pseudomembranous colitis?

Ulcerative Colitis

1. Arthritis, ankylosing spondylitis, sclerosing cholangitis, hepatitis, cholangiocarcinoma, pyoderma gangrenosum, erythema nodosum, uveitis, episcleritis.

2. Filiform (regenerative mucosa) and postinflammatory pseudopolyps are seen.

3. Yes, backwash ileitis secondary to a gaping ileocecal valve but only affecting a small segment, in contrast to Crohn.

4. *Clostridium difficile* overgrowth secondary to antibiotic administration, usually clindamycin.

Reference

Kirschner BS: Ulcerative colitis and Crohn's disease in children. Diagnosis and management. *Gastroenterol Clin N Am* 24(1):99–117, 1995.

Cross-Reference

Pediatric Radiology: THE REQUISITES, 2nd edn, pp 118–119.

Comment

Ulcerative colitis (UC) is an idiopathic disease that presents with diarrhea, rectal bleeding (30%), and failure to thrive (15%). Peak incidence is in young adults but UC may occur in teens and children, although rarely in infants. The disease primarily affects the mucosa of the rectum, and progresses proximally. Complications include toxic megacolon, obstruction secondary to strictures, and 5–30 times increased risk of malignancy.

Radiographically, plain films will often show large bowel wall thickening with a suspicious loss of haustrations. Note that if you see a large dilated bowel this may represent toxic megacolon, a contraindication to barium study. Double contrast barium enema will show a granular mucosa beginning at the rectum and extending proximally. Collar button ulcers (ulcers that appear as buttons on profile) are seen in more advanced disease. A shortened, featureless "lead pipe" appearance is often seen in chronic disease. Regenerating mucosa may give the appearance of pseudopolyposis. Differential diagnostic considerations include infectious colitis, necrotizing enterocolitis, Hirschsprung and allergic colitis. Infections agents include *Campylobacter, C. dificile, E. coli, Shigella, Salmonella,* and *Yersina.*

The death rate is 2% per year after the first 10 years due to increased incidence of adenocarcinoma. End stage disease is treated with total colectomy.

Notes

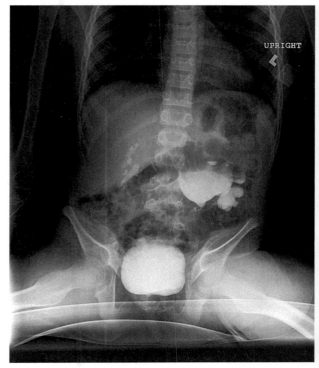

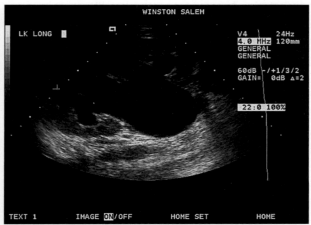

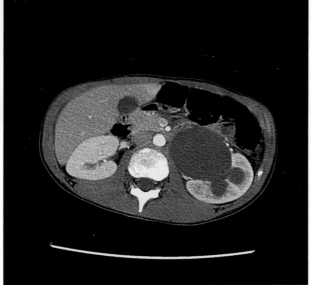

1. What is the differential diagnosis?
2. What percentage of this entity is bilateral?
3. What is the triad of prune belly syndrome?
4. What is the etiology of papillary necrosis?

Ureteropelvic Junction (UPJ) Obstruction

1. Calyceal diverticulum, Fraley syndrome, congenital megacalyces.

2. 20% of cases are bilateral. UPJ obstruction most commonly occurs on the left.

3. Abnormal anterior abdominal wall musculature, cryptorchidism, and dilated urinary tract.

4. Mnemonic "POSTCARD": **P**yelonephritis, **O**bstruction, **S**ickle cell disease, **T**B, **C**irrhosis, **A**nalgesics, **R**enal vein thrombosis, **D**iabetes.

Reference

Grignon A, Filiatrault D, Homsy Y, Robitaille P, Filion R, Boutin H, Leblond R: Ureteropelvic junction stenosis: antenatal ultrasonographic diagnosis, postnatal investigation, and follow-up. *Radiology* 160(3):649–651, 1986.

Cross-Reference

Pediatric Radiology: THE REQUISITES, pp 161–162.

Comment

Ureteropelvic junction obstruction is caused by the mechanical compression of either an aberrant vessel or fibrous band. UPJ obstruction is the most common cause of urinary obstruction in the pediatric age group.

Neonates present with an abdominal mass. In contrast, young children may present with hematuria due to a weakened dilated pelvis thought to be more sensitive to trauma. In either case an ultrasound ought to be performed first. In neonates, renal ultrasound will demonstrate a dilated pelvis with a preserved renal cortex (differentiates from multicystic dysplastic kidney). Renal scintigraphy may be followed up to confirm the diagnosis by demonstrating the site of stricture as well as the relative function of the kidney. Next stop in the department is fluoroscopy to ascertain that the problem is coming from above rather than below. Reflux may be the causative agent in hydronephrosis and must be ruled out by voiding cystourethrogram. In mild obstructions neonates are followed by ultrasound at 6 months. Substantial obstruction will go to surgery for excision and reanastomosis (pyeloplasty).

The older age group will go to ultrasound in order to examine the kidneys as well as the bladder, paying close attention to the presence of an ectopic ureterocele as well as primary megaureter. Some cases may regress, while others require surgery for those patients with significant obstruction.

Notes

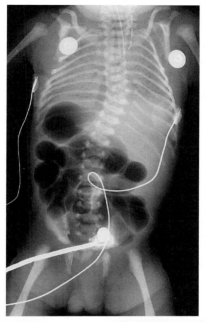

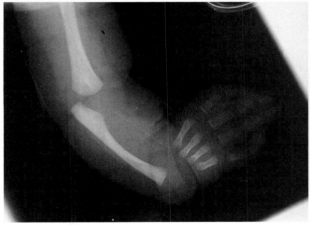

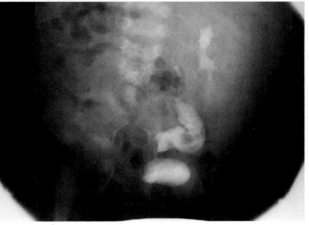

1. What comprises the acronym VACTERL?
2. What is Fanconi anemia?
3. What is Fanconi syndrome?
4. Who was Fanconi?

VACTERL

1. **V**ertebral abnormalities, **A**nal atresia, **C**ardiac abnormalities, **T**racheoesophageal fistula and/or **E**sophageal atresia, **R**enal agenesis, and **L**imb defects.

2. An aplastic anemia associated with numerous physical abnormalities present at birth, including limb, renal, hyperpigmentation, and microcephaly.

3. A hereditary disorder of renal tubular function with resultant renal osteodystrophy resistant to vitamin D, glycosuria, aminoaciduria, and hyperphosphaturia.

4. Guido Fanconi (1882–1979) was a Swiss pediatrician. He was one of the first pediatricians to advocate IV fluid to treat dehydration in children as well as promoting the use of fruit to treat diarrhea, a forerunner to pectin as an antidiarrheal agent.

References

McGahan JP, Leeba JM, Lindfors KK: Prenatal sonographic diagnosis of VATER association. *J Clin Ultrasound* 16(8): 588–591, 1988.

Quan L, Smith DW: The VATER association. Vertebral defects, Anal atresia, T-E fistula with esophageal atresia, Radial and Renal dysplasia: a spectrum of associated defects. *J Pediatr* 82(1):104–107, 1973.

Cross-Reference

Pediatric Radiology: THE REQUISITES, p 210.

Comment

Unilateral absence of the fibula is the most common hypoplasia of the skeletal system. Next most common in order include the radius, femur, and ulna. Radial deviation of the hand is usually seen accompanying radial ray absence. Radial ray absence is seen in Holt–Oram syndrome, the VACTERL association, Fanconi anemia, and trisomies 13 and 18.

The femur may be hypoplastic or absent, a spectrum of femoral abnormalities grouped together as proximal femoral focal deficiency. Most cases are unilateral, more common in boys, having right-sided predominance, and may be associated with aplasia or hypoplasia elsewhere in the same limb. These anomalies may also occur as part of the caudal regression syndrome.

Notes

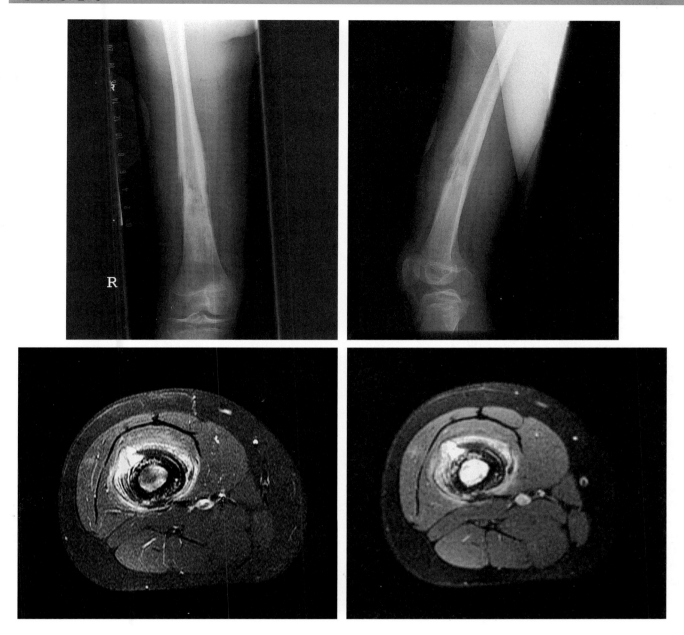

1. Can osteomyolitis mimic this entity?
2. What is the differential diagnosis?
3. What is the MR appearance?
4. What is the role of MR?

Ewing Sarcoma

1. Yes.

2. Osteosarcoma, osteomyelitis, and lymphoma. Always think of Ewing when considering a diagnosis of osteomyelitis.

3. Dark on T1, bright on T2, and often a prominent soft tissue component.

4. MR is used for staging purposes determining bone involvement, compartment involvement, and joint involvement.

Reference

Meyer JS, Dormans JP: Differential diagnosis of pediatric musculoskeletal masses. *Magn Reson Imaging Clin N Am* 6(3):561–577, 1998.

Cross-Reference

Pediatric Radiology: THE REQUISITES, p 228.

Comment

No one is quite sure of the etiology of Ewing sarcoma, although current thinking suggests a neural origin. The neoplasm is named after a Pittsburgh-born pathologist, James Ewing (1866–1943). A round cell tumor, histologically similar to primitive neuroectodermal tumors, is thought to arise from an oncogene translocation. Of the bone neoplasms, Ewing sarcoma affects the youngest age group, 10–15 years. Presentation includes fever, pain, swelling, and anemia. Long bones of the lower extremities and the sacrum are common targets with less common involvement in the scapula, pelvis, and vertebral bodies. Ewing sarcoma is medullary based but may enlarge to break through the cortex and grow outside the bone, producing an extraosseous soft tissue mass.

Radiographically, this lesion appears as a lytic diaphyseal or metadiaphyseal lesion as opposed to osteosarcoma, which favors the metaphysis. I was disappointed to find no explanation as to why Ewing sarcoma prefers the diaphysis to the metaphysis, although one reference did suggest that it may have to do with the relative population of neural-ectodermal elements present. Unlike osteosarcoma though, a sclerotic component is much less common. The permeative or moth-eaten appearance is seen in conjunction with cortical erosion, periosteal reaction, and a soft tissue mass. The periostitis may produce the classic laminated onion skin appearance.

MR will help demonstrate both the intra- and extraosseous extent of the tumor as well as quantitate the response to chemotherapy. Chemotherapy in addition to surgery and radiation have 5-year survival rates of 75% with long-term cures seen in half the patients.

Notes

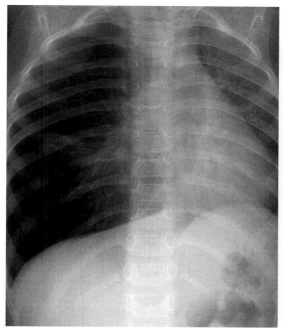 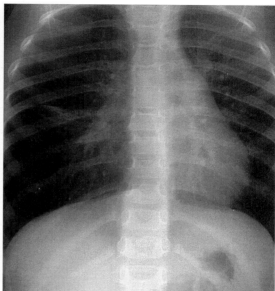

Inspiration   *Expiration*

1. Distinguish between foreign bodies in the esophagus vs. trachea.
2. What percentage of foreign bodies pass unaided?
3. What is ordered radiographically for suspected foreign body?
4. What is the differential diagnosis?

Foreign Body Aspiration

1. On frontal radiograph, coins in the esophagus will appear en face, while coins in the trachea will be seen on end (en profil).

2. 25% of objects larger than a quarter will not pass the ileocecal valve.

3. AP of the chest, abdomen, and lateral soft tissue of the neck ("mouth to anus view").

4. Foreign body, mucus plugging, Swyer-James, hypoplastic lung, pulmonary sling (R), CLE.

Reference

Swischuk LE: *Emergency Imaging of the Acutely Ill or Injured Child*, 4th edn. Baltimore: Williams & Wilkins, 2000.

Cross-Reference

Pediatric Radiology: THE REQUISITES, 2nd edn, pp 17, 98–100.

Comment

A presentation of stridor may be seen in either tracheal or esophageal foreign body aspiration or ingestion. Foreign bodies lodged within the upper respiratory system will cause partial or complete respiratory obstruction. Foreign bodies lodged within the esophagus may cause direct tracheal compression, abscess, or inflammation.

There are four sites of anatomic narrowing in the esophagus: (1) thoracic inlet below the level of the cricopharyngeal muscle (75%), (2) where the aortic arch or (3) left mainstem bronchus cross the esophagus (20%), and (4) at the GE junction (5%). Foreign bodies in the airway are most commonly seen on the right (55%), followed by the left (33%), bilaterally (7%), and the trachea (5%).

Coin-shaped foreign bodies in the esophagus are seen en face on frontal films. Alternatively, if in the trachea, frontal films will demonstrate an end-on appearance. Retrieval via a fluoroscopically guided esophageal Foley catheter placement with balloon inflation distal to the object has met with success but carries the risk of aspiration. Endoscopic removal is most widely recommended. The presence of esophageal edema indicates more than 24 hours of foreign body ingestion and may complicate retrieval with perforation or fistula formation.

Imaging airway foreign bodies with conventional radiographs may demonstrate hyperinflation, air trapping, atelectasis, consolidation, pneumothorax, pneumomediastinum, or bronchiectasis. The mechanism is a check valve with normal inspiration and obstructed expiration. The trick is to image the patient during expiration, most easily performed via fluoroscopy. The presence of a nonradiopaque foreign body may be inferred on fluoroscopy from mediastinal shift during expiration with resolution during inspiration (if the heart moves to the left on expiration the foreign body is on the right side).

Notes

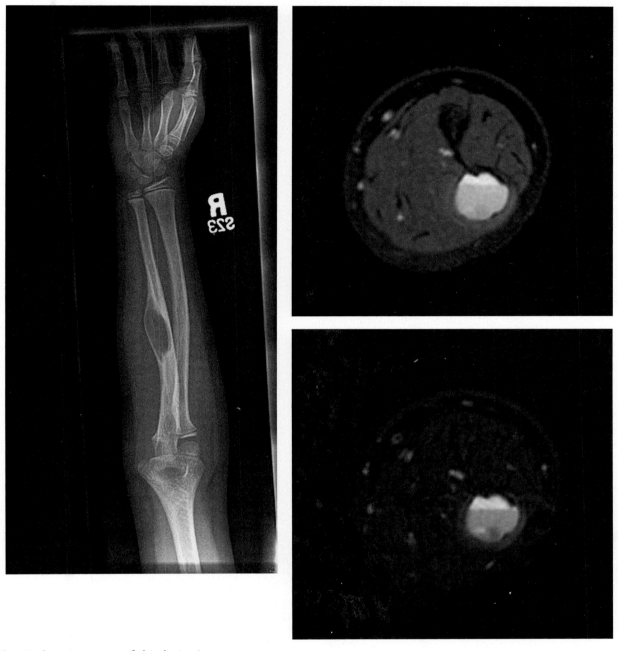

1. What is the age range of this lesion?
2. Where in tubular bones is this lesion most often found: diaphysis, metaphysis, or epiphysis?
3. Are these lesions most often seen within the posterior elements or the vertebral body?
4. What more sinister lesion is associated with fluid-fluid levels?

Aneurysmal Bone Cyst (ABC)

1. Between 5 and 20.

2. ABCs are eccentrically located and seen almost exclusively within the metaphysis.

3. Posterior elements.

4. Telangiectatic osteosarcoma.

References

Pediatric case of the day. Aneurysmal bone cyst. *Am J Roentgenol* 158:1372–1373, 1992.

Kransdorf MJ, Sweet DE: Aneurysmal bone cyst: concept, controversy, clinical presentation, and imaging. *Am J Roentgenol* 1995;164:573–580.

Cross-Reference

Pediatric Radiology: THE REQUISITES, p 286.

Comment

Aneurysmal bone cysts are expansile non-neoplastic lesions containing thin-walled blood filled cystic cavities. Two types exist. The majority, 70%, of cases are thought to result from previous trauma, while 30% are associated with a preexisting bone tumor. Giant cell is considered most common, while chondroblastoma, fibrous dysplasia, and osteoblastoma have been seen as well. Clinically, patients report acute pain with rapid onset and progression.

Radiographically, ABCs appear as eccentric, lucent, expansile lesions that may even balloon out the overlying intact cortex. A narrow zone of transition is present with no periosteal reaction. The periosteum may be elevated, suggesting a more sinister lesion. The growth plates may be involved as well. Fifty per cent of these lesions occur in long tubular bones with the posterior element of the spine and pelvis constituting the remainder. Lesions may lead to weakening and pathologic fracture of the bone. On MR and CT fluid–fluid lesions are noted. Helpful reminder: remember the orientation of the patient in the MR scanner.

Aneurysmal bone cysts have no malignant potential but may continue expanding requiring curettage and packing.

Notes

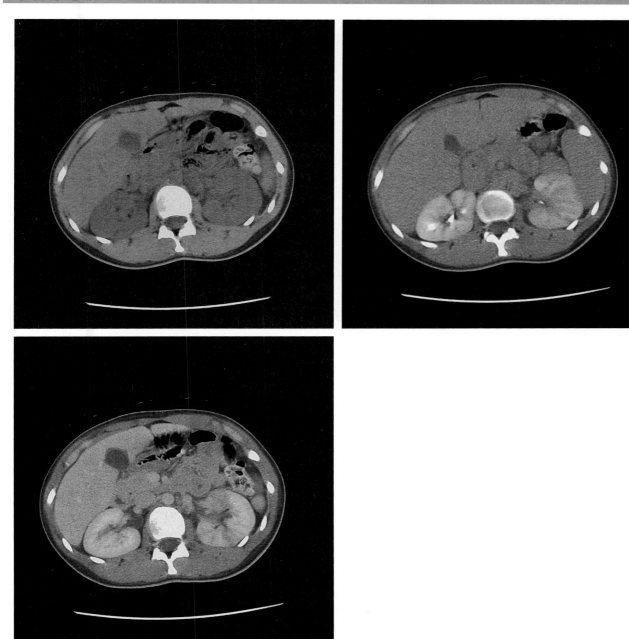

1. What is pyonephrosis and who cares?

2. What is the differential diagnosis for diffuse increased renal echogenicity?

3. Would you be surprised to see a striated nephrogram on CT?

4. Name several causes of a striated nephrogram.

Acute Pyelonephritis

1. You and your interventional team care! Pyonephrosis refers to an infected obstructed collecting system and requires urgent decompression and drainage through a percutaneous nephrostomy tube.

2. Nephrotic syndrome, glycogen storage, HUS, ADPKD, ARPKD, glomerulonephritis, pyelonephritis, lymphoma, leukemia.

3. No, a striated nephrogram may be seen in acute pyelonephritis.

4. Acute ureteral obstruction, pyelonephritis, ARPK, acute renal vein thrombosis, renal contusion, and radiation nephritis.

Reference

Ilyas M, Mastin ST, Richard GA: Age-related radiological imaging in children with acute pyelonephritis. *Pediatr Nephrol* 17(1):30–34, 2002.

Cross-Reference

Pediatric Radiology: THE REQUISITES, pp 182–183.

Comment

Acute pyelonephritis is a bacterial infection of the renal parenchyma with inflammation. Infection may enter the kidney from two different directions: retrograde ascending the urinary tract/collecting system or antegrade via the blood. Hematologic spread is limited to IV drug abusers, neonates with sepsis, and endocarditis patients. Ascending infection is usually (80%) accompanied by vesicoureteral reflux.

Acute pyelonephritis cannot be distinguished from simple cystitis by laboratory analysis alone. Acute pyelo, if left untreated, may lead to scarring with chronic renal failure and hypertension. Imaging is vital to localize the infection. Scintigraphy with 99mTc MAG3 is a sensitive tool (90%) in demonstrating parenchymal infection. Inflammatory change in the cortex leads to either vasoconstriction or abnormal metabolism of MAG3 yielding photopenic areas of focal pyelonephritis. Ultrasound demonstrates (1) focal or diffuse indistinct corticomedullary junction with abnormal echogenicity; (2) impaired renal movement with respiration; (3) size discrepancy >1 cm. Power Doppler has shown promise in detecting acute pyelonephritis with focal areas of ischemia detected as loss of flow.

Contrast-enhanced CT, more often used in the older age groups, demonstrates the classic wedge-shaped striated nephrogram. Delayed and diminished enhancement of the affected areas with focal or diffuse enlargement is characteristic. Perinephric stranding of fat is a sensitive sign for pyelo. Complications such as perinephric abscess or pyonephrosis are well seen on CT.

Uncomplicated pyelonephritis is treated with antibiotics. Complicated cases may require percutaneous drainage, percutaneous nephrostomy, or surgery.

Notes

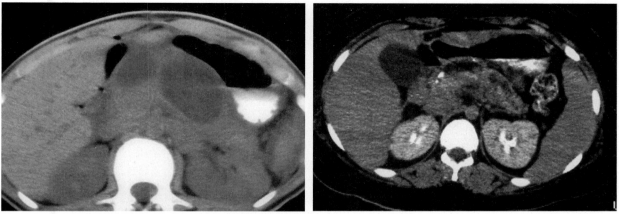

Patient 3.

Patient 2.

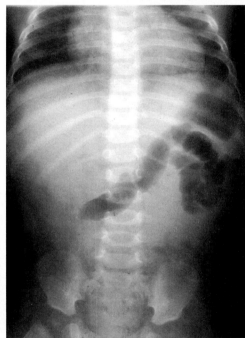

Patient 1.

1. What is the indication for invasive therapy?
2. What are the approaches?
3. Does it matter if the lesion is in contact with the pancreatic duct?
4. Is CT indicated for pancreatitis?

Acute Pancreatitis/Pseudocyst/Sentinel Loop

1. If the pseudocyst is stable in size or getting larger it must be drained.

2. Transgastric or transperitoneal.

3. Yes, drainage will take longer.

4. No, only the complications of pancreatitis, of which pseudocyst formation is one.

Reference

Jaffe RB, Arata JA Jr, Matlak ME: Percutaneous drainage of traumatic pancreatic pseudocysts in children. *Am J Roentgenol* 152(3):591–595, 1989.

Cross-Reference

Pediatric Radiology: THE REQUISITES, 2nd edn, p 140.

Comment

The most common cause for acute pancreatitis in children is blunt trauma. Minor as well as major trauma have been implicated. Other causes include medication (steroids, azathioprine, thiazides, sulfonamides), hemolytic uremic syndrome, sepsis, common bile duct obstruction secondary to gallbladder stones, and hereditary pancreatitis. Clinical presentation includes upper abdominal pain, nausea, and vomiting. Elevation of amylase and lipase are often seen but normal values do not rule out pancreatitis.

Conventional radiographs are relatively insensitive with the exception of a sentinel loop, a focal ileus of small bowel adjacent to the inflamed pancreas. Ultrasound may vary from a negative study to focal or diffuse abnormal findings. Focal findings consist of isoechoic or hypoechoic enlargement, while diffuse changes appear as an overall decrease in echogenicity relative to the normal liver. Necrosis cannot be discerned by ultrasound; contrast-enhanced CT is the gold standard. Necrosis on CT appears as nonenhancing foci of low attenuation with peripancreatic inflammatory stranding. Pseudocysts will demonstrate large nonenhancing collections with a thick well-defined capsule that is composed of dense fibrous tissue.

Therapies include percutaneous drainage of pseudocysts via image guidance or surgery.

Notes

Patient 1.

Patient 2.

1. What is the etiology of the first patient?
2. What is the differential diagnosis of the first patient?
3. What is the treatment? (Patient 2)
4. Which film is an emergency?

Acute Epiglottitis vs. Croup

1. *Haemophilus influenzae* Type B, *Pneumococcus,* group A *Streptococcus.*

2. Angioneurotic edema, epiglottic cysts, hematoma.

3. Stat intubation.

4. Epiglottitis is an emergency. (Patient 2)

Reference

Strife JL: Pediatric airway obstruction: imaging in the 1990s. In: Kirks DR, ed. *Emergency Pediatric Radiology. A problem-oriented approach.* Reston, VA: American Roentgen Ray Society, 1995, pp 225–232.

Cross-Reference

Pediatric Radiology: THE REQUISITES, 2nd edn, pp 13–14.

Comment

The incidence of acute epiglottitis has markedly decreased with the use of the *Haemophilus influenzae* vaccine. Epiglottitis, unlike croup, is rapid in onset. The patient sits upright, head extended, attempting to decrease airway resistance. Intubation may be necessary if the patient progresses to complete obstruction. In suspected cases, it is necessary for the experienced clinician to accompany the patient to the radiology department. Radiographically, the hypopharynx is enlarged, with swelling of the epiglottis and aryepiglottic folds. The aryepiglottic fold edema is responsible for the stridor. The characteristic "thumb" sign is used to describe an enlarged and thickened epiglottis. A common fake-out is the omega or curved epiglottis that on profile appears to have an increased A-P diameter. Closer inspection will demonstrate an additional line representing the true posterior wall, indicating a normal thickness rather than epiglottic enlargement.

Acute laryngotracheobronchitis (croup) is a self-limiting, seasonal disease presenting with a barking cough. The condition involves global inflammation of the upper respiratory tract most pronounced in the subglottic region. Radiographically, distention of the hypopharynx (a reflexive attempt at decreasing airway resistance), normal epiglottis, and symmetric subglottic narrowing are seen on the lateral. The AP shows the classic "steeple sign" or symmetric narrowing of the subglottic region.

Notes

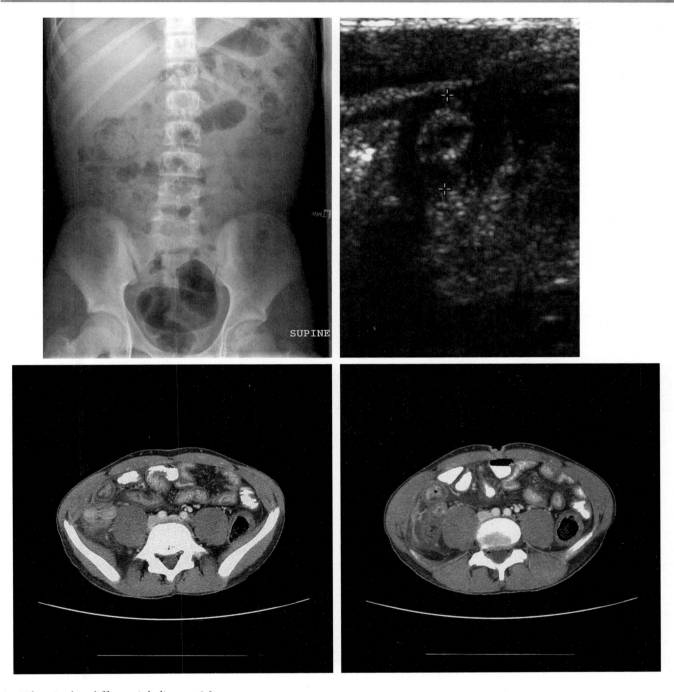

1. What is the differential diagnosis?
2. What question might you ask the clinician to narrow the diagnosis?
3. Do ultrasound findings change over time?
4. What are the indirect signs on ultrasound?

Appendicitis

1. Typhlitis, Crohn, constipation secondary to cystic fibrosis, renal calculi, right ovarian torsion, mesenteric adenitis.

2. Is there blood in the urine? Renal stones may mimic acute appendicitis.

3. Yes, post rupture the appendix will be difficult to find.

4. Periappendiceal collection, increased Doppler flow signal in enlarged appendix.

References

Fefferman NR, Roche KJ, Pinkney LP, Ambrosino MM, Genieser NB: Suspected appendicitis in children: focused CT technique for evaluation. *Radiology* 220(3):691–695, 2001.

Callahan MJ, Rodriguez DP, Taylor GA: CT of appendicitis in children. *Radiology* 224(2):325–332, 2002.

Cross-Reference

Pediatric Radiology: THE REQUISITES, 2nd edn, pp 122–123.

Comment

Traditionally a clinical diagnosis, radiologists increasingly have been called upon to image the right lower quadrant to improve diagnostic accuracy in suspected appendicitis.

What causes appendicitis? Current theory points to obstruction of the appendiceal lumen with secondary retention of secretion, overdistention, bacterial overgrowth, and vascular compromise (necrosis secondary to overdistention). A necrotic appendix will burst and cause peritonitis with or without abscess formation.

Presentation for classic appendicitis begins with periumbilical pain that later localizes to the right lower quadrant, anorexia, vomiting that causes temporary relief of pain, and diarrhea. Physical findings include rebound tenderness (peritoneum in the setting of peritonitis is exquisitely sensitive to stretching). Point tenderness to palpation at McBurney's point is considered the most sensitive physical sign. Young children *do not* present classically and can slip by surgery only to perforate, and cause substantial increased morbidity.

Radiographically, conventional radiographs may be normal. The presence of an appendicolith is seen in 5% of cases and indicates the presence of prior or chronic inflammation, a sign that greatly increases the probability of appendicitis. Prophylactic appendectomy is indicated in this case as the risk of future perforation is great. Other signs on plain films include small bowel and cecal air fluid levels, cecal wall thickening, splinting (the appearance of scoliosis convex left).

The next imaging step is ultrasound. A normal appendix is most often not visualized. Positive findings include a noncompressible appendix greater than 6 mm, appendiceal wall thickness greater than 2 mm, or an appendicolith. Differential diagnostic considerations are dependent on gender as girls may have ovarian torsion and require a full ultrasound pelvic examination to establish flow to the ovaries as well as ruling out other gynecologic etiologies.

CT is a powerful tool in determining the focus of inflammation with direct visualization of the appendix, neighboring structures, and the inflammatory changes in the surrounding fat. Always look for the center of inflammation and don't forget to look at the mesentery for enlarged nodes (mesenteric adenitis).

Notes

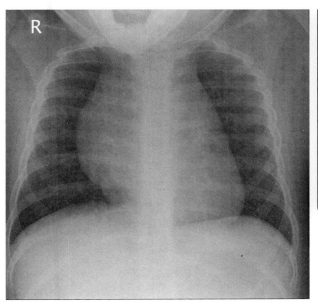
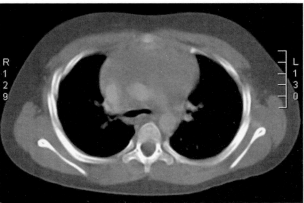

1. What is the differential diagnosis?
2. What is the most common AIDS-related neoplasm in children?
3. What is the differential diagnosis of this finding with a parenchymal opacity?
4. What if this lesion were cystic on CT?

C A S E 13

Anterior Mediastinal Mass

1. Thymus, thymoma, thymic carcinoma, teratoma, lymphoma, thyroid.

2. Non-Hodgkin lymphoma.

3. Tuberculosis, sarcoidosis, and histoplasmosis. Remember in older patients that neoplasm may present as a parenchymal opacity.

4. If this lesion were cystic, lymphangioma.

Reference

Merten DF: Diagnostic imaging of mediastinal masses in children. *Am J Roentgenol* 158:825–832:1992.

Cross-Reference

Pediatric Radiology: THE REQUISITES, 2nd edn, pp 45–50.

Comment

The chest is filled with a variety of tissues making differential diagnosis demanding. The key to generating a focused and useful differential is localization of the mass. If you can tell where it is you can probably tell what it is! The mediastinum is a midline grouping of soft tissue structures that are bounded by the lungs much like bookends, the diaphragm below and the thoracic inlet or scapulae above. The anterior mediastinum extends from the anterior diaphragm to the thoracic inlet and from the anterior chest wall to the anterior surface of the heart and great vessels. So now that we've localized our lesion to be in the anterior mediastinum we can use the T's: **T**hymus, **T**hymoma, **T**hymic carcinoma, **T**eratoma, **T**errible lymphoma, **T**hyroid (ectopic).

The thymus is normally seen in children up to 3 years of age but may be seen in older kids up to 9. Its primary function is maturation of T-lymphocytes. A thymoma is a fluid- or fat-filled thymus often associated with myasthenia gravis or red cell aplasia. Therapy for myasthenia includes thymectomy. Thymic carcinoma is exceedingly rare in the pediatric age group. Teratomas are formed from primordial germ cells slated for the gonadal ridges that are believed to migrate cephalad along the midline. These pluripotent germ cells will contain elements of the three germ cell layers. Teratomas may contain soft tissue, fat, and calcification, allowing for differentiation from other mediastinal masses. Benign teratomas tend to displace rather than invade normal mediastinal structures. Lymphoma is divided into Hodgkin and non-Hodgkin. Hodgkin represents only 5% of cases, NHL the remaining 95%. Hodgkin often involves the anterior mediastinum. Pediatric NHL, in contrast to adult NHL, is extranodal.

Ectopic thyroid may be seen to extend below the thoracic inlet.

Notes

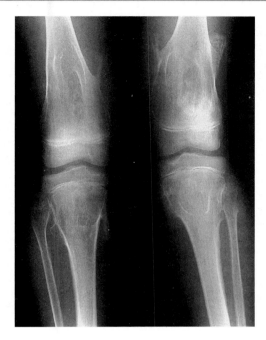

1. Does this entity have a male or female predominance?
2. Is this a heritable disorder?
3. There are two morphologic types. What are they?
4. The majority of lesions are of which morphologic type?

Hereditary Multiple Exostoses

1. Male.

2. Yes, it is autosomal dominant.

3. Pedunculated and sessile (broad based).

4. Sessile.

Reference

Murphey MD, Choi JJ, Kransdorf MJ, Flemming DJ, Gannon FH: Imaging of osteochondroma: variants and complications with radiologic-pathologic correlation. *Radiographics* 20:1407–1434, 2000.

Cross-Reference

Pediatric Radiology: THE REQUISITES, p 208.

Comment

Unlike enchondromas, in which the growth plate leaves behind a rest of cartilage, osteochondromas are formed from a segment of growth plate that separates and lays down cartilage off the normal axis of development. Clinically, patients present with a hard, slowly enlarging mass in proximity to a joint. Pain may be due to compression of a neurovascular bundle or irritation of a bursa. There is a 1–2% lifetime incidence of malignant degeneration into chondrosarcoma. Osteochondromas may also develop from radiation therapy.

Radiographically, osteochondromas are seen to grow on bony stalks diagonally away from the growth plate usually arising from the metaphysis of tubular long bones. The mushroom-shaped lesions contain a cartilaginous cap that ought to measure less than 2 cm in thickness. Greater than 2 cm suggests malignancy. Additional signs of malignancy include an indistinct bony margin, an area of lucency, and heterogeneous septal versus peripheral gadolinium enhancement. Sessile or broad-based osteochondromas that involve the metaphyseal region may appear as an undertubulated bone dysplasia.

Therapy is directed at resection-only cases in which there is either pain or malignant degeneration.

Notes

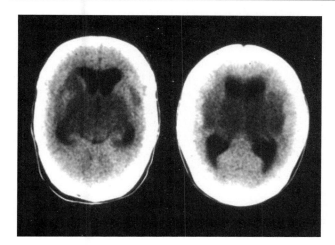

1. Does a normal study rule out this diagnosis?
2. What is the etiology for hydrocephalus in patients with this entity?
3. What percentage of neonates will develop related ventriculitis?
4. What are the causes of cavernous sinus thrombosis?

Group B Streptococcal Meningitis

1. No, there can still be meningitis without radiologic findings. Meningitis is a clinical diagnosis.

2. Exudate may accumulate in the foramen of Megendi or Luschka, causing intraventricular obstructive hydrocephalus. Exuadate may develop over the convexities and basal cisterns, causing extraventricular obstructive hydrocephalus.

3. 90%.

4. Paranasal sinus infection, dental abscess, orbital infection, meningitis.

Reference

Cockrill HH Jr, Dreisbach J, Lowe B, Yamauchi T: Computed tomography in leptomeningeal infections. *Am J Roentgenol* 130(3):511–515, 1978.

Cross-Reference

Pediatric Radiology: THE REQUISITES, pp 276–278.

Comment

The bacteria that cause meningitis vary with age. Meningitis in neonates is caused in a majority of cases by *Escherichia coli* and group B streptococci. Meningitis in childhood is often due to *Haemophilus influenzae*, while in adolescents and young adults *Neisseria* meningitidis is most common. The elderly are prone to *Streptococcus pneumoniae* and *Listeria monocytogenes*. Group B streptococci is a neonatal infection that may either be caused by ascending infection in the setting of premature rupture of membranes or at birth as the newborn travels through the infected birth canal. Early-onset disease is characterized by sepsis or pneumonia, and diagnosed in the first 6 days of life, accounting for approximately 80% of neonatal group B streptococcal infections. Late-onset disease presents at 7 or more days of life and manifests as sepsis or meningitis.

Meningitis is a clinical diagnosis based on sign, symptoms, and the lumbar puncture. Meningitis presents as fever, irritability, and seizures. Cases that do not show expected improvement following antibiotic treatment are imaged. Complications of meningitis include hydrocephalus, venous thrombosis, cavernous sinus thrombosis, venous infarction, arterial infarction, effusions, cerebritis and abscess, ventriculitis, and deafness.

On imaging acute neonatal meningitis may demonstrate edema with ischemic or hemorrhagic infarction. Infarction is secondary to either venous or arterial thrombosis. Ependymal or meningeal enhancement may be seen. Areas of cerebritis or rim-enhancing abscess are not uncommon. Venous sinus thrombosis will demonstrate loss of a flow void in the sinus with T1

hyperintensity (subacute blood). Patients with suspected venous sinus thrombosis ought to undergo MR venography. Ultrasound will show signs of ventriculitis; increased intraventricular echoes, wall thickening, and increased echogenicity just deep to the ependymal layer. Long-term sequelae on imaging appear as encephalomalacia, hydrocephalus, atrophy, and calcification.

Notes

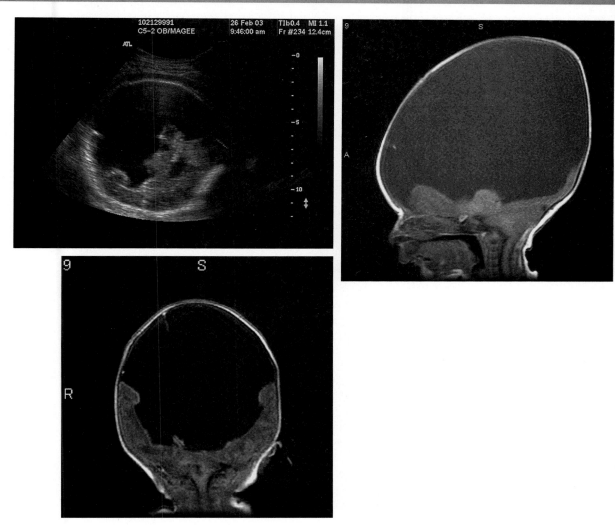

1. Is the falx present?
2. Why is an absent falx an important finding?
3. Is there tissue seen laterally?
4. Why is the absence of cortical tissue an important finding?

Hydranencephaly

1. Yes.

2. A present falx rules out holoprosencephaly.

3. No.

4. Absence of cortical tissue rules out hydrocephalus.

Reference

Poe LB, Coleman LL, Mahmud F: Congenital central nervous system anomalies.
Radiographics 9(5):801–826, 1989.

Cross-Reference

Pediatric Radiology: THE REQUISITES, p 271.

Comment

Hydranencephaly is a disorder considered to be an *in utero* ischemic event involving the anterior circulation. Thrombosis is thought to occur in the second trimester secondary to an infectious agent. The posterior fossa and basal ganglia are not involved as the posterior circulation is not affected. Hydranencephaly is normally picked up during prenatal ultrasound. If ultrasound has not been performed the baby will present clinically with irritability and motor abnormalities.

Sonographically, hydranencephaly will contain enormous lateral ventricles filled with fluid and a thin sac overlying the expected location of the parietal, temporal, and frontal lobes. The sac represents the meninges, which are fed by branches of the external carotid artery. No brain parenchyma is seen, as it has been destroyed due to infarction. The falx is present, unlike in semi and alobar holoprosencephaly, a useful differentiator. To differentiate from hydrocephalus look for the thin mantle of cortical tissue not present in hydranencephaly.

Prognosis is uniform with death in infancy.

Notes

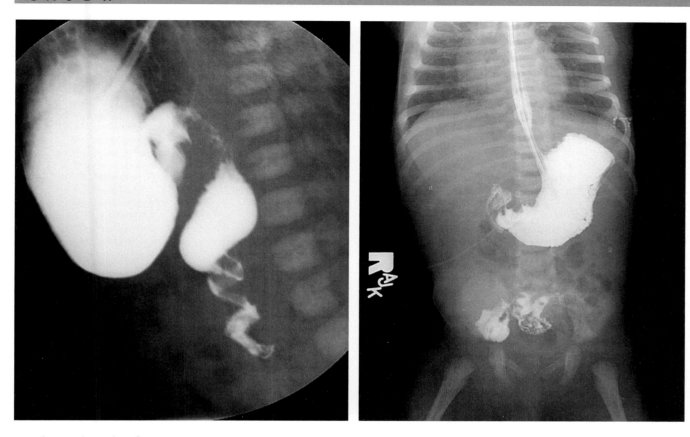

1. What is the rule of 3s?

2. What entities are associated with gastroesophageal reflux?

3. On ultrasound a large hypoechoic subhepatic cyst is most likely consistent with what diagnosis?

4. What is the most likely cause of portal hypertension in a neonate?

Midgut Volvulus

1. Therapeutic enema for intussusception. Three tries for three minutes with the bag three feet from the table.

2. Down syndrome, cystic fibrosis, and neurologically impaired states.

3. Choledochal cyst.

4. Idiopathic.

Reference

Yang CJ, Lu CH, Murakami J, Franken EA Jr: General case of the day. Midgut volvulus with necrotic small bowel. *Radiographics* 7(3):605–607, 1987.

Cross-Reference

Pediatric Radiology: THE REQUISITES, 2nd edn, pp 84–87.

Comment

The key to understanding midgut volvulus is gut development. Originating as a short tube the GI tract elongates and rotates around an axis, the superior mesenteric artery (SMA). The 270° of rotation commonly quoted refers to the duojejunal loop that begins midline above the SMA and rotates to the left upper quadrant where it is tethered to the ligament of Treitz. If the bowel does not undergo this normal deployment, the malpositioned intestine may be prone to twisting on its mesenteric access. The twisted gut or volvulus will strangulate by compressing its own blood supply. Complete loss of small bowel is incompatible with life, therefore it is essential that midgut volvulus be ruled out by the radiologist.

Midgut volvulus can occur at any age but is far more common in the infant. The symptom is primarily bilious vomiting. Older children may present with failure to thrive, diarrhea, and malabsorption (due to chronic venous and lymphatic obstruction). Alternatively, people with malrotation may live their entire lives without symptoms. Radiographically a plain film of the abdomen may demonstrate partial or complete duodenal obstruction evidenced by a dilated stomach and duodenum with a relative paucity of air distally. A barium study is used for confirmation of midgut volvulus except in severely sick infants. The upper GI could best be characterized as the hunt for the ligament of Treitz. If the ligament is visualized in its normal position, left of the spine and at roughly the level of the bulb, then volvulus is ruled out. An abnormal exam may show the characteristic corkscrew appearance of the spirally wound small bowel around the SMA.

Therapy is an emergent trip to the OR to "un-volv" the bowel and anchor the gut in order to avoid recurrence.

Notes

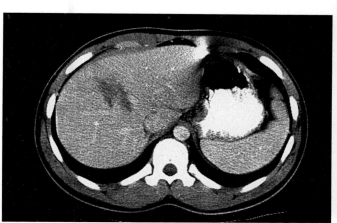

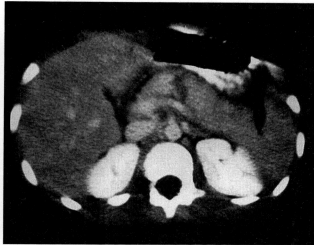

Patient 1.

Patient 2.

1. Which lobe is most often injured?
2. What space does deep peritoneal lavage sample?
3. In what space is fluid detected by ultrasound?
4. What retroperitoneal organs are at risk in blunt trauma?

Abdominal Organ Laceration

1. The right lobe, as it is in contact with the ribs and spine.

2. Only the peritoneal space.

3. The peritoneal space.

4. Pancreas, duodenum, and kidneys are retroperitoneal.

Reference

Arkovitz MS, Johnson N, Garcia VF: Pancreatic trauma in children: mechanisms of injury. *J Trauma* 42(1): 49–53, 1997.

Cross-Reference

Pediatric Radiology: THE REQUISITES, 2nd edn, p 146.

Comment

The liver is the second most commonly injured organ in blunt trauma after the spleen. Liver injury is best characterized with contrast-enhanced CT. Lacerations, intraparenchymal hemorrhage, and subcapsular hematoma are common in severe blunt injuries. Lacerations appear as branching hypodensities on contrast scans. Those lacerations that extend to two surfaces are termed fractures. Lacerations in the region of the porta hepatis may involve the cava or hepatic veins, potentially leading to rapid exsanguination. Intrahepatic hematomas appear as oval, poorly marginated hypodense regions, with regions of hyperdensity that represent clots of active extravasation. Subcapsular collections are hypodense with a crescentic shape along the margin. Blood may also dissect into the retroperitoneum through the bare area of the liver. A substantial bleed could easily be missed by a falsely negative ultrasound examination as the peritoneal cavity may be clear of blood.

Injury to the pancreas is far less common than hepatic injury and occurs as a result of compression between the abdominal wall and vertebral column. Kids in accidents involving handlebar injuries are good candidates for pancreatic injury. Contrast-enhanced CT will demonstrate lacerations as low attenuated lesions. Examination of the pancreatic duct is critical as transection of the duct or ductal fistulae must be repaired. Ultrasound may demonstrate peripancreatic fluid or pseudocysts as CT is often nondiagnostic in children.

Notes

Patient 1.

Patient 2.

1. What is an insufficiency fracture?
2. What is a fatigue fracture?
3. What is genu recurvatum?
4. How often is this entity bilateral?

Osgood–Schlatter vs. Sinding-Larsen–Johansson

1. A fracture due to normal stress on abnormal bone.

2. A fracture due to abnormal stress on normal bone.

3. Genu recurvatum is a condition in which there is hyperextension of the knees. Some degree of genu recurvatum is normal in females.

4. In 30% of cases.

References

Rosenberg ZS, Kawelblum M, Cheung YY, Beltran J, Lehman WB, Grant AD: Osgood-Schlatter lesion: fracture or tendinitis? Scintigraphic, CT, and MR imaging features. *Radiology* 185(3):853–858, 1992.

Medlar RC, Lyne ED. Sinding-Larsen–Johansson disease. Its etiology and natural history. *J Bone Joint Surg Am* 60(8):1113–1116, 1978.

Cross-Reference

Pediatric Radiology: THE REQUISITES, p 246.

Comment

Osgood–Schlatter disease is due to repetitive microtrauma of the patellar ligament at its tibial tuberosity insertion. Continual small microtears and cartilaginous avulsions lead to a clinical presentation of pain and swelling in boys 8–13 and girls 10–15 (M:F equals 5:1).

Radiographically, bony changes appear as fragmentation at the tibial tuberosity, although the appearance of fragmentation may only represent a normal ossification center. The distinguisher is the loss of the normal soft tissue appearance of Hoffa's fat pad, the region just posterior to the patellar tendon. Soft tissue changes demonstrates indistinctness of Hoffa's fat pad and loss of sharpness at its inferior edge, thickening of the patellar tendon, and soft tissue swelling anterior to the insertion. Naturally, you won't see many of these changes on a normal lateral radiograph of the knee. Low kVP is essential for bringing out the soft tissue contrast. MR demonstrates high signal in the tendon as well as bone marrow edema at the tibial insertion. Remember, this entity is a clinical diagnosis. Sequelae include nonunion, patellar subluxation chondromalacia, avulsion of the patellar tendon, and genu recurvatum.

Not to be outdone by the tibial tuberosity, the inferior pole of the patella, the patella tendon origin is susceptible as well to microtears and microavulsions due to repetitive trauma. Small ossification centers may be yanked off the bone and pulled inferiorly, leading to eventual fusion and elongation of the patella. Normal accessory ossification centers (bipartite patella) are found in the superolateral aspect of the patella, not inferiorly. This process is known by the eponym Sinding-Larsen–Johansson disease.

Notes

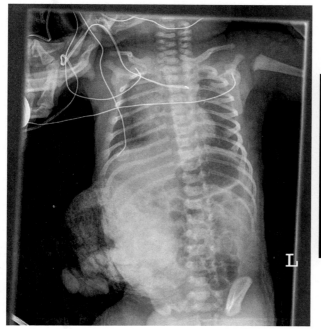

Patient 1.

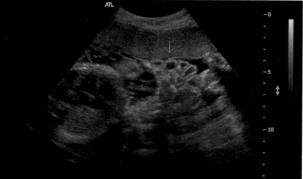

Patient 2.

1. Are osteomas related to Gardner syndrome or Peutz–Jeghers?
2. Would you perform an upper GI on this patient?
3. What is the therapy?
4. A normal barium enema in a newborn excludes malrotation, true or false?

Omphalocele/Gastroschisis

1. Gardner.

2. No, as the motility in gastroschisis is abnormal secondary to myenteric plexus damage from exposure to amniotic fluid.

3. The trick is to get the bowel back in the cavity; unfortunately the cavity has "shrunken" thereby requiring that the bowel be slowly "ratcheted" in by the use of a silo.

4. False.

Reference

Emanuel PG, Garcia GI, and Angtuaco TL: Prenatal detection of anterior abdominal wall defects with US. *Radiographics* 15:517–530, 1995.

Cross-Reference

Pediatric Radiology: THE REQUISITES, 2nd edn, pp 107–108.

Comment

The bowel leaves the abdominal cavity at the seventh week due to crowding by the liver and kidneys. Normally the homeless bowel reports back to the abdomen at 10 weeks fully rotated. In omphalocele, the bowel does not return but rather remains outside the abdominal cavity covered by two layers of peritoneum and connected to the umbilicus at the apex. The peritoneal covering ruptures in 10–20% of cases. Omphalocele is associated with prematurity as well as cardiac abnormalities, renal abnormalities, and Beckwith–Wiedemann syndrome (omphalocele, macroglossia, gigantism, and pancreatic hyperplasia with hypoglycemia).

Plain film findings will show a large soft tissue mass protruding from the abdomen, a finding easily conveyed to you by the technologist who took the film. The trick here is to diagnose it on ultrasound. Ultrasound features include; midline anterior abdominal wall defect, herniated sac of visceral contents, ascites, and the umbilical cord inserting at the apex of the sac. Therapy is surgical gut stuffing.

Gastroschisis, the other congenital anterior wall defect, is merely a rent or hole through which the abdominal contents herniate. The rent is most probably ischemic in origin and occurs after the bowel has returned into the body, hence there is no protective membrane as in omphalocele. The prognosis is much more favorable than omphalocele as there is a lower incidence of associated abnormalities. On ultrasound a small defect is seen located to the right side of the umbilical cord in 90% of cases. Plain film demonstrates a soft tissue mass protruding from the anterior wall.

Contrast study may show sluggish peristalsis, as there is presumed damage to the myenteric plexus from prolonged bathing in amniotic fluid.

	Gastroschisis	**Omphalocele**
Location	Right-sided defect	midline defect
Size of defect	Small (2–4 cm)	Large (2–10 cm)
Umbilical cord insertion	Anterior abdominal wall	On omphalocele
Membrane	No	Yes (3 layers)
Liver involved	No	Yes
Bowel involved	Common	Uncommon
Ascites	No	Yes
Other abnormalities	Rare	Common

Notes

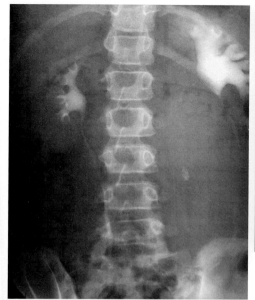

Patient 1.

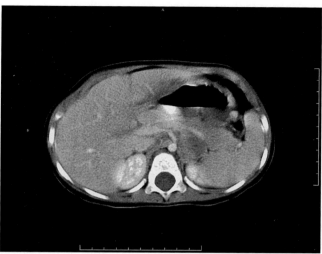

Patient 2.

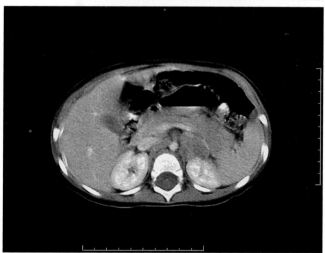

Patient 2.

1. What is the blood supply of the adrenal gland?

2. What age has the highest incidence of this entity?

3. Is "dumbbell" extradural extension more common in the abdomen or chest?

4. Name two associated paraneoplastic syndromes.

Neuroblastoma

1. Three arteries: superior adrenal, a branch from the inferior phrenic; middle adrenal, a branch off the aorta; and the inferior adrenal, a branch off the renal artery.

2. 2 months to 2 years.

3. Chest.

4. Opsoclonus/myoclonus ("dancing eyes and dancing feet") and cerebellar ataxia; watery diarrhea with hypokalemia syndrome (WDHK) (excess of vasoactive peptide).

Reference

David R, Lamki N, Fan S, Singleton EB, et al.: The many faces of neuroblastoma. *Radiographics* 9:859–882, 1989.

Cross-Reference

Pediatric Radiology: THE REQUISITES, pp 177–179.

Comment

Neuroblastoma arises from the overamplification of the myc oncogene in crest cells that reside within the adrenal medulla or the sympathetic nerve ganglia. Two-thirds of the tumors are located in the abdomen (the majority from the adrenals) and one-third are located within the chest, head, and neck region. Two variants, the ganglioneuroma and the intermediate ganglioneuroblastoma, differ by degree of cellular maturation.

Clinically, neuroblastoma will grow unnoticed until it invades adjacent structures or metastasizes. Irritability, weight loss, fever, and anemia are the nonspecific presentations. An abdominal neuroblastoma may present as a palpable mass. Ninety-five per cent of patients excrete excess vanillylmandelic acid (VMA) in the urine. Two-thirds of patients have disseminated disease at the time of presentation with metastatic involvement of the skeleton, bone marrow, liver, lymph nodes, and skin reported.

Radiographs will demonstrate a posterior mediastinal chest mass that will often erode bone (check the adjacent ribs). Abdominal radiographs will show an abdominal mass. Computed tomography may show an inferiorly displaced and compressed functional kidney. In contrast, Wilms tumor is more likely to distort the kidney parenchymal architecture due to its intraparenchymal location. Ultrasound demonstrates an abdominal mass with mixed echogenicity. MR, the mainstay of neuroblastoma imaging, describes the extent and morphology of the lesion.

Calcification is detected in 85% of cases, and only in 5% of Wilms tumors. Paravertebral extension, local organ invasion, and encasement of the celiac axis are easily detected with computed tomography of MR. In addition to vascular encasement, MR will best demonstrate invasion into the spinal canal as well as bony involvement.

Notes

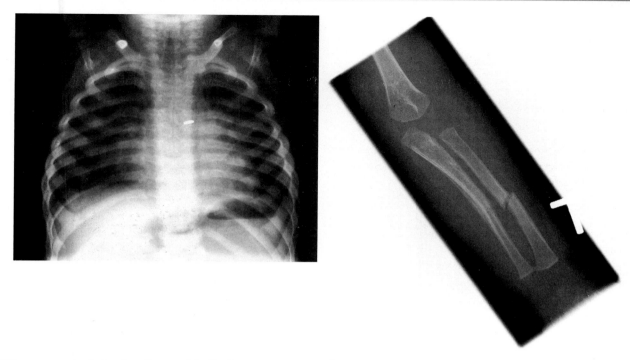

1. What musculoskeletal radiographic finding is seen in malnutrition?

2. State several cutaneous lesions seen in this entity?

3. What may be the ocular findings?

4. Should head CT be performed?

Posterior Rib Fracture

1. Osteomalacia.

2. Ecchymoses, abrasions, bites, burns.

3. Retinal hemorrhages.

4. Yes, to evaluate intercranial trauma if other injuries are present.

Reference

Kleinman, PK: *Diagnostic Imaging of Child Abuse,* 2nd edn. Philadelphia: Mosby, 1998.

Cross-Reference

Pediatric Radiology: THE REQUISITES, 2nd edn, pp 249–250.

Comment

An estimated 1.5 million children per year in the United States are abused. Between 1000 and 5000 die annually as a consequence, in almost all cases under 2 years old. Patients often present with signs of neglect and malnutrition. They may be withdrawn and quiet.

The skeletal survey is obtained for children under 2–3 years as a reliable history is neither feasible nor obtainable. Children over 2–3 receive a bone scan as skeletal surveys at this age impart substantial radiation. Follow-up radiographs are selected for confirmation of positive nuclide scans. Additional modalities such as CT for skull, cerebral, and abdominal injury as well as MR for the brain may be employed.

Characteristic imaging findings include:

1. Metaphyseal fractures, also called "bucket handle" or "corner fractures," which are most common in the distal femur, distal humerus, wrist and ankle. These fractures are most specific for child abuse. The mechanism is periosteal avulsion with microfracture of the growing bone at its metaphyseal insertion.

2. Fractures in different stages of healing:

    0–3 days: Soft tissue swelling

    3–7 days: Resolution of soft tissue swelling

    10–14 days: Periosteal new bone formation

    2–6 weeks: Callus formation and remodeling

    3–12 months: Further remodeling

3. Spiral fractures in infants, particularly in the femur, humerus, and tibia.

4. Fractures caused by unusual mechanisms: posterior ribs, spinous processes, or fractures of metacarpals and metatarsals.

5. Multiple skull fractures or fractures in unusual locations: scapular/spinous process/metatarsal/carpal fractures. A head CT revealing a parietooccipital subdural hematoma is classic.

The radiologist, when confronted with findings consistent with child abuse, is obligated to communicate both in writing and verbally with the referring clinician!

Notes

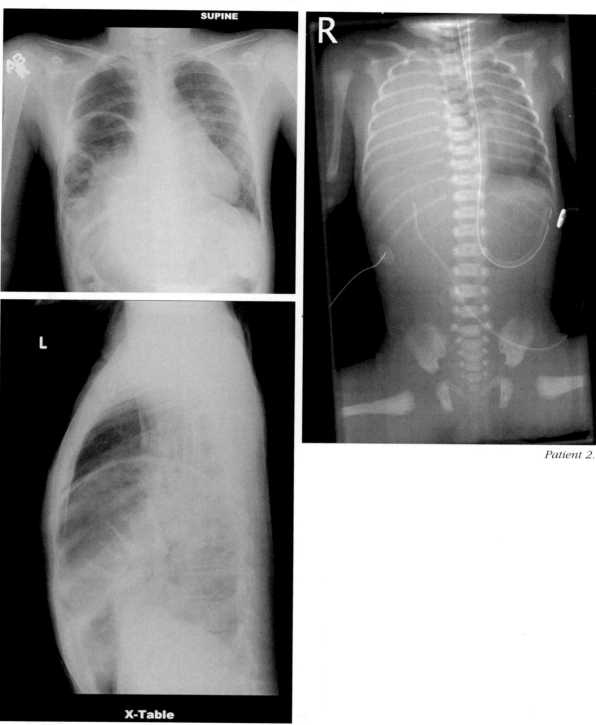

Patient 1.

Patient 2.

Patient 1.

1. Which entity is more common, the one present in Patient 1 or the one present in Patient 2?

2. What is the clinical presentation?

3. What is the incidence?

4. What is the differential diagnosis?

Diaphragmatic Hernia: Bochdalek vs. Morgagni

1. Yes. Patient 1 shows Bochdalek hernia.

2. Scaphoid abdomen.

3. 1:1000.

4. Congenital cystic adenomatoid malformation and congenital pulmonary cystic disease.

Reference

Panicek DM, Heitzman ER, Randall PA, et al.: The continuum of pulmonary anomalies. *Radiographics* 7:747–772, 1987.

Cross-Reference

Pediatric Radiology: THE REQUISITES, 2nd edn, pp 24–25, 43, 101, 104–105.

Comment

Ninety per cent of congenital hernias are **B**ochdalek (**b**ack of diaphragm, **b**ig **b**abies), and a herniation through the foramen of **M**orgagni occurring in 3% to 5% (**m**iddle of diaphragm, **m**ature, **m**inuscule baby). Morgagni hernias most commonly occur on the right side—the heart "protects" the left anterior chest.

Congenital diaphragmatic hernias lead to lung hypoplasia as the lung cannot adequately develop in a hemithorax filled with bowel. The GI tract begins to develop at roughly 7 weeks by lengthening within the coelomic cavity, or primitive nonpartitioned chest and abdomen. As lengthening occurs, the tube exceeds the capacity of the cavity and begins developing externally. At around 12 weeks the tube migrates back within the coelomic cavity. The hole that the primitive gut travels through is known as the pleuroperitoneal canal. Timing is critical! Concurrently, the diaphragm begins to develop, dividing the chest from the abdomen. A good analogy is to think of the diaphragm as a gate. If the gut migrates back before the diaphragm fully develops an excess of GI tract will be caught in the thorax. Alternatively, if the diaphragm is slow to develop, the "hungry-for-real-estate" bowel will take up residence within the thorax.

Imaging of the hernia ordinarily occurs at prenatal ultrasound yielding a "bright chest" filled with echogenic bowel. On conventional radiographs early neonatal films will demonstrate a soft tissue density that will give way to the classic air-filled bowel loops. Few loops will be seen within the abdomen, which on physical exam appears scaphoid due to the relative loss of abdominal contents.

Associated anomalies include neural tube defects, malrotation, and cardiovascular anomalies. Therapy includes surgical repositioning of the bowel and extracorporeal membrane oxygenation therapy. Prognosis and mortality (45%) have remained poor over the last few decades.

Notes

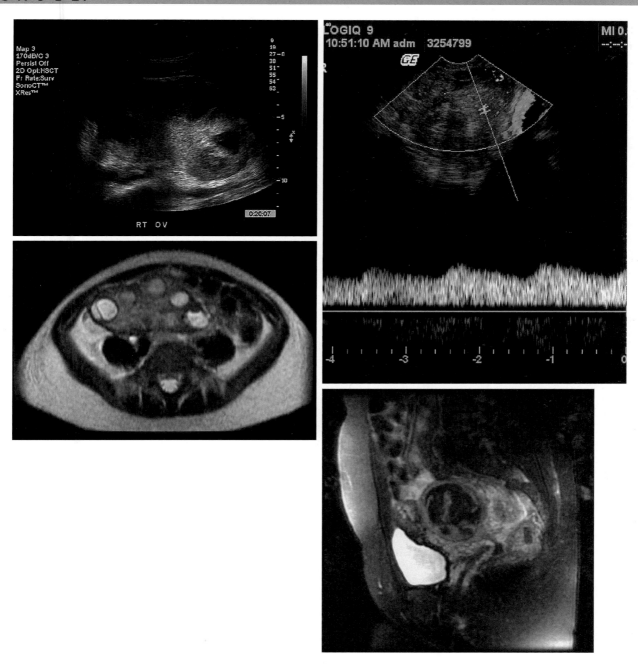

1. Is this entity an emergency?

2. Adnexal masses tend to stabilize ovaries, reducing the risk of this entity: true or false?

3. The follicles will commonly appear larger than expected in this entity: true or false?

4. The appearance on enhanced CT will demonstrate a homogenous attenuation: true or false?

Ovarian Torsion

1. Yes.

2. False. Masses greatly increase the risk of torsion.

3. True. Congestion causes increase pressures and fluid diffuses into the follicles.

4. False. The ovary is more likely to be heterogeneous due to variable perfusion.

References

Fleischer AC, Brader KR: Sonographic depiction of ovarian vascularity and flow: current improvements and future applications. *J Ultrasound Med* 20(3): 241–250, 2001.

Fleischer AC, Stein SM, Cullinan JA, Warner MA: Color Doppler sonography of adnexal torsion. *J Ultrasound Med* 14(7):523–528, 1995.

Cross-Reference

Pediatric Radiology: THE REQUISITES, p 188.

Comment

Ovarian torsion is a clinically uncommon occurrence that leads to the all-too-common rule-out torsion ultrasound requisition. The football-shaped ovary is connected to the broad ligament via the anterior "football laces" while the medial aspect is suspended by the ovarian ligament. The lateral and posterior aspects are free to flap in the intraperitoneal breeze. The blood supply splits between the uterine artery and the ovarian artery via the aorta or right renal artery. Twisting on the long axis of the ovary can occur, causing compression and occlusion of the ovarian vessels. Ovarian cysts are commonly found in torsion cases, suggesting that a large floppy ovarian cyst may predispose to a nonspontaneously reducing twisting event. The low-pressure venous system is the first to occlude, causing edema and ovarian enlargement. As the vascular compromise grows, ischemic changes increase with transudative fluid leaking out of the dying cells, creating prominent follicles as well as free fluid in the cul-de-sac. Eventually arterial thrombosis with ovarian infarction occurs. Obviously, the trick is to get to the ovary before necrosis.

Clinically, ovarian torsion presents with nonspecific findings such as lower abdominal pain, nausea, vomiting, and low-grade fever. Palpable masses are present in two-thirds of those patients that undergo physical examination.

Ultrasound findings include enlargement of the ovary with prominent follicles and a hypoechoic echotexture. Doppler ultrasound may demonstrate the presence of arterial flow but this may be secondary to recruited arteries from the uterine artery. Differential considerations include hemorrhagic ovarian cyst, ovarian teratoma, and an appendiceal abscess.

Therapy is surgical "untorsing" of the ovary.

Notes

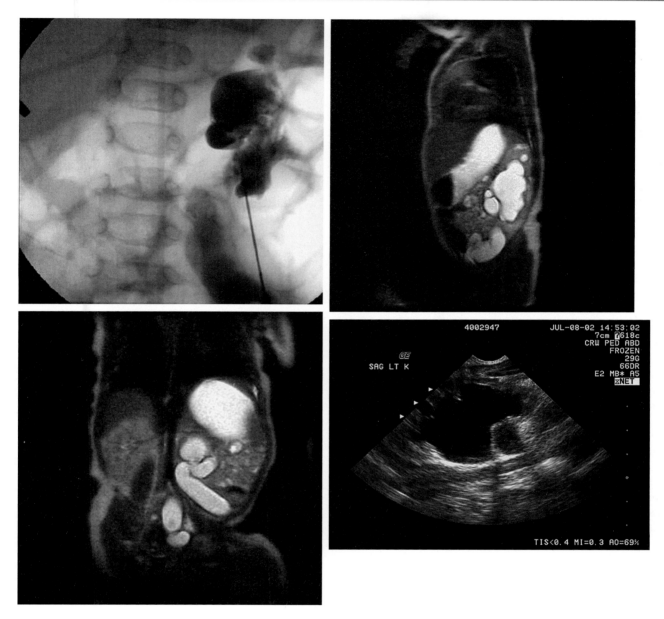

1. Name some associated anomalies of this entity.

2. How often is this entity an isolated finding?

3. Do yolk sac tumors or seminomas have associated elevated alpha-fetoprotein (AFP) levels?

4. How is a functional obstruction distinguished from dilatation?

C A S E 25

Primary Megaureter

1. Calyceal diverticulum, papillary necrosis, reflux, ureterocele, ureteral duplication, renal ectopia, ureteropelvic junction obstruction.

2. Primary megaureter is an isolated finding in 95% of cases.

3. Yolk sac tumors have elevated AFP levels.

4. Furosemide scintigraphy or Whitaker test.

Reference

Kirks DR, ed.: *Practical Pediatric Imaging: Diagnostic Radiology of Infants and Children,* 3rd edn. Philadelphia: Lippincott Williams & Wilkins, 1997, pp 776–778.

Cross-Reference

Pediatric Radiology: THE REQUISITES, pp 164–165.

Comment

Megaureter results from a shortened aperistaltic fibrotic segment just proximal to the ureterovesicular junction that causes a functional obstruction (a permanent "ureteral ileus") with resultant hydronephrosis. Most commonly patients are asymptomatic (detection through prenatal ultrasound), although they may present with pain, urinary tract infection, or a mass.

Prenatal ultrasound may show a markedly dilated ureter with peristaltic activity down to the distal aperistaltic segment. A voiding cystourethrogram is necessary to rule out VUR. Excretory urography and renal scintigraphy are used to demonstrate ureteric anatomy and renal function. Treatment is surgical with excision of the fibrotic distal portion, reanastomosis, and resultant normalization of the urine flow.

Notes

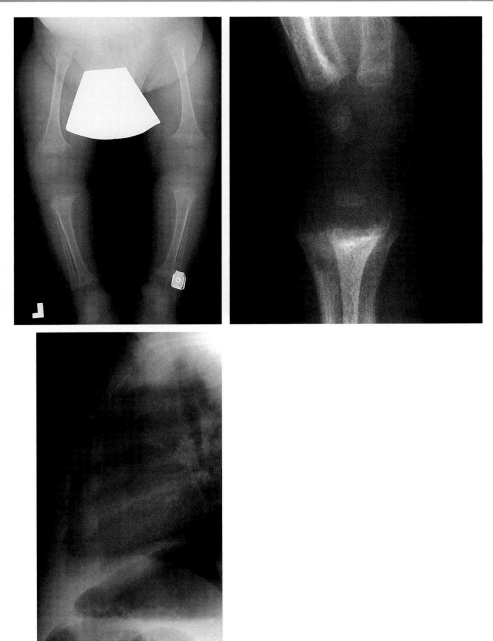

1. What is the difference between adsorption and absorption?
2. What are the radiographic features of this entity?
3. At what age is this entity diagnosed?
4. What are the demographics of this entity?

Rickets

1. Adsorption is the attachment of one substance onto the surface of another. Absorption is to take in or assimilate. Resorption is the loss of a substance through physiologic or pathologic means.

2. Widened physis, cupping, fraying and irregularity of the distal metaphysis, osteopenia, anterior rib splaying (rachitic rosary).

3. Usually before 2 years.

4. Patients who have nutritional vitamin D deficiency, lack of sunlight, neonatal hepatitis, anticonvulsant medications, sprue, defect in D synthesis, inherited renal tubular acidosis, familial vitamin D resistance.

Reference

States LJ: Imaging of metabolic bone disease and marrow disorders in children. *Radiol Clin N Am* 39(4):749–772, 2001.

Cross-Reference

Pediatric Radiology: THE REQUISITES, p 214.

Comment

Building bone and building skyscrapers share many similarities. Bone is made of an organic matrix that is reinforced by the inorganic calcium containing hydroxyapatite salt, much the same way as buildings are framed by steel and reinforced by concrete. One can think of bone disorders as either affecting the mineral component (concrete), or the organic matrix (steel girders). A short discussion of osteogenesis will prove useful.

Two kinds of bone formation exist, intramembranous and enchondral ossification. Mesenchymal cells are the precursors of both forms. Intramembranous ossification, as seen in flat bones, occurs with the direct transformation of mesenchymal cells into osteoblasts. Alternatively, enchondral ossification, the tubular or long bone method, employs a chondroblast or cartilage producing middle man that is responsible for the cartilaginous growth plate.

Enchondral ossification begins with conversion of the mesenchymal osteoprogenitors into chondrocytes that lay down a cartilaginous template for eventual bone deposition. The chondrocytes at the center diaphysis die, releasing calcium that joins with serum phosphate to mineralize the cartilage (provisional calcification). Osteoclasts are signaled by the mineralized cartilaginous matrix and begin to remove it, causing the ingrowth of vessels and arrival of the osteoblasts. Osteoblasts substitute collagen matrix for the removed mineralized cartilaginous matrix. The matrix then mineralizes with hydroxyapatite and mature bone is born. This describes the primary ossification center. The same process produces lengthening at the secondary ossification centers (growth plates) or at the end of long bones.

Rickets is caused by some disturbance in the building blocks of hydroxyapatite crystals, calcium, and phosphate. Vitamin D and parathyroid hormone are the major players in the homeostasis of serum calcium and phosphate. Vitamin D increases Ca intestinal absorption, increases PO_4 and Ca renal absorption. Parathormone increases serum Ca by bone resorption, renal resorption, and intestinal resorption; however, it decreases phosphate resorption in the kidney, spilling phosphate into the urine. A deficiency of normal vitamin D will decrease calcium levels, prompting parathormone to maintain serum calcium levels by initiating osteoclasts to pull Ca from the bones. Unopposed parathormone will cause phosphate wasting as there is no vitamin D to direct phosphate resorption in the kidney. It is this loss of phosphate, more so than calcium, that appears to be responsible for rickets. With low phosphate there is no provisional calcification, no osteoclast resorption of the cartilaginous matrix and no stop to the chondrocyte matrix production. Therefore a widened, disorganized, nonmineralized growth plate is seen in rickets. The cartilage grows its way into the marrow cavity, producing the appearance of frayed metaphyses. Rickets is both an abnormality of steel (disorganized cartilage matrix template) and an abnormality of concrete (absent provisional calcification necessary for bone synthesis).

Osteomalacia occurs as a result of poorly mineralized new osteoid laid down during routine bone remodeling. Vitamin D is also required for proper mineralization of remodeling bone during adult life. The poorly mineralized, newly laid down matrix is soft and easily deformable without the support of the hydroxyapatite "concrete." Softening of the bone will occur with bowing and coarsening of the matrix.

Notes

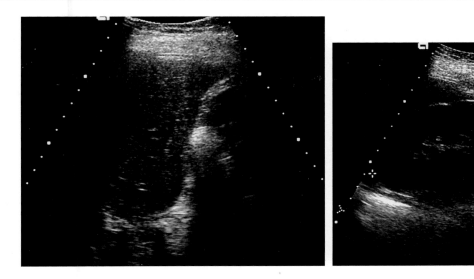

1. What is the etiology of oligohydramnios?
2. What is the etiology of polyhydramnios?
3. What structures develop from the Mullerian duct?
4. What structures develop from the Wolffian duct?

Renal Agenesis

1. **DRIPPC: D**emise, **R**enal abnormalities, **I**UGR, **P**remature rupture of membranes, **P**ost dates, **C**hromosomal abnormalities.

2. Idiopathic, diabetes, hypertension, neural tube defects, proximal GI obstruction, chest masses, twin—twin transfusion, nonimmune hydrops.

3. Mullerian duct forms the entire female genitalia except the distal third of the vagina.

4. Wolffian duct is the anlage for the vas deferens, seminal vesicles, and epididymis.

References

Daneman A, Alton DJ: Radiographic manifestations of renal anomalies. *Radiol Clin N Am* 29(2):351–363, 1991.

Romero R, Cullen M, Grannum P, et al.: Antenatal diagnosis of renal anomalies with ultrasound. III. Bilateral renal agenesis. *Am J Obstet Gynecol* 151(1):38–43, 1985.

Cross-Reference

Pediatric Radiology: THE REQUISITES, p 155.

Comment

Formation of the urinary system involves northward migration of the primitive collecting system (ureteric bud) and subsequent fusion to the primitive kidneys (the metanephrogenic cap portion of the nephrogenic blastema). The kidneys differentiate secondary to induction by the ureteric bud and then "ascend" to their position in the upper abdomen. It is not a true ascension but rather caudal growth of the body around the kidneys. Urine is produced early in the first trimester with excretion into the amniotic fluid, which is then swallowed and absorbed by the small intestine.

Renal agenesis occurs in two varieties, unilateral (1:1000) or bilateral (1:8000). Bilateral agenesis is incompatible with life; infants usually die either following birth or a few months thereafter. The etiology points toward failure of induction by the ureteric bud, as it does not come into contact with the nephrogenic blastema in instances of renal agenesis. Bilateral agenesis results in oligohydramnios, prematurity, Potter facies, with low-set, floppy ears, prominent epicanthal folds, micrognathia and pulmonary hypoplasia. Oligohydramnios in the absence of ruptured membranes ought to point you toward renal evaluation in utero via ultrasound. Naturally, the kidneys are not visualized. The adrenals, however, are present as they develop from a differing embryologic origin. The adrenals will be larger and have a discoid shape, so be careful not to mistake them for kidneys. Follow-up radionuclide imaging at birth demonstrates no functional renal tissue.

Unilateral renal agenesis occurs by the same mechanism, failure of the ureteric bud formation or degeneration. The solitary (contralateral) kidney undergoes compensatory hypertrophy following birth. The ipsilateral adrenal gland is present in 85% of cases. Renal agenesis may be seen associated with genital malformation: in girls, hydrometrocolpos, vaginal atresia, and vaginal septum; in boys, associations include cryptorchidism, hypospadias, and absent testes.

Notes

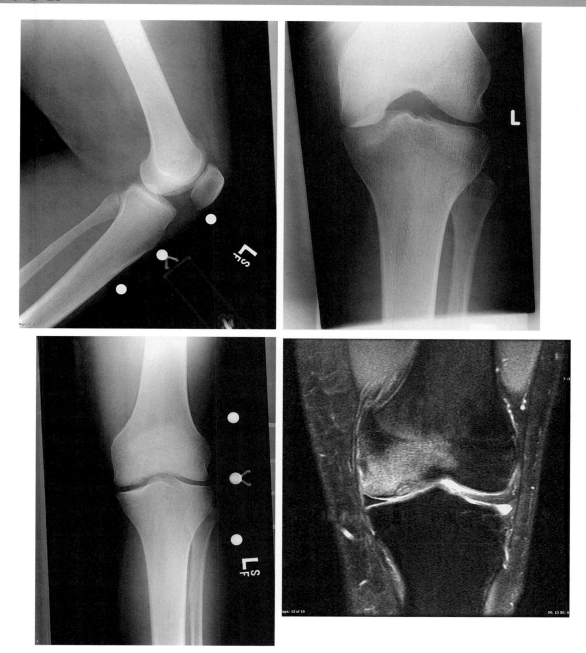

1. Males are more commonly affected. True or false?

2. Adults heal better due to physeal closure. True or false?

3. The age group is commonly 4–15 years. True or false?

4. The most common site is the lateral aspect of the medial femoral condyle. True or false?

Osteochondritis Dissecans

1. True. M:F equals 3:1.

2. False. Children heal far better with stable lesions than adults, who often require surgery. The physis has nothing to do with it.

3. True. The age is commonly 4–15 years.

4. True: the "intracondylar aspect" of the weight-bearing medial condyle.

Reference

Kier R, McCarthy S, Dietz MJ, Rudicel S: MR appearance of painful conditions of the ankle. *Radiographics* 11:401–414, 1991.

Cross-Reference

Pediatric Radiology: THE REQUISITES, p 243.

Comment

Osteochondritis dissecans is thought to arise in children due to repetitive microtrauma, the most common site is the lateral aspect of the medial femoral condyle (the side the makes up the notch). Other sites include patella, talar dome, and capitellum. A trauma history is elicited in 50% of cases. Long-term complications include osteonecrosis and degenerative arthritis. The process may involve cartilage, subchondral bone, or both.

Radiographically, a lucent defect with irregular edges will be seen in those fractures involving subchondral bone. Naturally, cartilage defects will only be detected on MR. Lesions may range from a rent in the cartilage to a partial or completely separated osteochondral loose body. MR is used to characterize the lesions as either stable (conservative management) or unstable (requiring surgery). Stable lesions are bone bruises with mild subchondral collapse and intact cartilage. Unstable lesions demonstrate bright T2 signal (joint fluid) interdigitating between the fragment and the parent bone and are far less likely to heal on their own, thus necessitating surgery.

Notes

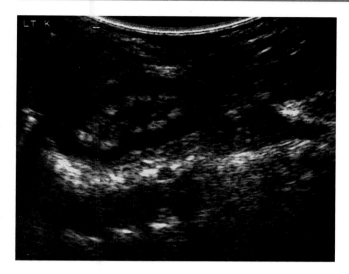

1. What is Alport syndrome?

2. What percent of stones are radiopaque?

3. What stone cannot be seen on CT?

4. How are uric acid stones treated? How are oxalate stones treated?

Nephrocalcinosis

1. Hereditary chronic nephritis, hearing loss, sensation loss and visual loss

2. 85%.

3. A stone formed from the HIV protease inhibitor class.

4. Uric acid stones are treated by raising the pH of the blood and secondarily the urine. Oxalate stones are treated by hydration, dietary oxalate restriction, and ureteroscopic removal, depending on the size and location of the stone.

References

Dyer RB, Chen MY, Zagoria RJ: Abnormal calcifications in the urinary tract. *Radiographics* 18:1405–1424, 1998.

Fowler KA, Locken JA, Duchesne JH, et al.: US for detecting renal calculi with nonenhanced CT as a reference standard. *Radiology* 222(1):109–113, 2002.

Cross-Reference

Pediatric Radiology: THE REQUISITES, pp 170–171.

Comment

Renal calcifications can occur in three locations, the cortex, the medulla, and the collecting system. Cortical nephrocalcinosis is caused by chronic glomerulonephritis, cortical ischemic necrosis (ethylene glycol—antifreeze, straight up), hyperoxalosis, chronic hypercalcemia, oxalosis and Alport syndrome. Cortical nephrocalcinosis, calcification at the glomerulus is rare compared with calcification of the renal tubules or medullary calcinosis.

Medullary calcinosis appears as fine or coarsened calcific densities in the medullary portion of the kidney. They seldom shadow on ultrasound. The causes of medullary calcinosis are a pimp classic. Renal tubular acidosis (RTA) (distal Type I) demonstrates low citrate levels that normally act as urolithiasis inhibitors. RTA patients are unable to secrete adequate amounts of hydrogen into the collecting tubule. This higher pH produces a compensatory hypercalciuria that in the setting of low citrate levels produces diffuse calcification in normal-sized kidneys. Medullary sponge kidney (MSK) or benign renal tubular ectasia produces tubular calcification due to areas of stasis. Radially arrayed calcification emanating from the papilla is characteristic for MSK. Ultrasound will illustrate hyperechoic deposits of calcium in the renal pyramids, diuretics, hyperparathyroidism, milk-alkali syndrome, Cushing syndrome, papillary necrosis, and chronic pyelonephritis.

Urolithiasis is idiopathic in 30% of cases. Other causes of stones include chronic UTI, urinary stasis, proximal RTA, and enteric causes such as interruption of the enteropathic circulation (oxalate stones), and dehydration secondary to diarrhea will produce uric acid stones. Lasix therapy for surfactant deficiency in neonates commonly causes stone formation. CT will localize the stone, measure the stone (urology will extract stones too large to pass), and rule out other potential pathologies that present with flank pain.

Notes

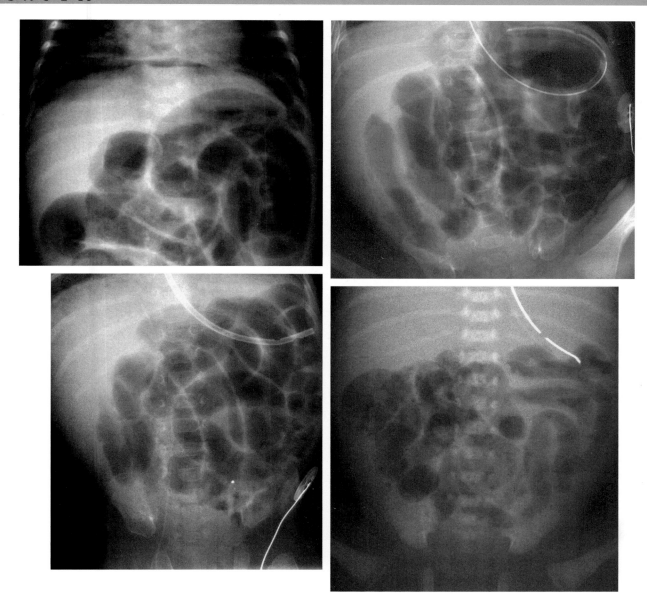

1. What are predisposing factors for the above entity?

2. Air in the liver indicates lethality, true or false?

3. This entity occurs most commonly in the left upper quadrant, true or false?

4. Barium study is often therapeutic, true or false?

Necrotizing Enterocolitis (NEC)

1. Premature rupture of membranes, preeclampsia, diabetes mellitus, multiparity, early feeding formula, umbilical artery/venous catheter (all are controversial however).

2. False.

3. False. Most commonly in the right lower quadrant, right colon or ileum.

4. Absolutely false. Under no circumstances should an upper GI or barium enema be performed!

Reference

Buonomo C: The radiology of necrotizing enterocolitis. *Radiol Clin N Am* 37(6):1187–1198, vii, 1999.

Cross-Reference

Pediatric Radiology: THE REQUISITES, 2nd edn, pp 83–84.

Comment

The midnight babygram usually means NEC watch. Necrotizing enterocolitis is an entity common to pre-emies that is thought to be caused by bowel ischemia. Decreased blood perfusion to the bowel wall may lead to edema, as well as "fixed dilated" loops giving way to loss of integrity with air dissecting into the ischemic wall.

Necrotizing enterocolitis presents with bloody diarrhea, abdominal distention, signs of sepsis, vomiting, apnea or lethargy in premature infants weighing less than 2500 g at the third to fourth day of life. Bowel ischemia from low flow has been hypothesized to result from hypoxia, stress, low blood pressure, and/or infection. Gas that enters the compromised wall may travel through the venous system to the liver. At this late stage, metabolic acidosis with disseminated intravascular coagulation may be present.

The work-up for NEC involves serial abdominal film every 12–24 hours with the addition of a decubitus film for the detection of free air or a fixed loop. The radiograph, taken at the time of presentation, will demonstrate a jumbled bowel appearance with areas of dilation and collapse. Gas may be seen within the bowel wall in either a bubbly or linear distribution. The gas may track into the bowel wall veins leading to the portal venous system. Portal venous gas may appear as fine branching lucencies, a diffuse mottled appearance, or as a focal central collection within the liver. Ultrasound may be helpful in detecting portal venous gas due to the conspicuity of dirty shadowing. Although debate has centered on the significance of portal venous gas as an indication for surgery, all agree that frank perforation with resultant pneumoperitoneum buys a trip to the OR. In less severe cases a conservative therapy of bowel rest and antibiotics is used until clinical and radiographic normalization occurs.

Notes

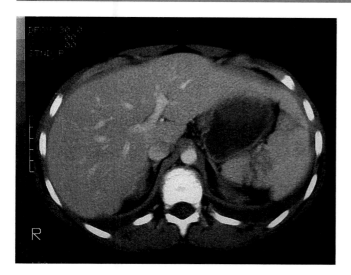

1. What is the sentinel clot sign?

2. What is the grading of this entity?

3. Are clefts usually seen medially or laterally?

4. How many HUs for sentinel clot? How many for hemoperitoneum?

Splenic Rupture

1. The attenuation of hemoperitoneum is highest adjacent to the injured organ.

2. I. Localized capsular disruption; small subcapsular hematoma.

   II. Small parenchymal laceration; parenchymal hematoma <3 cm.

   III. Fractures extending to hilum; parenchymal hematomas >3 cm.

   IV. Shattered spleen; vascular disruption.

3. Clefts are seen medially, small lacerations are usually noted laterally.

4. Sentinel clot = 60 HU, hemoperitoneum = 35–45 HU.

Reference

Paterson A, Frush DP, Donnelly LF, et al.: A pattern-oriented approach to splenic imaging in infants and children. *Radiographics* 19:1465–1485, 1999.

Cross-Reference

Pediatric Radiology: THE REQUISITES, 2nd edn, p 145.

Comment

The spleen is the most commonly injured abdominal organ with 10%–20% of injuries subclinical. Contrast-enhanced CT, not ultrasound, is the modality of choice in screening for abdominal injury in blunt or penetrating trauma.

Injury to the spleen may range from laceration, intrasplenic hematoma, subcapsular hematoma, infarction, or complete obliteration. Splenic laceration appears as a hypodense (nonenhancing) linear area. Splenic bleeds confined to the parenchyma will show focal hyperdensity on I– scan, while on I+ the bleed will be relatively hypodense to the normal enhancing tissue. Crescentic collections are attributed to subcapsular hematomas, while infarcts are typically wedge-shaped hypodensities with a broad base at the margin of the organ.

Therapy for pediatric patients has grown increasingly conservative due to the increased awareness of the importance of normal splenic function as well as favorable outcomes following watchful waiting. Long-term sequelae of splenic injury include pseudocyst formation as well as splenosis.

Notes

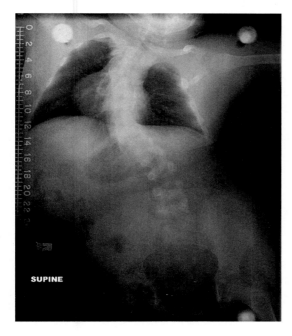

SUPINE

1. Name several common causes of this entity.

2. What are the most frequent patterns of the idiopathic form of this entity?

3. The congenital form is most commonly associated with what other abnormalities?

4. In contrast to the C shape in the idiopathic form, the S shape is seen in neuromuscular disorders, true or false?

Scoliosis

1. Idiopathic, hemivertebrae, myelodysplasia, cerebral palsy, neurofibromatosis, and postoperative deformity.

2. Convex right thoracic, convex right thoracic and convex left lumbar, convex right throracic and convex right lumbar.

3. Genitourinary, caudal, and spinal dysraphisms.

4. False. S = idiopathic, C = neuromuscular.

References

Greiner KA: Adolescent idiopathic scoliosis: radiologic decision-making. *Am Fam Physician* 5(9):1817–1822, 2002.

Afshani E, Kuhn JP: Common causes of low back pain in children. *Radiographics* 11:269–291, 1991.

Cross-Reference

Pediatric Radiology: THE REQUISITES, pp 295–296.

Comment

Scoliosis is the presence of one or more lateral curvatures of the spine. Scoliosis in children is most often idiopathic and is usually painless. The remaining 15% of cases are congenital, neuromuscular, post-traumatic, inflammatory, or neoplastic.

There are three types of idiopathic scoliosis: infantile, juvenile, and adolescent. Infantile scoliosis may either be progressive or nonprogressive. The nonprogressive form has a thoracic convex left curve that will not exceed 30°. The patients resolve spontaneously. The progressive form, however, progresses to curves greater than 35° (5°/year) and carries a poor prognosis as these patients are prone to scoliosis-related cardiorespiratory insufficiency. The juvenile form, most common in girls 4–9 years, demonstrates a right thoracic convexity, is progressive, and carries a poor prognosis.

The most common form, adolescent idiopathic scoliosis, is presumed to have a genetic component transmitted via autosomal dominance. There is a strong family occurrence with girls outnumbering boys 8:1. Typically there is a convex right thoracic curve that usually will not exceed 30°. These cases resolve spontaneously. Progression of the curvature occurs during growth spurts. The three main determinants for progression include gender, future growth potential, and the severity of curvature at diagnosis. Females have a tenfold risk for progression. The more severe the curve is the more likely it is to progress. Evaluation of future growth potential is determined by assessing the Tanner and Risser grade. The Tanner stages 2 and 3 occur just prior to the onset of the pubertal growth spurt, the period of greatest curvature progression. Estimation of further growth potential is made by measuring the percentage of iliac apophyseal fusion. The iliac apophysis fuses from anteromedial to posterolateral along the crest. A high thoracic level is associated with a worse prognosis. There is an association between idiopathic scoliosis and congenital heart disease.

Imaging depends on patient age and the cause of the curvature. Initial examination includes standing frontal and later radiographs of the entire spine obtained with a bone age evaluation. Findings on this examination determine the need for MRI or CT and the occasional skeletal survey in patients with suspected skeletal dysplasias or other syndromes. Measuring the magnitude of the curvature is performed with the method of Cobb. To use this method, draw lines parallel to the endplates of the two vertebral bodies that stray furthest from spinal axis, draw perpendicular lines and measure the angle at the intersection. Angles less than 10∞ are often neither clinically noted nor treated.

In 25% of cases of idiopathic scoliosis, the most common type, the curve may progress. Surgical correction of the scoliosis often is not contemplated until the Cobb angle exceeds 40° after skeletal maturity. In children with lesser degrees of scoliosis, initial treatment includes the use of a brace to counteract progression. Operative treatment may include internal fixation and bony fusion.

Notes

Patient 1.　　　　　　　　　　　　　　　　　　　*Patient 1.*

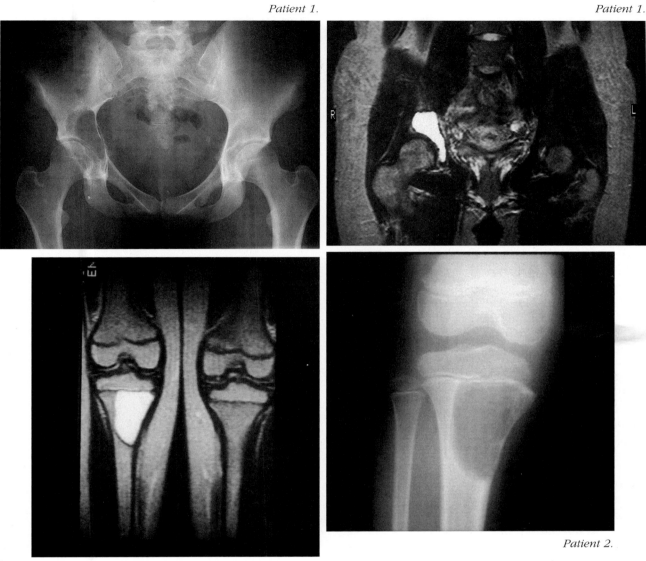

Patient 2.

Patient 2.

1. Do these lesions tend to be located centrally or eccentrically?

2. What is the appearance of this lesion on MR?

3. Is there a gender predominance?

4. What is the matrix?

Simple Bone Cyst

1. Simple bone cysts are found centrally.

2. Dark on T1 and uniformly bright on T2.

3. 2:1, male:female.

4. There is none. Cysts can fracture and hemorrhage, yielding heterogeneous signal intensity on MR sequences.

Reference

Lokiec F, Wientroub S: Simple bone cyst: etiology, classification, pathology, and treatment modalities. *J Pediatr Orthop B* 7(4):262–273, 1998.

Cross-Reference

Pediatric Radiology: THE REQUISITES, pp 236–237.

Comment

Simple or unicameral bone cysts are intramedullary fluid-filled lesions thought to occur due to venous outflow obstruction secondary to increased intramedullary pressure. Bone cysts are seen in 10–20-year-olds and present as pathologic fractures in 50% of cases. In time, the lesions fill in.

Radiographically, these lesions appear entirely lucent with a narrow zone of transition and no cortical breakthrough or periostitis. The cysts are located within the medullary cavity, most often in the proximal humerus and femur. Unlike the eccentric aneurysmal bone cyst, the unicameral bone cyst is in the center of the medullary cavity. Cysts may have an expansile appearance, expanding the cortex but never breaking through it. Unicameral bone cysts do not cross the growth plate. A part of the cyst wall may fracture and fall into the cyst, a so-called "fallen fragment sign." Fluid–fluid levels may then be seen on MR and CT.

Therapy is directed at preventing pathologic fractures in weight-bearing bones and includes steroid injection, curettage, and packing with bone fragments.

Notes

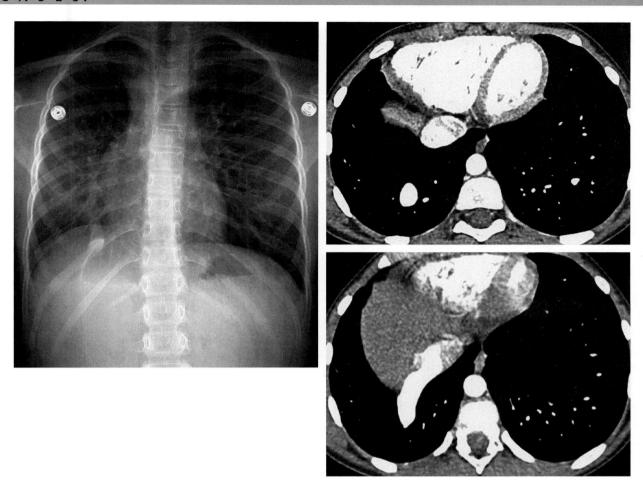

1. Are infections a common presentation?

2. Would bronchography be diagnostic?

3. Does this entity present more commonly on the right side?

4. What is the differential diagnosis?

C A S E 34

Scimitar Syndrome

1. Infections are not common as there is no sequestration present.

2. No, there is no abnormality of the bronchial tree.

3. Yes, it's more common on the right side.

4. Atelectasis, arteriovenous malformation, sequestration.

Reference

Woodring JH, Howard TA, Kanga JF: Congenital pulmonary venolobar syndrome revisited. *Radiographics* 86(5):607–613, 1994.

Cross-Reference

Pediatric Radiology: THE REQUISITES, 2nd edn, pp 23–24.

Comment

Scimitar syndrome consists of:

1. Hypoplasia or aplasia of one of more lobes of the right lung

2. Partial anomalous pulmonary venous return below the diaphragm

3. Absent or small pulmonary artery

4. Occasional rib and vertebral body anomalies

Scimitar or pulmonary venolobar syndrome is a constellation of congenital abnormalities including a small right lung, partial anomalous venous return, absent pulmonary artery, pulmonary sequestration, systemic arterialization of the lung, absent IVC, and accessory diaphragm. The syndrome may be inherited and has been associated with tetralogy of Fallot, truncus arteriosus, and hemivertebrae. Rather than draining to the left atrium, the oxygenated blood may enter the IVC, portal vein, hepatic vein, or right atrium. The pulmonary artery may be absent as well.

What distinguishes the venolobar syndrome from pulmonary sequestration is connection to the bronchial tree. The sequestration is separated from the pulmonary circulation as well as the airway, hence the propensity to present with infection. The scimitar syndrome contains only anomalous vasculature; the abnormally draining lobe is connected to the bronchial tree. As mentioned above, sequestration has been associated with venolobar syndrome.

Radiographically, a small right hemithorax demonstrates a crescent-shaped opacity (the pulmonary vein) that often parallels an indistinct right heart border. The vein is coursing toward either the IVC, portal, or hepatic veins. CT is used to evaluate venous drainage, absence of pulmonary arteries, sequestration, and IVC anomalies. CT will demonstrate a small right hemithorax with consolidations or bronchiectasis in severe cases.

The majority of patients are asymptomatic. Severe hypogenetic lung as well as sequestration may lead to recurrent pneumonias and bronchiectasis requiring surgery. Associated cardiac defects may present with congestive failure, necessitating surgical repair as well. In cases of severe shunting a surgical conduit may be required to link the pulmonary vein to the left atrium.

Notes

Patient 1.   Patient 1.

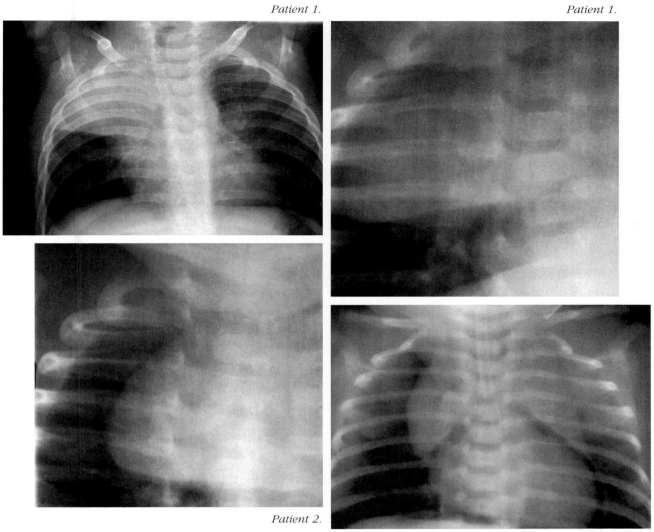

Patient 2.   Patient 2.

1. What is the differential diagnosis?

2. Name a common infectious etiologic agent seen in cystic fibrosis patients.

3. Name several causes of unilateral pulmonary edema.

4. Name three primary pulmonary malignancies.

Thymus vs. Pneumonia

1. Thymus, pneumonia, mediastinal mass, congenital cystic adenomatoid malformation.

2. *Pseudomonas aeruginosa.*

3. Rapid removal of air (chest tube for pneumothorax) or fluid (large pleural effusion), abnormal lymph drainage of one lung, pulmonary edema with child in decubitus position.

4. Bronchogenic carcinoma, leiomyosarcoma, and fibrosarcoma.

Reference

Griscom NT: Pneumonia in children and some variants. *Radiology* 167:297, 1988.

Cross-Reference

Pediatric Radiology: THE REQUISITES, 2nd edn, p 45.

Comment

In children, the thymus comprises the majority of the anterior mediastinum. Often nonvisualization of the thymus is a result of shrinkage secondary to stress or steroid therapy, and will rebound to its original size following resolution of the inciting condition. The thymus does not normally displace adjacent structures, and may be indented by ribs or the cardiac shadow. On fluoroscopy, the thymus is seen to elongate and narrow on inspiration; no surprise as the expanding lungs will push it more anteriorly. The much referred to "sail" sign merely represents the inferior border of the right thymic lobe tucking itself into the nearby minor fissure. On chest films the thymus is visible in children up to 3 years of age but may be seen in children as old as 9.

Three major features distinguish a thymic shadow from a pneumonia:

1. The thymus does not extend to the lung periphery

2. The thymus is seen more medially

3. The thymus is heterogenous with no air bronchograms

What does the thymus do? The T-cell is "born" in the bone marrow and shortly after migrates to the thymus. Rapid division with maturation (genetic splicing and recombination producing unique surface antibodies) takes place within the thymus for every single T-lymphocyte. The thymus will then present all of the body's "self-antigens" testing for reactivity. Nine out of ten T-cells will react to the body's own tissues as if they were foreign, necessitating destruction by the thymus. The bulk of this process begins at birth and lasts several months. Athymic infants will have no cellular immunity as the T-cells have no place to undergo this process of differentiation and selection. If the T-cell is lucky enough to graduate from the thymus its next port of call is the lymph node, where it will take up residence and wait for that "one-in-a-million antigen" with which to cross-react.

Notes

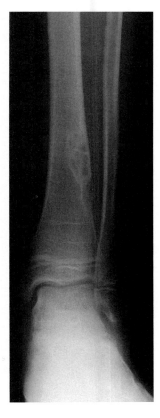

1. What percentage of the pediatric population is affected?

2. By what age do these lesions "disappear"?

3. Do these lesions grow?

4. Would you recommend biopsy?

Nonossifying Fibroma

1. Some reports claim up to 20% of the pediatric population have nonossifying fibromas (NOF).

2. These lesions fill in by age 30 years.

3. Yes, NOF may grow to become quite large before sclerosis and healing.

4. No, NOF is a benign lesion with very characteristic imaging findings.

Reference

Smith SE, Kransdorf MJ: Primary musculoskeletal tumors of fibrous origin. *Semin Musculoskelet Radiol* 4(1):73–88, 2000.

Cross-Reference

Pediatric Radiology: THE REQUISITES, pp 202–203.

Comment

A fibrous cortical defect is just that, a cortical defect composed of spindle-shaped connective tissue and giant cells. Unlike the similarly appearing fibrous dysplasia found in the medullary cavity, fibrous cortical defects originate in the cortex. A common benign entity, these lesions contain fibrous tissue and are thought to originate from abnormal physeal ossification. Larger lesions that extend into the medullary cavity are termed nonossifying fibromas and are seen more in adolescents.

Radiographically fibrous cortical defects appear as focal radiolucent areas in the cortex with an almost blister-like appearance. Mild cortical expansion with no periosteal reaction and a bubbly appearance are typical, while the larger nonossifying fibroma may appear with a sclerotic rim and trabeculation. These lesions are commonly found in tubular long bones and in those of the lower extremities, with a strange predilection for posteromedial surfaces. Although nonossifying fibromas have been known to fracture, these lesions usually fill in with osteoid, become mineralized, and resolve completely.

Notes

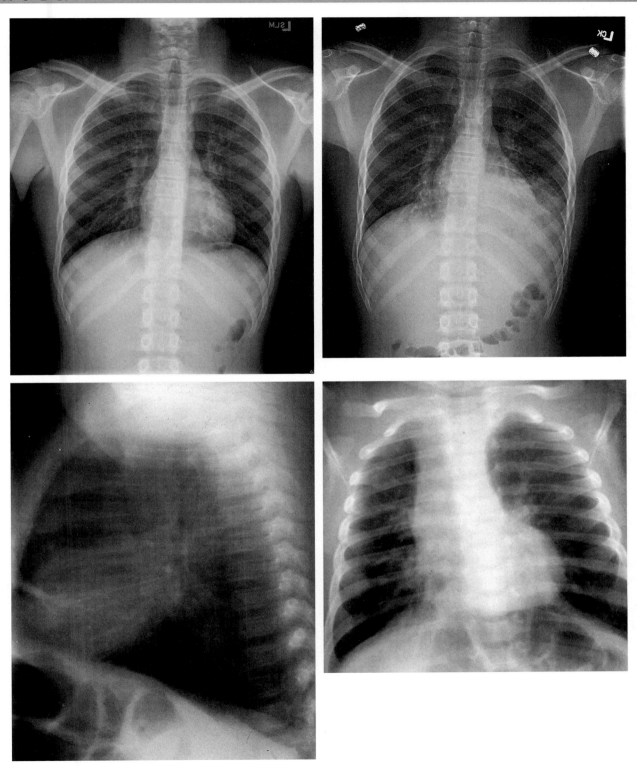

1. What is the differential diagnosis?

2. What percentage of patients with myasthenia gravis develop a thymoma?

3. What is bronchopneumonia?

4. What percentage of patients with thymoma develop myasthenia gravis?

C A S E 37

Mycoplasma Pneumonia vs. Viral Pneumonia

1. Viral pneumonia, miliary tuberculosis, and sarcoidosis.

2. 10–15%.

3. Pulmonary opacity due to peribronchial extension of inflammation: translation–airway into airspace disease.

4. 50%.

Reference

Betenay FAL, de Campo JF, McCrossin DB: Differentiating bacterial from viral pneumonias in children. *Pediatr Radiol* 18:453–454, 1988.

Cross-Reference

Pediatric Radiology: THE REQUISITES, 2nd edn, p 38.

Comment

Is it a bacterium? Is it a virus? No one is really sure. But what is known is that mycoplasma pneumonia is the most common cause of pneumonia in children over 5: 50% get tracheobronchitis, 30% pneumonia, and 10% each pharyngitis and otitis media. The presentation includes dry crackles, malaise, lethargy, dyspnea, cough, fever, and myalgias.

Chest films appear as segmental, subsegmental, or reticulonodular interstitial infiltrates. Lower lobe predominance with small transient effusions (20%) is also seen.

While bacterial pneumonias appear as discrete segmental to multilobar consolidation, viral pneumonias are far more subtle. Peribronchial thickening, hyperinflation, and scattered atelectasis are characteristics of viral lung infection. Peribronchial thickening or cuffing refers to the appearance of the bronchioles en face. The bronchi and bronchioles should appear as pencil-thin circles that are no larger in diameter than their corresponding vasculature. A thickened bronchiole that appears as a small doughnut is indicative of peribronchial cuffing. Peribronchial cuffing is more common in the pedi age group than adults, as the immature, small lungs have a lower surface to volume ratio. The reduced ratio greatly exaggerates airway resistance of even the smallest increases in bronchial mucus production, leading to hyperemia, edema, and air trapping. Hyperinflation, defined as flattened diaphragms, increased lucency, or more than 9–10 ribs on frontal films results. Scattered atelectasis is a result of disordered aeration with collapse of alveoli due to collateral flow of air.

Viral pneumonia in the under-2-year age group most commonly involves respiratory interstitial virus, parainfluenza viruses, and adenovirus. Patients present with cough and rhinitis. The appearance on chest films is bilateral hyperinflation, peribronchial thickening leading to increased hilar density. Bronchiolitis or inflammation of the bronchiole, as apposed to airway disease, is a seasonal entity (winter) commonly caused by respiratory syncytiovirus, giving a typical "viral" chest film appearance. While bronchiolitis affects the under-1-year age group, the term bronchitis is used in older children. Bronchitis, defined by strict clinical criteria, involves the same inflammatory airway picture seen in viral pneumonias as well as the so-called "dirty chest" film appearance due to peribronchial opacification.

Notes

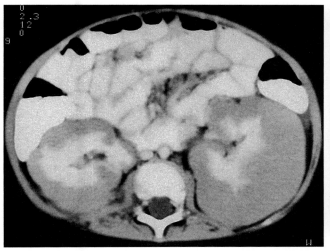

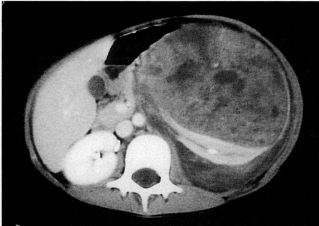

Patient 1.

Patient 2.

1. Who introduced paravertebral rib resection?

2. What is the peak incidence of this lesion? (Patient 2.)

3. What is the WAGR syndrome?

4. What is the differential diagnosis of bilateral renal enlargement?

C A S E 38

Intrarenal Masses: Nephroblastoma and Wilms Tumor

1. Max Wilms.

2. 4 months to 4 years.

3. **W**ilms tumor, **A**niridia, **G**enital anomalies, mental **R**etardation.

4. Nephroblastomatosis, nephrotic syndrome, polycystic kidney disease, glycogen storage, lymphoma/leukemia.

Reference
Lowe LH, Isuani BH, Heller RM, et al.: Pediatric renal masses: Wilms tumor and beyond. *Radiographics* 20:1585–1603, 2000.

Cross-Reference
Pediatric Radiology: THE REQUISITES, pp 174–177.

Comment
Nephroblastomatosis is an entity in which the kidney is peppered with primitive rests of metanephric tissue. These foci of renal tissue are intermixed with normal parenchyma in a predominantly subcapsular location. Nephroblastomatosis is considered a precursor to Wilms tumor. Congenital nephroblastomatosis leads to diffusely enlarged kidneys and is associated with trisomies 13 and 18 and with Beckwith–Wiedemann and Drash syndromes.

On ultrasound, the kidneys will appear diffusely enlarged with isoechoic or hyperechoic foci that represent the nephrogenic rests. CT will demonstrate homogenous, low attenuation and nonenhancement areas that represent the primitive nodules.

Wilms tumor, named after Max Wilms (1867–1918), a German surgeon who described it in 1899, is a malignant embryonic neoplasm. It accounts for about 10% of all childhood malignancies and represents the most common renal malignancy. Associated congenital abnormalities occur in 15% of all children with Wilms tumor. One per cent of patients have sporadic aniridia. Other associations include Beckwith—Weidemann, and isolated hemihypertrophy.

Wilms tumor is derived from abnormal cell development. The tumor may contain abnormal glomeruli, tubules, muscle, bone, and fat. Prognosis is based on grade. Clinical presentation includes an asymptomatic abdominal mass but may include hematuria and hemorrhage from a trivial trauma.

As with most of pediatrics, imaging begins with sonography. Ultrasound will demonstrate a large sharply marginated echogenic intrarenal mass. Necrosis and hemorrhage may result in mixed hypoechoic and hyperechoic areas with the tumor. Doppler evaluation of the IVC is helpful to rule out tumor extension. CT plays a central role evaluating the extent of tumor, vascular involvement, nodal involvement, liver mets, and the contralateral kidney (10% bilateral). On CT, Wilms will appear as a spherical, large, intrarenal mass with a well-defined rim. Enhanced studies will demonstrate decreased enhancement relative to normal renal tissue with areas of necrosis. Calcification is detected in approximately 10% of cases. Similar to renal cell carcinoma in adults, Wilms may extend into the renal veins and vena cava. MR is gaining acceptance as the new characterization modality due to multiplanar and vascular imaging. The tumor will appear dark on T1 and bright on T2. Areas of heterogeneity indicate necrosis, while focal regions of high T1 signal suggest hemorrhage.

Notes

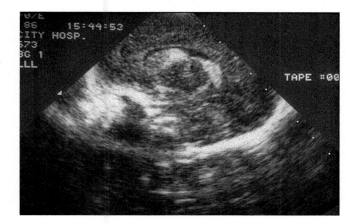

1. Is this entity seen in full-term infants?

2. What tracts run close to the germinal matrix?

3. What is spastic dysplasia?

4. What is the "flare" sign?

Germinal Matrix Hemorrhage

1. Rarely. It is primarily a disease of prematurity.

2. Corticospinal tract, making impaired motor function the most common clinical sequelae.

3. Bilateral spasticity with the upper limbs affected more than the lower.

4. Areas of abnormal increased globular echogenecity seen within the germinal matrix.

Reference

Blankenberg FG, Loh NN, Bracci P, et al.: Sonography, CT, and MR imaging: a prospective comparison of neonates with suspected intracranial ischemia and hemorrhage. *Am J Neuroradiol* 21(1):213–218, 2000.

Cross-Reference

Pediatric Radiology: THE REQUISITES, p 280.

Comment

Germinal matrix hemorrhage (GMH) is a common event in premature infants less than 32 weeks gestational age. What is the germinal matrix? The germinal matrix is the site of fetal brain cell genesis and is supplied by a fine lace-like network of delicate blood vessels. The germinal matrix is located in the subependymal layers just between the caudate and the thalamus, anterior to the caudothalamic groove. The vessels are sensitive to small changes in pressure and electrolyte abnormalities. Causes of GMH include hypoxia, hypertension, hypercapnia, hypernatremia, rapid volume increase, and pneumothorax. Germinal matrix bleeds begin in the subependymal location and may rupture into the ventricle or, less commonly, extend into the parenchyma. More serious bleeds will develop periventricular leukomalacia (PVL)—white-matter ischemia that leads to coagulation necrosis, phagocytosis, and eventual cyst formation.

All patients born under 32 weeks should be screened for GMH and then later at 4 weeks for PVL. On ultrasound, hemorrhage will appear as an echogenic focus anterior to the caudothalamic groove. A severity grading system aids in predicting outcome. Grade I is subependymal hemorrhage only. Grade II is intraventricular hemorrhage without hydrocephalus, while grade III demonstrates intraventricular hemorrhage with hydrocephalus. Blood within the ventricle will often lead to ventriculitis demonstrated by thickening of the echogenic subependymal layer. Progressive hydrocephalus requires shunting. Grade IV represents intraparenchymal hemorrhage and usually occurs in the frontal or parietal lobes. Intraparenchymal hemorrhage is thought to be due to an initial germinal matrix bleed that compresses adjacent veins, leading to parenchymal venous infarction. Evolving hemorrhage will lose its echogenic appearance and eventually become echolucent. The cysts measure on the order of 1 mm to 2 cm. Cysts found at birth suggest fetal hemorrhage or ischemia. Following substantial bleeds, PVL will show white-matter echogenecity that develops into cystic changes.

Notes

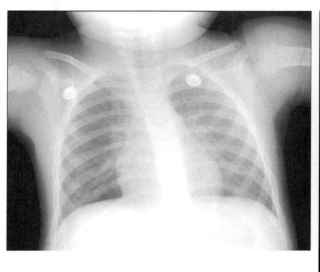

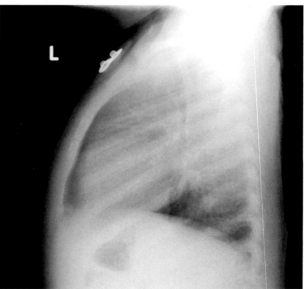

Noncyanotic patient

1. Is there increased or decreased pulmonary vascularity?

2. If the vascularity was normal what is your differential?

3. If the vascularity was increased what is your differential?

4. If this patient were cyanotic what diagnosis might you entertain?

C A S E 40

Atrial Septal Defect (ASD)

1. It is increased.

2. Acyanotic with normal vascularity: aortic stenosis, pulmonic stenosis, coarctation, and interrupted aortic arch.

3. Endocardial cushion defect, ASD, patent ductus arteriosus (enlarged LA and enlarged aorta), and ventricular septal defect (VSD) (enlarged LA and normal aorta).

4. Total anomalous pulmonary venous return.

Reference

Allen H: *Moss and Adams Heart Disease in Infants, Children and Adolescents: Including the Fetus and Young Adult,* 6th edn. Baltimore: Lippincott Williams & Wilkins, 2001, pp 603–617.

Cross-Reference

Pediatric Radiology: THE REQUISITES, 2nd edn, pp 57–58.

Comment

Atrial septal defect is roughly a third as common as VSD and accounts for 10% of congenital heart lesions. ASDs are most often isolated lesions and have a gender predominance for females by 4:1. ASDs are associated with Holt–Oram, Lutembacher, and Down syndromes. The atrial septum forms at 4 weeks with a small hole present (ostium primum) at the interface with the endocardial cushion. This first hole closes and a second hole forms at the roof of the septum (ostium secundum). A second membrane then forms in front of the primum septum with a similarly situated fenestration of its own. The two septa with their two ostia form the foramen ovale. ASDs may occur due to malformation of any of these elements; the clinical impact depends upon the location and size of the defect.

The most common defect is the ostium secundum, thought to be due to either excessive resorption or inadequate formation of the septum primum. A large left-to-right shunt develops. Ostium primum ASD is associated with endocardial cushion defects. Sinus venous ASD is located at the entrance of the superior vena cava (SVC) and is always associated with partial anomalous pulmonary venous return. The right upper pulmonary vein ought to drain into the left atrium, not the SVC.

The high pressure in the left atrium relative to the right atrium causes flow across the defect and increased pulmonary circulation with a similar appearance to VSD. However, unlike VSD, the left atrium is not enlarged as it decompresses into the RA through the septal defect. Clinically, most patients are asymptomatic and only discovered on physical exam as a mid-systolic murmur is heard. EKG will show right-sided enlargement.

Radiographically, small ASDs show no findings on chest films. Moderate to large ASD will demonstrate right atrial and right ventricular enlargement with increased pulmonary vasculature. RV enlargement is detectable by abnormal filling of the retrosternal air space on the lateral film and "disappearance" of the right superior mediastinum (rotation due to RV enlargement). Increased vascularity will only be detectable if the pulmonary circulation is twice the systemic circulation. The pulmonary vessels are enlarged and detectable in the lung periphery. If the diameter of the right descending pulmonary artery is greater than the trachea, think shunt vascularity. There is no enlargement of the left atrium, ventricle, or aorta. A sinus venosus ASD will contain a right upper lobe pulmonary vein in a horizontal rather than its normal oblique course as it anomalously drains into the SVC. In addition a bifid manubrium is sometimes associated with Down syndrome and is a helpful pickup on the lateral to push you toward an endocardial cushion defect. Also, look under the diaphragm for a double bubble/duodenal atresia.

The prognosis is excellent. These patients may undergo either transcatheter closure or surgical correction.

Notes

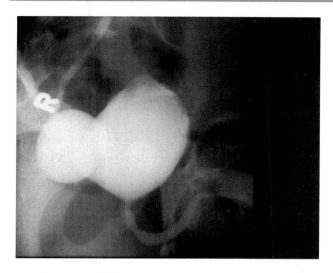

1. Is there a risk for malignancy?
2. What is the name of this entity if it was less than 2 cm?
3. Is there an increased risk for stone formation?
4. Is there an increased risk for infection?

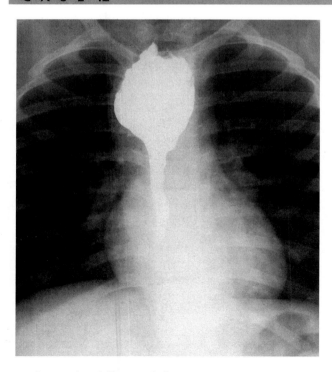

1. What is the differential diagnosis?
2. What are the two esophageal diverticula?
3. What is a feline esophagus?
4. What are transverse folds?

Bladder Diverticulum

1. 2% of patients will develop carcinoma.

2. A saccule.

3. Yes, there is an increased risk for stone formation.

4. Yes, there is an increased risk for infection.

Reference

Fernbach SK, Feinstein FA, Schmidt MB: Pediatric voiding cystourethrography: a pictorial guide. *Radiographics* 20:155–168, 2000.

Cross-Reference

Pediatric Radiology: THE REQUISITES, p 155.

Comment

Diverticula are mucosal outpouchings through the muscular layer of the bladder wall. Those congenital bladder defects located adjacent to or involving the ureterovesicular junction are referred to as Hutch diverticula. Alternatively, diverticula may result from outlet obstruction (posterior urethral valve) whereby the mucosa extrudes between hypertrophied muscular bundles. Post-surgical suprapubic tube recipients may also develop diverticula.

Bladder diverticula may cause obstruction if they involve the ureters or produce a mass effect on the bladder. A Hutch diverticulum may put traction on the ureterovesicular junction, opening up the orifice and permitting reflux to potentially infect and scar the ipsilateral kidney. Diverticula lead to stasis, infection, and stone formation.

Ultrasound will clearly show a large diverticula provided that it is filled at the time of the examination. Fake-outs include ascites, ovarian cysts, and seminal vesicle cysts. As the transfer of urine is made from the bladder to the diverticulum a Doppler signal may be detected, allowing for definitive diagnosis. Unfortunately, diverticula are renowned for not reading textbooks and a diverticular jet effect is often not found. A voiding cystourethrogram will demonstrate diverticula during the pressure of micturition. Diverticula cannot be ruled out without a dynamic voiding spot film.

Bladder diverticula are commonly resected if greater than 3 cm or if producing symptomatology.

Notes

Esophagitis

1. Gastroesophageal reflux, caustic esophagitis, Barrett esophagus, tracheoesophageal fistula (TEF) repair following radiation therapy.

2. Traction caused by infection and pulsion in the elderly.

3. It's the tube that connects a cat's mouth to the cat's stomach.

4. A normal finding in cats, transverse folds are seen in the very young and have no significance beyond conference pimping. Fixed transverse folds must not be confused with "feline" folds. Fixed folds are specific for severe esophagitis.

Reference

Swischuk LE, Fawcett HD, Hayden CK, et al.: Gastroesophageal reflux: how much imaging is required? *Radiographics* 8:1137–1145, 1988.

Cross-Reference

Pediatric Radiology: THE REQUISITES, 2nd edn, p 82.

Comment

Esophagitis is most commonly caused by gastroesophageal reflux (GER). Infection with *Candida*, herpes simplex virus, and cytomegalovirus in immunocompromised patients is the second most common cause. Gastroesophageal reflux can occur with or without a hiatus hernia but it most commonly occurs in association with immaturity of the gastroesophageal junction. GER is considered normal up to 1 year provided there are no pathologic consequences. GER that persists longer may cause inflammatory changes or strictures in the distal esophagus. Lye ingestion is the most common cause of strictures of the distal esophagus (30% of ingestion cases demonstrating stricturing). A TEF/atresia repair may also lead to stricture formation.

Radiographically, a strictured esophagus will demonstrate tapering and narrowing in the middle or lower third segment secondary to caustic ingestion. Barium studies will demonstrate mucosal ulceration and loss of peristalsis with eventual stricture formation.

Notes

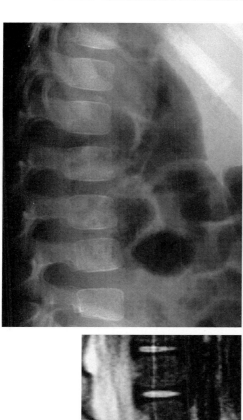
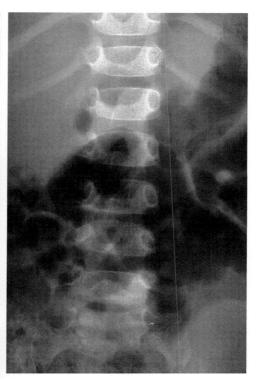
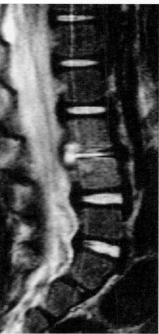

1. At what age does the intervertebral disc lose its blood supply?

2. What is the most common etiology of this entity?

3. What are the most commonly affected levels?

4. Is there involvement of the posterior elements?

Discitis

1. 20 years.

2. Bacterial infection by *Staphylococcus aureas*.

3. L2-3 and L3-4.

4. The posterior elements are spared.

Reference
Mahboubi S, Morris MC: Imaging of spinal infections in children. *Radiol Clin N Am* 39(2):215–222, 2001.

Cross-Reference
Pediatric Radiology: THE REQUISITES, p 291.

Comment
The distinction between adult and pediatric discitis lies in the point of origin of the infection. Hematagenous spread in adults seeds the bony vertebral endplates, while hematogenous spread in children seeds the vascularized disc or vascularized cartilaginous endplates. The intervertebral disc normally contains vascular supply up until the age of 20 years, while the cartilaginous endplates remain vascularized until 7 years. The take-home message is that discitis may precede osteomyelitis.

On radiographs early discitis appears normal; however, within 2–4 weeks, disc space narrowing is present. Further involvement of the neighboring vertebral bodies is demonstrated by demineralization and irregularity of the adjacent endplates. Eventually remineralization is restored in the healing phase, although there remains permanent endplate irregularity and loss of disc height. More severe infection may lead to vertebral collapse and scoliosis. The disc may reconstitute over time.

On MR, the disc appears narrowed and may either be bright or dark on T2-weighted images. Hyperintense T2 signal in the adjacent vertebral bodies is consistent with osteomyelitis. This variability may be related to antibiotic treatment of the primary infection. Post-contrast T1-weighted images will yield enhancement of the disc and involved adjacent vertebral bodies, prevertebral, and/or epidural soft tissues.

Tuberculosis, unlike staphylococcal injection, may travel longitudinally via the subligamentous space. These infections will demonstrate involvement of multiple vertebral body levels with sparing of the disc spaces between them.

Therapy for discitis includes bed rest and intravenous antibiotics. Some patients are treated based on clinical and imaging findings, while others undergo open or image-guided needle biopsy.

Notes

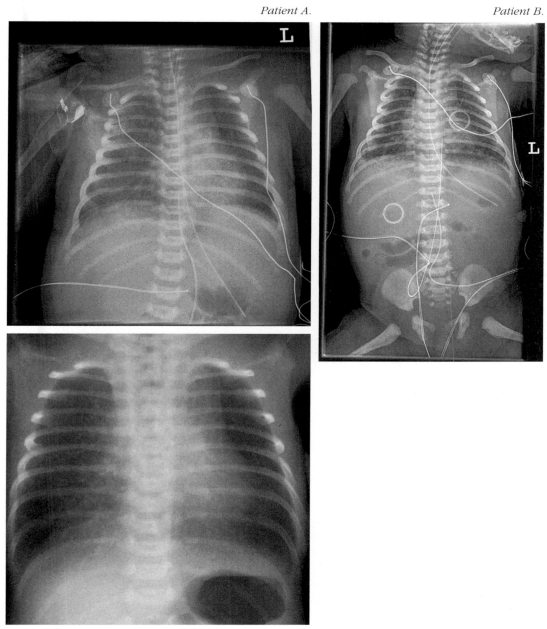

Patient A.

Patient B.

Patient C.

1. Differential diagnosis A.

2. Differential diagnosis B.

3. Differential diagnosis C.

4. What newborn chest disorder is associated with ground glass opacities?

Transient Tachypnea of the Newborn (TTN)/Meconium/Neonatal Pneumonia

1. TTN: cyanotic CHD with congestive heart failure, hypervolemia, pneumonia, meconium aspiration.

2. Meconium: TTN, neonatal pneumonia, pulmonary hemorrhage, note endotracheal tube.

3. Neonatal pneumonia: TTN, meconium aspiration.

4. Surfactant deficiency.

Reference

Kirks DR: *Practical Pediatric Imaging: Diagnostic Radiology of Infants and Children.* 3rd edn. Philadelphia, New York: Lippincott-Raven, 1998, pp 711–717.

Cross-Reference

Pediatric Radiology: THE REQUISITES, 2nd edn, pp 34–35.

Comment

It's late and you are on call. The technologist hands you a small film, a preemie. You can just make out the word "respirations" scrawled on the requisition by a sleep-deprived intern. The first thing you do is look at the lung volumes: are they small or large? If small, you'd think of surfactant deficiency. If large, transient tachypnea of the newborn, meconium aspiration, or neonatal pneumonia. These three common neonatal entities share the radiologic finding of increased lung volumes. Their time course is within the first 2 days of life. An accurate history is essential for imaging evaluation.

Transient tachypnea of the newborn is retention of lung fluid normally squeezed out by the vaginal birthing process. The rule of threes is useful in thinking of the etiology behind TTN or wet lung. One-third of the fluid is squeezed out through vaginal delivery, one-third resorbed by lymphatics, and one-third resorbed by capillaries. Naturally, babies delivered by c-section do not undergo this process and are at risk for TTN. Also at risk are newborns involved in prolonged labor, maternal anesthesia, or maternal diabetes. Fluid in the lung presents clinically with mild cyanosis, retraction, and grunting, as early as 6 hours with resolution by 2 days.

Radiographically, findings include hyperinflated lungs, enlarged heart, interstitial edema, fissure fluid, and small pleural effusions. Treatment is conservative and supportive.

Meconium aspiration (the first bacteria-free bowel movement below the vocal cords), is thought to be caused by a vagal reflex secondary to perinatal stress. Think of the aspirate as a great number of foreign bodies yielding a typical check valve mechanism with hyperinflation and associated chemical pneumonitis. On chest film, one sees a course nodular appearance with bilateral asymmetric areas of atelectasis and hyperaeration. Twenty-five per cent of patients develop pneumomediastinum or pneumothorax as a complication. Treatment is supportive with oxygen and antibiotics. Hypercarbia may lead to lowered pH and persistence of fetal circulation.

Neonatal pneumonia is contracted through an infected mother either during pregnancy or at delivery. Prolonged labor, premature rupture of membranes, placental infection, and ascending infection from the perineum are predisposing factors. Respiratory distress with tachypnea and metabolic acidosis is the most common clinical scenario. Most commonly, group B hemolytic streptococcal infection is acquired at birth via a colonized vagina (25% of all women). Other bugs include *Klebsiella* and *Staphylococcus* often presenting with empyema. Staphylococcal infection is especially susceptible to pneumatocele formation, so beware of developing pneumothoracies.

Radiographically, a patchy, asymmetric, radiating, bilateral, interstitial infiltrate is commonly seen. A nodular pattern may predominate in diffuse hazy lungs. Pleural effusions are common. Antibiotic therapy is essential, as mortality rates in untreated infants are high.

	Surfactant deficiency disorder	Transient tachypnea of the newborn	Meconium aspiration	Neonatal pneumonia
Typical patient	Premature	Term/c-section	post-term stained below cords	Premature rupture of membranes
Time course	<6 hours	24–48 hours	12–24 hours	<6 hours
Lung volume	Decreased	Increased	Increased	Increased
Imaging	Ground glass	Interstitial edema	Coarse, nodular, asymmetric	Perihilar streaking

Notes

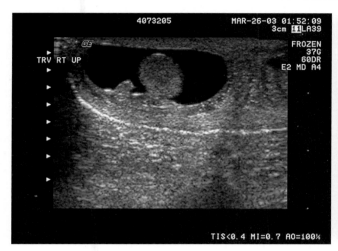 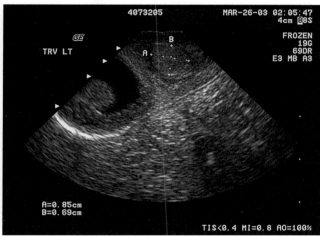

1. What are the most common age groups affected by this entity?

2. What is the halo sign?

3. What is the nubbin sign?

4. What might increased flow to the testis suggest?

C A S E 45

Testicular Torsion

1. Infants under 1 year and adolescents.

2. Nuclear scan with increased flow to the Dartos fascia and decreased central uptake (>24 h).

3. Nuclear scan with increased activity medial to the iliac artery at the site of the twist.

4. Orchitis or recent detorsed testis.

Reference

Pavlica P, Barozzi L: Imaging of the acute scrotum. *Eur Radiol* 11(2):220–228, 2001.

Cross-Reference

Pediatric Radiology: THE REQUISITES, p 193.

Comment

The testis is suspended within the scrotum by the spermatic cord. The tunica vaginalis is a serosal layer that extended from the peritoneal cavity to the scrotum enveloping the anterior superior portion of the testicle. The bell-clapper deformity occurs when the tunica vaginalis completely encircles the testis superiorly involving the epididymis as well. The term bell-clapper refers to the tunica as the part of the Liberty bell that has that famous crack in it. The testis is that metallic ball that does the striking. In bell-clapper deformity the testis can now rotate on the spermatic cord, twisting and compressing its blood supply. This is the basic mechanism in adolescence. Alternatively, neonate torsion involves twisting of both the tunica and testis.

Torsion causes acute pain in adolescents and adults but not in neonates. Neonate torsion has a poor prognosis. Time is the big factor in discovering the torsion and surgically reducing it. There is an 80–100% salvage rate after 5–6 hours of the onset of pain, 70% after 6–12, 20% after 12 hours.

Two modalities are used for the detection of torsion, scintigraphy and ultrasound. Scintigraphy is performed by injecting 99mTC pertechnetate followed by dynamic phase and blood pool imaging. Acute torsion is demonstrated by asymmetric blood pool imaging. Later, in the natural history of torsion, a halo sign will be detected by scintigraphy secondary to scrotal hyperemia. This neighborhood has a dual blood supply. The testes are fed by the testicular arteries via the aorta/right renal vein, while the scrotum receives blood from the internal and external iliaci. Don't get fooled by epididymitis! Increased flow will be seen on the painful side, so be careful that you know which side is affected. You might mistakenly call the normal side positive for torsion.

Ultrasound is used as well for the detection of testicular torsion. The angry edematous testis will appear mildly larger and more hypoechoic than the happy one. The echotexture will coarsen and become hypoechoic. Color and power Doppler examination will demonstrate absence of flow within the testicular parenchyma of a torsed testicle. Skin thickening, hydrocele formation, and an enlarged epididymis are common extratesticular findings.

Therapy is surgical with an emergent attempt at reducing the torsion. Patients will also undergo contralateral exploration as the bell-clapper deformity is more often bilateral, thereby prompting fixation of the testis to the scrotum.

Notes

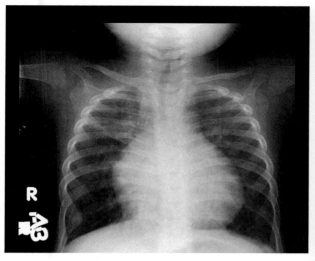

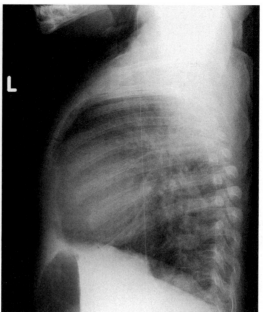

Noncyanotic patient

1. Is there increased or decreased pulmonary vascularity?
2. If the vascularity was normal what is your differential?
3. If the vascularity was increased what is your differential?
4. What percentage of these patients spontaneously resolve?

Ventricular Septal Defect (VSD)

1. It is increased.

2. Acyanotic with normal vascularity: aortic stenosis, pulmonic stenosis, coarctation, and interrupted aortic arch.

3. Endocardial cushion defect, atrial septal defect, patent ductus arteriosus (PDA) (enlarged LA and enlarged aorta), and VSD (enlarged LA and normal aorta).

4. Spontaneous closure in VSD occurs in 90% by 12 months.

Reference

Allen HD, Gutgesell HP, Clark EB, et al.: *Moss and Adams Heart Disease in Infants, Children and Adolescents: Including the Fetus and Young Adult,* 6th edn. Baltimore: Lippincott Williams & Wilkins, 2000, pp 636–651.

Cross-Reference

Pediatric Radiology: THE REQUISITES, 2nd edn, p 57.

Comment

Ventricular septal defect is the most common congenital heart defect, accounting for 30% of all cases. VSD is the most common defect associated with other congenital anomalies, although it may occur as an isolated entity as well. Translation: patients with anomalies such as coarctation, PDA, tetralogy of Fallot, truncus, double outlet right ventricle, and trisomies are prone to having VSD. A VSD may involve four different septal locations: the membranous, muscular, anterior, or posterior regions. The vast majority (80%) are perimembranous.

Pressure differences between the low-resistance right ventricle and the high-resistance left ventricle create a net movement of blood to the right side—a left-to-right shunt. The increased load on the right heart is transmitted to engorged pulmonary arteries. The increased pressure and shear forces on the arteriole endothelial cells cause destruction with decreased nitric oxide production, resultant vasoconstriction and eventual fibrin and smooth muscle deposition. This formation of fibrin and smooth muscle impedes the diffusion of oxygen from the alveoli into the capillaries. As this process occurs, right-sided heart pressures continue to rise, eventually producing reversal of flow and a right-to-left shunt. The right-to-left shunt will manifest clinically as cyanosis, a rare finding today as these patients are treated before this late-stage sign develops.

Clinical presentation is variable and dependent on the size of the defect. A large defect will produce congestive heart failure at 1–3 months following the normal physiologic drop in pulmonary resistance at this time. The pressure at the capillaries is transmitted to the left atrium, leading to pulmonary venous hypertension and pulmonary edema. Congestive heart failure, dyspnea, sweating, tachycardia, and a loud pansystolic murmur at the left sternal border are the findings on exam.

Small defects will present with a normal chest radiograph. Increased vascularity will only be detectable if the pulmonary circulation is twice the systemic circulation. Shunt vascularity differs from pulmonary edema as the vessels maintain their sharpness, in contrast to pulmonary venous hypertension in which interstitial edema leads to indistinct vessel borders. In addition, pulmonary vessels are enlarged and detectable in the lung periphery. If the diameter of the right descending pulmonary artery is greater than the trachea think shunt vascularity. This being said, the detection of shunt vascularity is quite difficult.

Larger defects cause increased flow to the pulmonary arteries and shunt vascularity. The increased pulmonary circulation enlarges the left atrium but not the left ventricle as the ventricle decompresses into the RV through the VSD. Left atrial enlargement is best detectable on the lateral film. A normal LA will comprise the upper half of the posterior cardiac border and be even with the posterior tracheal wall. An LA that extends beyond a line drawn from the posterior tracheal wall is indicative of enlargement. Eisenmenger physiology appears when there is constriction of peripheral pulmonary vessels due to persistent high pulmonary artery pressures resulting in a reversal of flow through the defect. The chest film is characterized by prominent central vessels with tapering and right-sided cardiac enlargement. The aorta is normal in these cases.

Patients with VSD symptomatology undergo echocardiography for characterization of the shunt flow and defect size. Prognosis is excellent for these patients as a third of VSDs close spontaneously. Patients with large shunts require correction either by surgery or with transcatheterization closure.

Notes

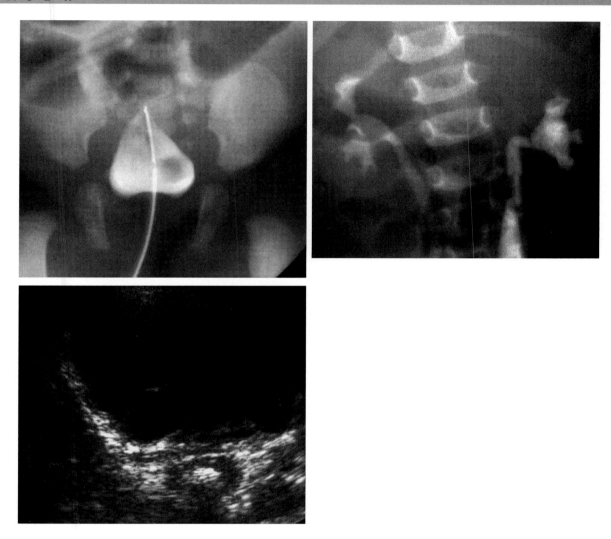

1. Where is the location of the urethral opening in male hypospadias?
2. What is the etiology of hypospadias?
3. What is the incidence of hypospadias?
4. What entities are associated with hypospadias?

Ureterocele

1. Ventral aspect of the penis, scrotum, or perineum.

2. Defective midline fusion of the genital folds is the etiology of male hypospadias.

3. The incidence of hypospadias is 1:300.

4. Cryptorchidism, inguinal hernias, UTIs.

Reference

Fernbach SK, Feinstein KA, Schmidt MB: Pediatric voiding cystourethrography: a pictorial guide. *Radiographics* 20:155–168, 2000.

Cross-Reference

Pediatric Radiology: THE REQUISITES, pp 163–164.

Comment

Ureteroceles are congenital dilations of the intramucosal portion of the ureter. Ureteroceles are divided into two varieties, ectopic or simple. Ectopic ureteroceles demonstrate an abnormal location at their bladder insertions and are nearly always associated with a duplex or dual ureteral drainage of the kidney. Presentation commonly includes UTIs, hematuria, or in association with prenatally detected hydronephrosis. For embryologic reasons, ectopic ureteroceles may insert distal to the external bladder sphincter in females, in contrast to males, in which the ectopic ureter inserts proximal to the external sphincter. Anatomic differences yield differing presentations; in boys, epididymitis or hydronephrosis is seen. In girls, incontinence or UTIs are common.

Radiographically, a filling defect can be seen on both voiding cystourethrogram and excretory urography (intravenous urogram, intravenous pyelogram). The associated upper pole draining ureter may demonstrate several characteristic findings: increased distance between the top of the nephrogram and the top of the collecting system, abnormal axis, concave upper border of the renal pelvis, fewer calyces than expected, lateral displacement of the kidney and ureter as a result of the obstructed dilated ectopic upper pole ureter, tortuous course of the ureter and/or filling defect in the bladder. Ultrasound will make the diagnosis in the majority of cases, confirmed by a nuclear medicine renogram.

Simple ureteroceles refer to cystic dilatation and invagination at the expected insertion point into the bladder. It is primarily a finding picked up incidentally during adulthood. The "cobra" sign is seen on cystogram with a dark halo outlining the invaginated intramural portion of the bilateral ureterocele.

Treatment ranges from transurethral unroofing of the ureterocele to heminephroureterectomy.

Notes

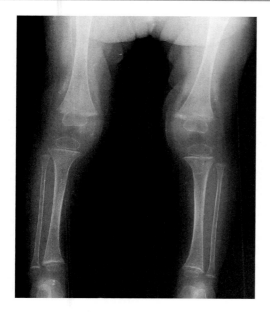

1. What are the causes of rickets?

2. What are causes of vitamin D deficiency?

3. A patient is treated with vitamin D for rickets but shows no improvement. Why?

4. What is this entity?

C A S E 48

Scurvy

1. Rickets is caused by vitamin D deficiency.

2. Inadequate exposure to sunlight, lack of dietary intake, poor maternal nutrition, dark skin pigmentation.

3. The patient has a congenital end organ resistance to vitamin D.

4. Scurvy, *not* rickets.

Reference
Boeve WJ, Martijn A: Case report 406: Scurvy. *Skeletal Radiol* 16(1):67–69, 1987.

Cross-Reference
Pediatric Radiology: THE REQUISITES, p 216.

Comment
Bone is made of an organic matrix strengthened by a deposited mineral crystal, hydroxyapatite. The organic matrix is primarily composed of collagen fibers synthesized by osteoblasts. Ascorbic acid or vitamin C is essential for activating an enzyme that hydroxylates procollagen for stable helical crosslinking. Collagen synthesis is impaired in vitamin C deficiency, affecting wound healing, blood vessel integrity, and osteoid matrix formation.

In Scurvy, the initial steps of osteogenesis are intact with normal chondrocyte activity laying down a cartilaginous template for eventual bone deposition. Osteoblasts, however, are unable to lay down bone matrix. Osteoclast resorption of the provisionally calcified cartilage arrests. The zone of provisional calcification continues to grow unopposed by osteoclast resorption, yielding the dense metaphyseal line (Frankel). On the other side of the growth plate a dense pencil ring of calcification corresponds to the mineralized zone of provisional calcification on the epiphysis. Cartilage overgrowth ensues and will grow laterally as well as back into the metaphysis, giving a widened appearance. Diffuse demineralization is seen on radiographs, although the mechanism is poorly understood. Periosteal reaction is common secondary to subperiosteal bleeding from vessel fragility. This rare disease never occurs before 6 months of age as the infant uses prenatally transmitted stores of vitamin C.

Notes

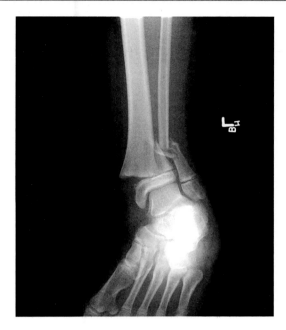

1. What are causes of growth plate arrest?
2. What imaging modalities would one use to evaluate for growth plate injury?
3. What are the sequelae of growth plate arrest?
4. Why image-suspected physeal bridging?

Salter–Harris II Fracture

1. Fracture involving the physis and infection.

2. Thin-section CT with coronal and sagittal reformats or a cartilage-sensitive MR sequence such as spoiled gradient echo (S-GRE).

3. Premature closure may lead to limb shortening due to growth arrest or angular deformity.

4. The bridge may be resected allowing for normal physeal physiology and longitudinal growth.

Reference

Carey J, Spence L, Blickman H, Eustace S: MRI of pediatric growth plate injury: correlation with plain film radiographs and clinical outcome. *Skeletal Radiol* 27(5):250–255, 1998.

Cross-Reference

Pediatric Radiology: THE REQUISITES, pp 238–239.

Comment

Growth plate injuries occur in a third of pediatric fractures. Bone is far stronger than the cartilaginous physis and very susceptible to injury. The fracture line will travel between the germinal layers (epiphyseal side) and the zone of provisional calcification (metaphyseal side). So why did Salter, an orthopedist, and Harris, a radiologist, bother with devising a classification system? The system is devised to predict the likelihood of normal healing. SH 1–V carries a progressively worse prognosis.

Metaphyseal involvement in growth plate injuries is present in three quarters of cases as it is structurally weakest owing to a thin cortex and predominance of cancellous bone—the SH II. Type I involves a traction injury and is very hard to detect unless there is displacement of the epiphysis. Type III injury is the reciprocal of type II in which the fracture is through the epiphysis and physis. Type IV involves the epiphysis, growth plate, and metaphysis. Type V is a result of compressive forces on the physis due to axial loading on the epiphysis.

MR has been playing an ever increasing role in suspected physeal injuries as well as evaluation of suspected growth plate arrest. MR is substantially more sensitive than plane films in detecting growth plate injuries. Radiographs often understage physeal injuries. Growth plate arrest, the major complication of growth plate injuries, will lead to limb shortening or angular deformity. A cartilage-sensitive gradient echo sequence will define the physis and demonstrate a physeal bar. Physeal bars or bridges connect the ephiphysis and metaphysis prematurely during development. Growth plate size is important to establish, as therapy is determined by size. Bridges smaller than 50% may be resected, while bridges greater than 50% undergo ephiphysiololysis of both the involved and contralateral growth plate.

Notes

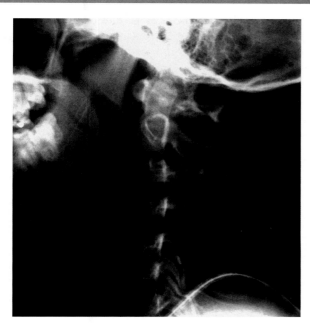

1. Which two flexion injuries are unstable?
2. Which two extension injuries are unstable?
3. Which compression injury is unstable?
4. Which complex injuries are unstable?

Pseudosubluxation vs. Abnormal C-spine

1. Bilateral facet dislocation. Flexion tear drop fracture.

2. Hangman's fracture, hyperextension dislocation fracture.

3. Jefferson fracture.

4. Odontoid fracture, atlantooccipital dissociation. Note that absence of any of these fractures does not imply stability! Don't be a Leonard Berlin case report.

Reference

LE Swischuk: Anterior displacement of C2 in children: physiologic or pathologic. *Radiology* 122:759–763, 1977.

Cross-Reference

Pediatric Radiology: THE REQUISITES, p 297.

Comment

In accurately assessing the pediatric cervical spine in the setting of trauma, knowledge of the biomechanical differences between the adult and pediatric spine is critical. In adults, the fulcrum on which the cervical spine flexes is at C5–C6. In contrast, in children it is at the level of C2–C3 or C3–C4. Normal flexion on the lateral c-spine may suggest anterior subluxation of C2 on C3, which is actually normal and thought to be due to generalized ligamentous laxity. Additionally, normal buckling of both the trachea and prevertebral soft tissues may yield the misleading appearance of prevertebral soft tissue swelling. The width of the prevertebral soft tissues should not be greater than half the vertebral body width from C2 to C4. A good strategy to avoid this pitfall is use of the spinolaminar line. The spinolaminar line is defined as point of fusion of the laminae to form the posterior arch. Less than 2 mm of subluxation is considered physiologic. Naturally, one ought to still look at the anterior longitudinal, posterior longitudinal, and spinous process lines at every level. It is important to evaluate the atlantodental distance, as adults can be normal up to 2 mm, while children may be normal up to 4 mm.

Evaluation of the atlanto-occipital relationship is vital to detecting atlanto-occipital dissociation (AOD), a terrible injury that leads to severe neurologic impairment. AODs are usually the result of motor vehicle vs. pedestrian type accidents. In the vast majority of cases the skull base slides anteriorly relative to the atlas. The Powers ratio is used to detect and quantify the dissociation. A good way to think of the Powers ratio is just by drawing a line from the front of the foramen magnum (basion) to the back of C1(inner aspect) and dividing it by a line drawn from the back of the foramen magnum (opisthion) to the front of C1(inner aspect). Normal ought to be less than 0.

Notes

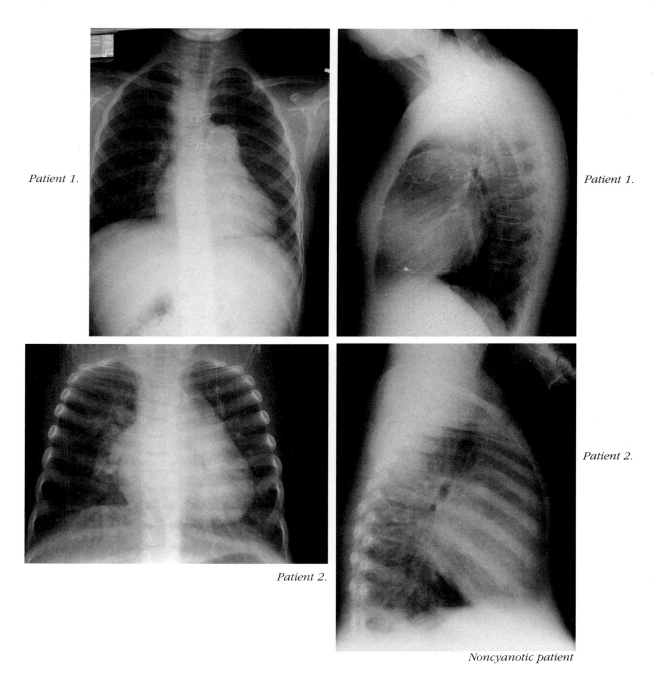

Patient 1.

Patient 1.

Patient 2.

Patient 2.

Noncyanotic patient

1. Is there increased or decreased pulmonary vascularity?
2. If the vascularity was normal what is your differential?
3. If the vascularity was increased what is your differential?
4. Is the aorta enlarged?

Patent Ductus Arteriosus (PDA)

1. It is increased.

2. Acyanotic with normal vascularity: aortic stenosis, pulmonic stenosis, coarctation, and interrupted aortic arch.

3. Endocardial cushion defect, atrial septal defect, PDA (enlarged LA and enlarged aorta), and ventricular septal defect (VSD) (enlarged LA and normal aorta).

4. Yes, this is the finding that allows you to distinguish PDA from VSD.

Reference

Allen HD, Gutgesell HP, Clark EB, et al.: *Moss and Adams Heart Disease in Infants, Children and Adolescents: Including the Fetus and Young Adult,* 6th edn. Baltimore: Lippincott Williams & Wilkins, 2000, pp 652–669.

Cross-Reference

Pediatric Radiology: THE REQUISITES, 2nd edn, p 59.

Comment

Patent ductus arteriosus is an abnormal persistence of the normal fetal circulation. During fetal life, blood is shunted from the collapsed fluid-filled fetal lungs into the systemic circulation by the aorta via the ductus arteriosus. The duct knows to close at birth due to arterial oxygen saturation levels as well as vasoactive substances. Prostaglandins dilate the ductus, while prostaglandin antagonists such as indomethacin constrict and close the vascular conduit. The ductus arteriosus will normally close functionally at 24 hours with anatomic closure at 4 weeks. Failure of closure is poorly understood. Ninety per cent of cases are isolated with no other congenital heart malformation.

Clinically, patients present with a left-to-right shunt and classic washing-machine-like murmur. Premature infants may present with left ventricle failure (tachycardia and tachypnea). Term infants often present with congestive heart failure or failure to thrive at an older age. Wide pulse pressure and bounding peripheral pressures are due to the heart's attempt to compensate for the blood that is diverted from the aorta into the pulmonary circulation.

At birth the pulmonary resistance drops and blood is shunted from the aorta through the ductus into the pulmonary artery. As in all the left-to-right shunts, increased pulmonary blood flow and shunt vascularity are present. Enlargement of the pulmonary arteries, pulmonary veins, left atrium, left ventricle, and aorta are also present. A normal LA will comprise the upper half of the posterior cardiac border and be even with the posterior tracheal wall. An LA that extends beyond a line drawn from the posterior tracheal wall is indicative of enlargement. The LV comprises the lower half of the posterior cardiac board on the lateral view. The posterior heart border ought to cross the IVC 2 cm above the diaphragm. An intersection below this point suggests LV enlargement. Increased vascularity will only be detectable if the pulmonary circulation is twice the systemic circulation. Shunt vascularity differs from pulmonary edema as the vessels maintain their sharpness, in contrast to pulmonary venous hypertension in which interstitial edema silhouettes the distinct vessel borders. In addition, pulmonary vessels are enlarged and detectable in the lung periphery. If the diameter of the right descending pulmonary artery is greater than the trachea, think shunt vascularity. An appearance very similar to VSD, the PDA distinguishes itself by an enlarged aorta. The right side remains uninvolved. Small shunts demonstrate normal chest films while moderate to large PDAs will show these findings. Findings are subtle in the newborn preemie and include modest cardiac enlargement over a series of films and interstitial edema.

Premature infants are treated with indomethacin for closure unless contraindicated (intracranial hemorrhage). Alternatives include surgical closure of endovascular coil placement in the older age group.

Notes

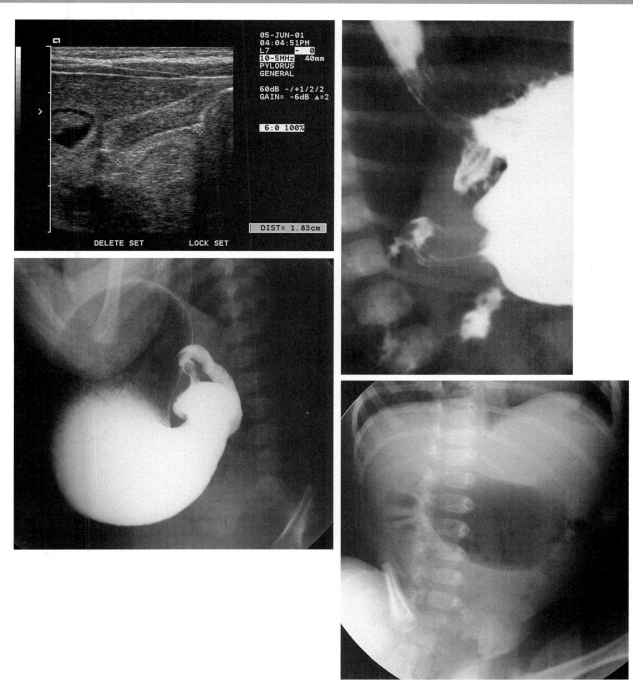

1. Is there seasonal variance in this disorder?

2. What is the incidence?

3. Is there a gender predominance?

4. Is this a surgical emergency?

Hypertrophic Pyloric Stenosis

1. Maybe, perceived as more common in fall and winter.

2. 1 in 500.

3. M:F 4:1.

4. No, the most pressing problem is fluid imbalance. The patient will require IV fluids and an NG tube in preparation for surgery.

Reference

Merten DF: Practical approaches to pediatric gastrointestinal radiology. *Radiol Clin N Am* 31(6):1395–1407, 1993.

Cross-Reference

Pediatric Radiology: THE REQUISITES, 2nd edn, pp 87–88.

Comment

Hypertrophic pyloric stenosis (HPS) presents with non-bilious vomiting in the range of 2–6 weeks of age. HPS is hypertrophy of the circular muscle fibers of the pylorus thought to be due to abnormal innervation. Although HPS has been considered a clinical diagnosis, it is common practice to confirm it with imaging.

Ultrasound is the initial test of choice. The bullseye is simple to spot with the patient turned slightly to his right. The thickness of the pylorus should measure 3 mm or more for a diagnosis of HPS. A thickness of 3 mm refers to the distance from echogenic mucosa to serosa (the radius or the circular pylorus) and a pyloric channel length of more than 16 mm. The most accurate measurement is taken on longitudinal scan, as a short access scan will yield a falsely elevated measurement unless the transducer is at a perfect right angle with the pylorus. If the ultrasound is negative the next step is an upper GI. The scout film may show a massively overdistended stomach with a paucity of air in the large and small bowel. The classic UGI findings include hyperperistalsis of the stomach, the antral "teat," a "double track" elongated pyloric channel and an "umbrella" duodenal cap.

Treatment is surgery, a Ramstedt pyloromyotomy, a very effective procedure involving incision and spreading of the hypertrophied muscle.

Notes

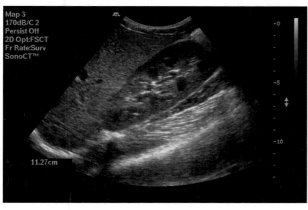 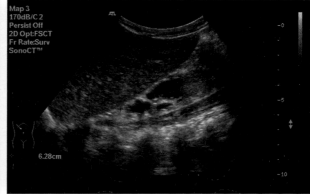

1. What is the name of the umbilical attachment of the bladder in the fetus?

2. Voiding through the umbilicus is secondary to what entity?

3. What is the incidence of horseshoe kidney?

4. What is bladder exstrophy?

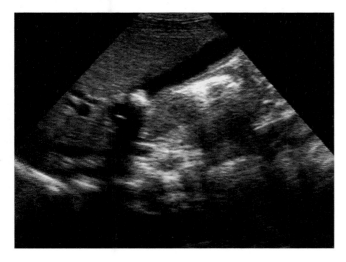

1. Is there an association with renal stones?

2. Associated ileus is common with this entity, true or false?

3. Is surgical intervention considered?

4. Is surgery curative?

C A S E 53

Renal Hypoplasia

1. Initially the allantois and then later the urachus.

2. Persistent canalization of the urachus.

3. 1:400 is the incidence of horseshoe kidney.

4. *Jeopardy style:* abdominal wall defect that allows for the bladder wall to be continuous with the skin.

Reference

Risdon RA, Young LW, Chrispin AR: Renal hypoplasia and dysplasia: a radiological and pathological correlation. *Pediatr Radiol* 3(4):213–225, 1975.

Cross-Reference

Pediatric Radiology: THE REQUISITES, p 155.

Comment

There are numerous varieties of hypoplasia: simple hypoplasia, segmental hypoplasia, and oligonephronic hypoplasia. Simple hypoplasia is merely a congenitally small or miniature kidney. Ectopia or malrotation is commonly seen and commonly complicated by recurrent infections and scarring. Segmental hypoplasia appears as a transverse groove over the margin or surface of cortex that corresponds with cortical thinning and focal dilatation of the collecting system. In the context of hypertension this finding is referred to as an Ask–Upmark kidney. Grooves with cortical thinning are associated with reflux usually involving the upper or lower pole. Oligonephronic hypoplasia is rare with extremely small kidneys. A reduced number of nephrons leads to eventual renal failure.

Notes

C A S E 54

Cholelithiasis

1. Yes, furosemide may cause both gallstones and renal stones.

2. False, gallstone ileus is rare in children.

3. Yes, as it is appropriate in many settings.

4. No, stones may rarely develop within the common duct.

Reference

Gubernick JA, Rosenberg HK, Ilaslan H, et al.: US approach to jaundice in infants and children. *Radiographics* 20:173–195, 2000.

Cross-Reference

Pediatric Radiology: THE REQUISITES, 2nd edn, p 133.

Comment

Three varieties of stones exist: cholesterol (supersaturated bile), pigmented (precipitated calcium bilirubinate), and mixed, the most common. Causes include hemolytic and nonhemolytic anemias, although many cases are idiopathic.

Neonates are prone to pigmented stones due to immaturity of bile conjugation, cholestasis secondary to poor feeds, and diuretic therapy with Lasix. Hemolysis secondary to sickle cell, thalassemia, or hereditary spherocytosis will yield pigmented stones secondary to stasis. Abnormal enterohepatic circulation is the proposed culprit for stone formation in inflammatory bowel disease. Cystic fibrosis, obesity, and short gut syndrome are associated with stone formation as well. Cholesterol stones are uncommon in children.

Plain films of the abdomen demonstrate stones up to 50% of the time. Ultrasound is the imaging champion of stones. Real-time imaging allows for discernment of the dependent rolling stone. The classic description is a mobile echogenic stone that shadows.

Notes

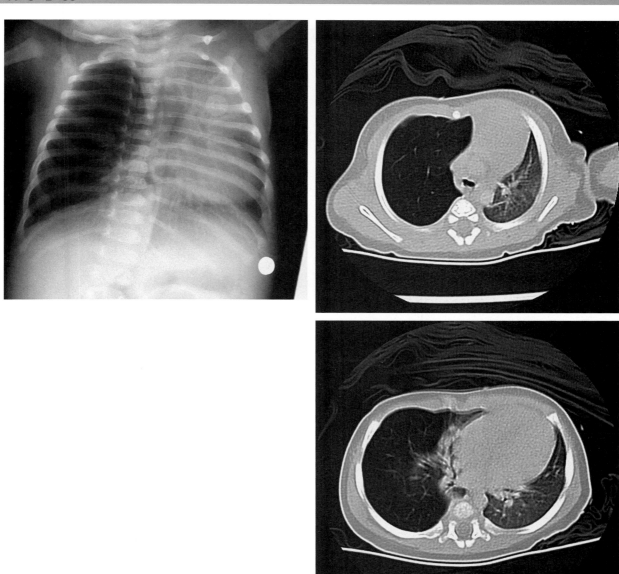

1. What is the differential diagnosis?
2. What other organ system is most often involved?
3. What are the findings on V/Q scan?
4. Is the patient a candidate for bronchoscopy?

Congenital Lobar Emphysema

1. Congenital cystic adenomatoid malformation, pulmonary sling, bronchogenic cyst.

2. Cardiovascular (patent ductus arteriosus, ventricular septal defect, tetrad of Fallot).

3. Decreased ventilation with decreased perfusion and delayed washout in the affected lobe.

4. Yes, to rule out an endobronchial lesion prior to surgery.

References

Siegel BA, Proto AV, eds.: *Pediatric Disease (Fourth Series) Test and Syllabus*. Reston, VA: American College of Radiology, 1993, pp 102–106.

Schwartz DS, Reyes-Mugica M, Keller MS: Imaging of surgical diseases of the newborn chest. Intrapleural mass lesions. *Radiol Clin N Am* 37(6):1067–1078, 1999.

Cross-Reference

Pediatric Radiology: THE REQUISITES, 2nd edn, pp 28–29.

Comment

Congenital lobar emphysema is thought to be due to defective cartilage or a compressive mass that prevents the outflow of fluid (neonatals) and then air (infants). Remember, that in utero the unexpanded lungs are filled with fluid that normally drain during the first breath of life. Due to the outflow obstruction, retained fluid is seen on the newborn chest radiograph as a dense lobar opacity.

Symptoms most often present in the neonatal period with respiratory distress and/or fever. Male:female incidence is 3:1. The left upper lobe is most commonly involved followed by the right middle lobe, right upper lobe, and then lower lobes (LUL > RML > RUL > R & LLLs). Initially an opacified lobe due to impaired bronchial drainage of in utero fluid presents most commonly in the LUL. The opacified lobe slowly clears through lymphatic resorption, yielding a reticular pattern. Eventually hyperlucency develops due to dilated alveoli containing trapped air and mass effect upon the nonaffected lobes. Therapy is surgical resection and carries an excellent prognosis.

Notes

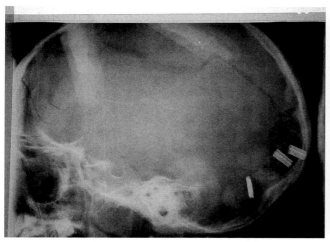

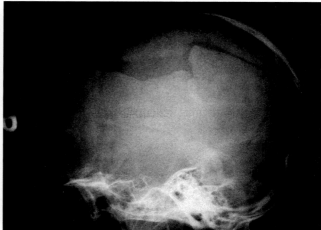

Status Post Head Injury

3 Weeks Post Injury

1. Where is this entity most commonly found?
2. Is surgery always indicated?
3. Where is the first place one should look when interpreting a head CT?
4. Skull series has a limited role in pediatric trauma, true or false?

Skull Fracture vs. Venous Channel vs. Growing Fracture

1. Parietal (45%), frontal (33%), occipital (11%), and temporal bone (10%).

2. No, only if there is a depressed skull fracture with overriding greater than the calvarial thickness.

3. The scout image should be assessed for skull fractures. Fractures parallel to the axial plane are easily missed.

4. True. The status of the underlying brain is paramount. CT with reconstructed or reformatted 3-D or surface-rendered images with bone windowing will supply the neurosurgeon with all the information needed.

Reference

Makkat S, Vandevenne JE, Parizel PM, et al.: Multiple growing fractures and cerebral venous anomaly after penetrating injuries: delayed diagnosis in a battered child. *Pediatr Radiol* 31(5):381–383, 2001.

Cross-Reference

Pediatric Radiology: THE REQUISITES, p 262.

Comment

Skull fractures are either caused by high-impact trauma or child abuse. So-called "nonaccidental" trauma is highly suspicious in cases that exhibit fractures that are bilateral, multiple, diastatic, or in different stages of healing. Far more important than the skull is the underlying brain— a normal skull film does not rule out brain injury. A depressed skull fracture may require surgical elevation. Although surgery will often request skull radiographs, given the reformatting capabilities of today's multidetector scanner this additional radiation is no longer indicated. Skull fractures heal within 3 to 6 months.

Radiographically, skull fractures will appear as linear and sometimes branching lucent lines often detected far from the site of impact. The trick is not to confuse a suture with a fracture. The best way to guard against this potentially embarrassing mistake is learning your sutures by taking note of them on normal CTs and nonindicated conventional radiographs. Sometimes bilaterality will not bail you out. Sclerotic appearing lines will often indicate the presence of an overriding skull fracture. If the overriding is greater than the calvarial thickness, surgical elevation is required. Depressed skull fractures account for 25% of all skull fractures and are more common in children older than two.

If a breach in the dura is made at the time of the fracture, pulsation of the CSF may hinder healing and actually expand the fracture site (the growing fracture). The fluid-filled arachnoid will herniate through the defect, creating a leptomeningeal cyst. The cyst will also press against the brain, causing displacement and associated encephalomalacia or parenchymal volume loss.

Notes

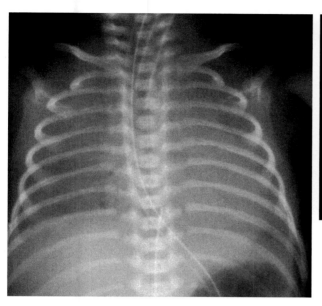

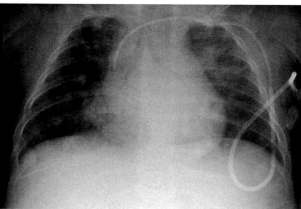

1. What are the sequelae?
2. Who is most commonly affected?
3. This is the second leading cause of death among liveborn infants, true or false?
4. What are the common acute complications?

Surfactant Deficiency Disease

1. Common long-term complications include bronchopulmonary dysplasia, hyperinflation, and recurrent respiratory tract infections.

2. Premature infants, 26–36 weeks weighing less than 2.5 kg.

3. False. It is the number one cause of death in liveborn infants.

4. Pneumothorax, pneumomediastinum, atelectasis, and mucus plugging.

Reference

Wood BP, Sinkin RA, Kendig JW, et al.: Exogenous lung surfactant: effect on radiographic appearance in premature infants. *Radiology* 165(1):11–13, 1987.

Cross-Reference

Pediatric Radiology: THE REQUISITES, 2nd edn, pp 30–34.

Comment

Respiratory distress syndrome presents within the first few hours of life in preemies under 36 weeks. The pathophysiology centers on the type II alveoli surfactant producing lung cells that begin to mature at 24 weeks. The surfactant prevents the alveoli from collapsing on expiration reducing the force required to open them on each inspiration. Surfactant can be measured in utero by the decrease in the lecithin/sphingomyelin ratio.

Imaging characteristics:

1. Low lung volumes

2. Ground glass appearance

3. Bell-shaped thorax

4. Poorly defined vessels

Following a typical SDD chest radiograph, the clinical team will move to intubate the patient giving positive expiratory end pressure or continuous positive airway pressure. Rupture of the air sacs due to high ventilation may lead to pulmonary interstitial emphysema. The air can escape in two directions: centrally, leading to pneumomediastinum, and peripherally, leading to tension pneumothorax. Pay special attention to development of a pneumomediastinum or pneumothorax. Unlike the chest film in upright adults, in supine infants, air will be seen medially (the highest point in a supine infant): the sharp mediastinum sign (get a lateral decubitus if you aren't sure!). Artificial surfactant may be administered via an endotracheal tube. This mechanism of delivery often leads to uneven dosage to the left and right lungs, yielding asymmetric ventilation on chest films.

Impaired air exchange in collapsed alveoli leads to hypercarbia, low oxygen tension, acidosis, and a persistent patent ductus arteriosus. The high-pressure arterial system then shunts blood into the low-pressure pulmonary system, left to right, causing vascular engorgement. These babies will be given artificial surfactant via an endotracheal tube.

Four weeks of positive pressure ventilation may lead to interstitial fibrosis with exudative necrosis and honeycombing on X-ray—bronchopulmonary dysplasia (BPD). This appears as interstitial fibrosis, cyst-like emphysematous changes, and increased lung volumes.

BPD Classification

Stages	Time course	Findings
Stage I	0–4 days	Ground glass
Stage II	4–10 days	Bilateral increased density from exudative necrosis
Stage III	10–20 days	Honeycombing—air sac overdistention in dysplastic interstitium
Stage IV	>30 days	Fibrosis and cystic emphysema—40–50% mortality

The prognosis includes restrictive changes and increased LRIs into the teen years. Ten per cent do show complete resolution.

	Surfactant deficiency disorder	Transient tachypnea of the newborn	Meconium aspiration	Neonatal pneumonia
Typical patient	Premature	Term/ c-section	Post-term Stained below cords	Premature rupture of membranes
Time course	<6 hours	24–48 hours	12–24 hours	>6 hours
Lung volume	Decreased	Increased	Increased	Increased
Imaging	Ground glass	Interstitial edema	Coarse, nodular, asymmetric	Perihilar streaking

Notes

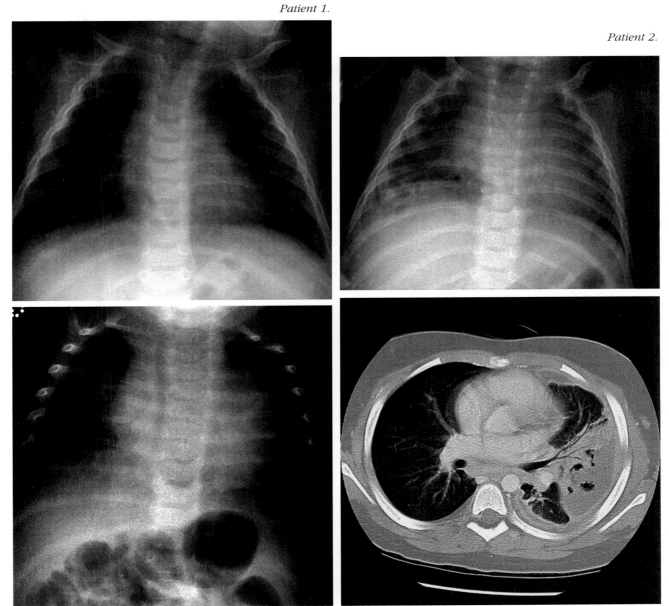

Patient 1.

Patient 2.

Patient 3.

Patient 2.

All Patients Share Same Diagnosis

1. Would it surprise you if the patient presented with abdominal pain?

2. What is the differential diagnosis for case B?

3. A 2-year-old with conjunctivitis, eosinophilia, otitis media, and elevated immunoglobulins might have what diagnosis?

4. What is the radiographic appearance of the diagnosis in question 3?

Staphylococcal Pneumonia

1. No, children with pneumonia may often present with abdominal pain.

2. Granuloma, aspergilloma, bronchogenic cyst, sequestration, collapse due to adenopathy.

3. Chlamydia.

4. Chlamydia appears as hyperinflation with perihilar, patchy, focal, airspace densities.

Reference

Osborne D, Kirks DR, Effmann EL: Pneumonia in the child. In: Putman CE, ed. *Pulmonary Diagnosis: Imaging and Other Techniques.* New York: Appleton-Century-Croft, 1981, pp 219–245.

Cross-Reference

Pediatric Radiology: THE REQUISITES, 2nd edn, pp 36–37.

Comment

Staphylococcal pneumonia is a serious infection associated with empyemas and pneumatoceles. Staph pneumonia is more commonly seen in infancy, while H flu occurs most commonly between 6–12 months, and strep 1 to 2 years. Fifty per cent of staphylococcal pneumonias will develop pneumatoceles. Pneumatoceles are thought to be a form of PIE and local emphysema caused by airway obstruction through a check valve mechanism. Pneumatoceles may pop and leak into the pleural space, causing pneumothorax. Pneumatoceles often resolve within 6 weeks.

While pneumatoceles are a late complication of staphylococcal pneumonia seen during the healing phase of the disease, empyema is generally seen at the onset. Empyemas are thick pus-containing pleural collections separate from the parenchyma that tend not to layer as simple effusions as due to either viscosity or loculation. The treatment for any pus collection is evacuation. Surgery will place a chest tube at the base of the pleural space to aspirate the collection, provided no fibrinous bands are seen on ultrasound.

Alternatively, a pulmonary abscess is a circumscribed thick-walled collection of pus within the lung parenchyma. Peripheral abscesses are tricky to distinguish from empyema. On CT, the abscess usually creates an acute angle with the chest wall, while an empyema will layer in an obtuse angle. Quite often an abscess will live in collapsed or consolidated lung and delineation of the abscess can be determined by contrast enhancement. The treatment for pulmonary abscess is often antibiotics, with thoracentesis used in complicated cases.

Round pneumonia is just a big ball of fluid-filled infected alveoli usually seen in the under-8-years age group. The shape is thought to be a result of poor communication between the pores of Kohn and the channels of Lambert, collateral channels between the alveoli. Children have poorly formed collateral pathways, smaller alveoli, and thinner septae leading to a more focal, well-defined infiltrate. The entity is often referred to as a pseudotumor due to its well-defined hard-edged morphology, which differs from the soft marginated adult pneumonic infiltrate pattern. The round pneumonias tend to be pleural based with lower lobe predominance. Round pneumonias are most commonly caused by pneumococcal not staphylococcal infections.

Notes

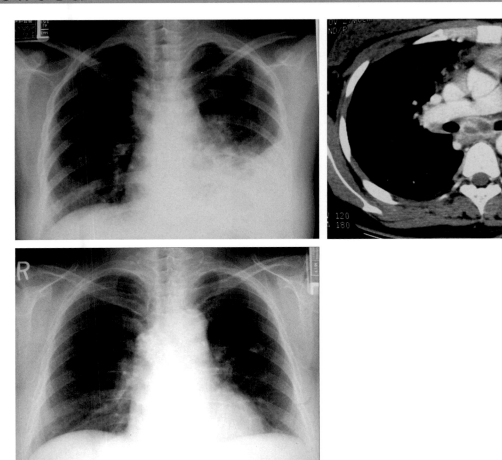

Status Post Antibiotic Therapy

1. What is the differential diagnosis?

2. "You ask me if I have a Ghon complex?"

3. What three findings suggest primary infection?

4. What are Simon's foci?

Primary Pulmonary Tuberculosis

1. Histoplasmosis, coccidioidomycosis, and viral pneumonia.

2. A primary lower lobe lesion with a calcified draining node seen on chest X-ray.

3. Lobar consolidation, hilar adenopathy, pleural effusion.

4. Apical calcifications.

References

Mosby's Medical, Nursing and Allied Health Dictionary, 4th edn. Scientific American Medicine.

Lamont AC, Cremin BJ, Pelteret RM: Radiological patterns of pulmonary tuberculosis in the paediatric age group. *Pediatr Radiol* 16:2–7, 1986.

Cross-Reference

Pediatric Radiology: THE REQUISITES, 2nd edn, pp 38–40.

Comment

Tuberculosis is a granulomatous disease. Granulomas are defined as accumulations of macrophages, lymphocytes, and giant cells into discrete chronic inflammatory granules. The causative agent is a mycobacterium, slow-growing, aerobic, nonpsporulating, nonmotile bacilli with a high cell-wall lipid content.

Infection is via airborne droplets of water containing mycobacterium from an infected coughing patient. The bacillus is inspired and falls into the lower lobes (preferentially the superior segment) due to gravity and increased airflow. The bacilli implant in the alveoli but do not secrete toxins, hence provoking little inflammatory response, and allowing for massive undetected growth. At around 6 weeks the bacilli find their way to the lymphatics spreading to the regional draining lymph node. High oxygen is preferred by the bacilli, leading to residence in the upper lobes, presumably through a hematogenous or lymphatic root. At about 6–8 weeks the immune system detects the bacilli and establishes cell-mediated immunity (engulfment by macrophages activated by lymphocytes as opposed to humoral immunity involving antibodies produced by B cells). This activation of cell-mediated immunity is what is measured by the tuberculin test.

The activated macrophages run to the site of the bacilli, clump together, and begin engulfing their acid-fast staining invaders, yielding formation of the granuloma. The majority of the bacilli are killed, leading to resolution of the process. If the immune system fails to clear all the bacilli, primary symptomatic tuberculosis may develop. Healed lesions may harbor dormant bacilli that under immune stress (immunosuppression, HIV, chemotherapy, childbirth, steroids) may become activated.

On chest film the findings of primary tuberculosis include consolidation, hilar or paratracheal adenopathy, and pleural effusions. Miliary tuberculosis appears on conventional radiographs as bilateral, multiple, small, nodules, and on high-resolution CT as nodular interstitial thickening.

Notes

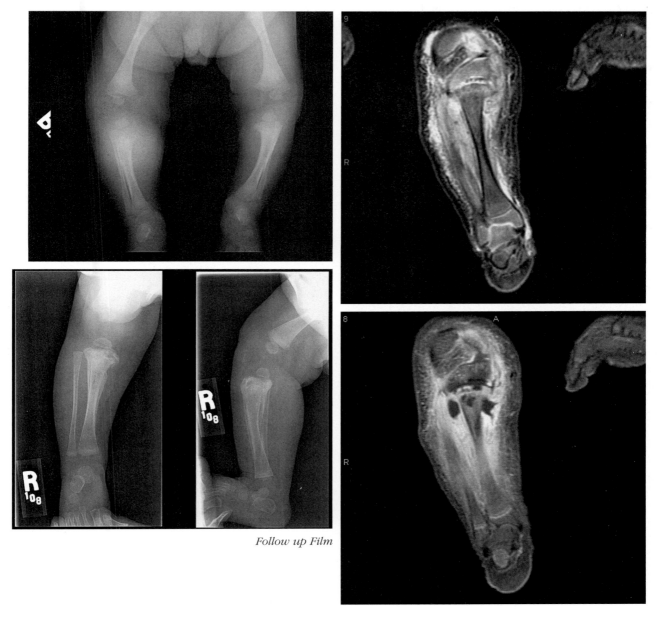

Follow up Film

1. What bones are commonly affected by this entity?
2. What is the differential for a small lucent nidus with surrounding periosteal new bone?
3. What is the etiologic agent?
4. What is a bony sequestrum?

Osteomyelitis

1. Distal and proximal femur, proximal and distal tibia, proximal and distal humerus, and fibula are involved in decreasing order.

2. Brodie's abscess, osteoid osteoma.

3. *Steptococcus* or *Staphylococcus.*

4. A piece of devitalized bone that may harbor latent infection. The bone is devitalized due to periosteal stripping by the infection. The periosteum is rich in vessels and accounts for much of the cortex's blood supply.

Reference

Oudjhane K, Azouz EM: Imaging of osteomyelitis in children. *Radiol Clin N Am* 39(2):251–266, 2001.

Cross-Reference

Pediatric Radiology: THE REQUISITES, p 261.

Comment

Osteomyelitis in children differs from adults due to anatomic differences. As the cartilaginous growth plate is avascular the arteries that feed the metaphysis course toward the physis, then bend away in a hairpin turn to dump into large sinusoidal veins. This unusual vascular model creates areas of slow flow where bacteria from the blood may thrive. The epiphysis is spared as there is no vascular connection with the metaphysis with one exception—under 18 months transphyseal arteries are present that link the two circulations.

Bacteria seed these slow-flowing veins and infect the marrow space, leading to increased medullary pressure and thrombosis. Unlike the rest of the body's tissues, bone volume does not increase with edema. Instead, the pressure drives the pus to burrow through and out of the cortex, elevating the periosteum in its wake. The elevated periosteum ossifies, forming a tunnel around the stream of pus flowing from the marrow cavity. Necrosis ensues as the periosteal blood supply to the cortex is disrupted in addition to intramedullary arterial destruction. The infection, no longer confined to the bone, may now invade soft tissues and joint spaces.

Hematologic spread most commonly involves fast-growing tubular bones. Flat bones are involved at juxta-articular locations due to the blood supply required for growth. Swelling, pain, and decreased range of motion are common presenting signs. Only a third of patients have an elevated white count, while only 40% demonstrate positive cultures. Antibiotics may give false negative cultures following aspiration.

Radiographic bone findings for osteomyelitis do not show up until 7–10 days after infection (30% of bone needs to be destroyed before detectable on radiography). Bone lucencies develop with trabecular destruction as well as periosteal new bone formation. Given today's aggressive antibiotic intervention it is uncommon to see involucra and sequestra formation as they are late findings.

Scintigraphy is positive after 24 hours and shows increased uptake. MRI will demonstrate changes within 24 hours as well. Bone marrow edema as well as an abscess collection will light up on fat-suppressed or short tau inversion recovery (STIR) imaging. Gadolinium will detect absence of perfusion in cases of necrosis. Extension to soft tissues as well as the growth plate are useful diagnostic questions that MR may answer. Infection of the physis may lead to growth arrest, hence early intervention is imperative.

Notes

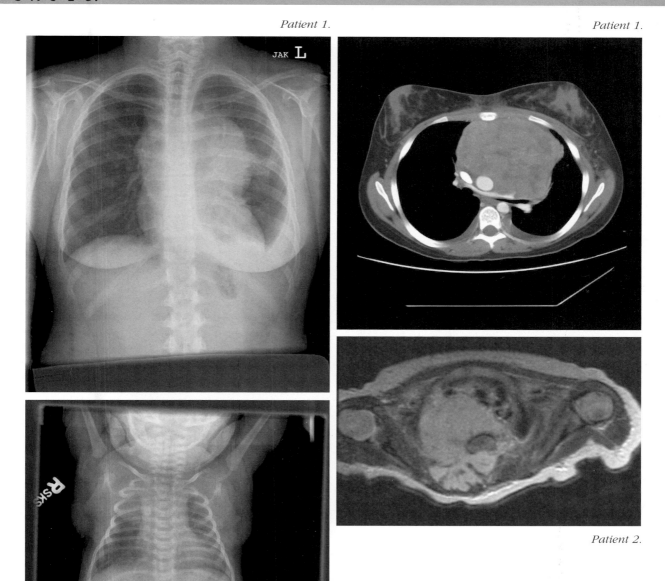

Patient 1.

Patient 1.

Patient 2.

Patient 2.

1. Where is the lesion?
2. What is the differential diagnosis?
3. What percentage of thymomas calcify?
4. What modalities are useful in the work-up?

C A S E 61

Lymphoma vs. Neuroblastoma, Middle/post. Mediastinal Masses

1. Posterior mediastinum.

2. Posterior mediastinal masses: neuroblastoma, ganglioneuroma, ganglioneuroblastoma, extramedullary hematopoiesis.

3. 25%.

4. CT, MR, Nuclear bone scan.

References

Reed JC, Hallet KK, Feigin DS: Neural tumors of the thorax: subject review from the AFIP. *Radiology* 126:9–17, 1978.

Hamrick-Turner JE, Saif MF, Powers CI, et al.: Imaging of childhood non-Hodgkin's lymphoma: assessment by histologic subtype. *Radiographics* 14:11–28, 1994.

Cross-Reference

Pediatric Radiology: THE REQUISITES, 2nd edn, pp 50–54.

Comment

The middle mediastinum extends from either the anterior or posterior surface of the heart to the anterior margin of the ribs depending on who you read, quote, or sit opposite from in Louisville. The middle mediastinum extends from diaphragm up to the thoracic inlet (the clavicles). Middle mediastinal masses include adenopathy, esophageal duplication cysts, hiatal hernia, bronchogenic cysts. Adenopathy in the middle mediastinum is seen in lymphoma. Lymphoma is divided into Hodgkin disease and everything else; everything else is known as non-Hodgkin lymphoma (NHL). Hodgkin accounts for 5% of all childhood lymphoma cases. Hodgkin is divided into four types in order of favorable prognosis: lymphocytic predominance, nodular sclerosing, mixed cellularity, and lymphocyte depleted. Staging involves the Ann Arbor classification and is based on the number of nodal sites and their location. Radiographically, superior, anterior, and middle mediastinal nodes may show involvement (enlargement). Nodes will be contiguous (unlike NHL). The lung may show direct extension with a mass lesion or pleural effusions.

By contrast NHL accounts for 95% of the lymphoma in kids. NHL is divided into two categories based on histology, lymphoblastic and nonlymphoblastic. Nonlymphoblastic is further subdivided into histiocytic and undifferentiated of which there are Burkitt and non-Burkitt types. All you need to know are four types: lymphoblastic (35%), histiocytic (15%), Burkitt (25%), and non-Burkitt (25%). Unlike its adult manifestation, NHL is primarily extranodal in distribution. Each type has a distribution predominance: lymphoblastic (chest), Burkitt and non-Burkitt (abdomen-ileocecal), histiocytic (anywhere but mediastinum). T-cell derived NHL is commonly found in the **T**horax, while the **B**elly demonstrates lineage of **B**-cells.

The CT appearance of NHL is varied and may demonstrate bulky mediastinal adenopathy or extranodal disease involving the spleen, liver, kidneys, and gastrointestinal tract with large foci of low attenuation or an infiltrative pattern. Systemic involvement is typical at the time of diagnosis, obviating the need for radiographic staging. All patients receive chemotherapy. Prognosis is determined by bone marrow and CNS involvement.

The posterior mediastinum is bounded by the anterior margin of the spine and superiorly by the cervical spine. Ninety per cent of these tumors are neurogenic, derived from the sympathetic chains that flank the thoracic vertebral bodies. The vast majority of these neurogenic tumors are neuroblastomas, while the rest are ganglioneuroblastoma or ganglioneuroma. Neuroblastoma, although malignant, holds a more favorable prognosis if diagnosed under the age of one. Clinical presentation includes fever, irritability, weight loss, and anemia. Neural symptoms from cord compression may cause paraplegia, extremity weakness and altered bowel and bladder dysfunction.

On conventional imaging a posterior mediastinal soft tissue density is seen on the chest film. Erosion of the adjacent ribs and foraminal enlargement points to the diagnosis. Further evaluation with CT will demonstrate the presence of calcification confirming neuroblastoma. MR evaluation of the spine will stage CNS involvement. Bone scan will stage the neuroblastoma. Therapy is surgical with prognosis varying depending on location, chest more favorable than abdomen.

Notes

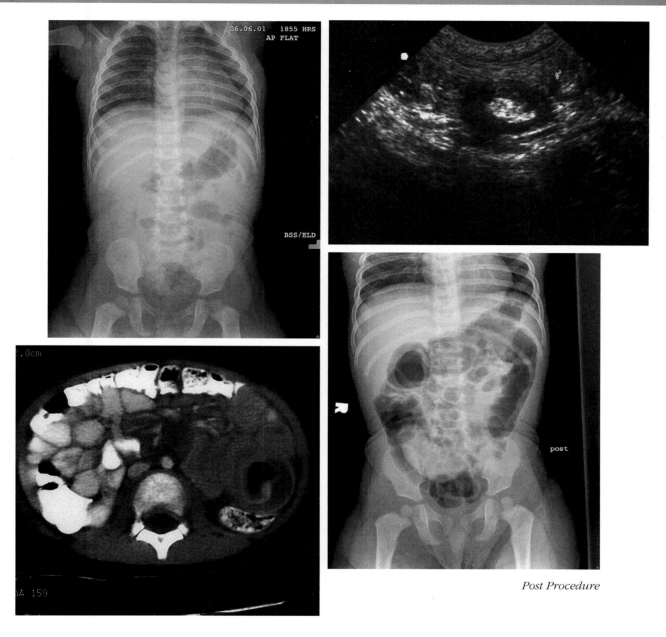

Post Procedure

1. Who was Lippershey?

2. What is the rule of 2s?

3. What is the differential diagnosis?

4. Where is the most common location for this entity?

Intussusception

1. A Dutch spectacle maker who invented the first telescope, 1608.

2. Meckel diverticulum, seen in 2% of autopsies, 2 feet from ileocecal valve; complications occur before 2 years of age in 2% of patients.

3. Viral gastroenteritis, peritonitis secondary to ruptured viscus, and sepsis.

4. Ileocolic, 90%.

Reference

Kornecki A, Daneman A, Navarro O, et al.: Spontaneous reduction of intussusception: clinical spectrum, management and outcome. *Pediatr Radiol* 30(1):58–63, 2000.

Cross-Reference

Pediatric Radiology: THE REQUISITES, 2nd edn, pp 88–91.

Comment

Intussusception can be described as telescoping or arializing bowel similar to the retractable antenna on old cordless phones or radios. Pediatric intussusception is thought to be a result of hypertrophied Peyer patches, small bowel lymphoid tissue, in the 5-month to 5-year age range. Passive maternal immunity begins to wear off at 3 to 5 months, triggering endogenous production of immune mediators and hence hypertrophied Peyer patches. Infants may have "lead" points associated with Meckel diverticulum, lymphoma, polyps, bowel wall hemorrhage (Henoch–Schönlein purpura), appendiceal inflammation, and inspissated stool in patients with cystic fibrosis. Lymphoma is the most common lead point in the over-5-years group.

Clinically, abdominal pain, vomiting, and less commonly blood per rectum, are encountered. Some patients have a prior upper respiratory tract infection. No discussion of intussusception is complete without mentioning the buzzwords currant jelly stool, a mixture of blood, mucus, and stool seen in 15%–20% of cases.

A conventional radiograph is most often normal, but a right lower quadrant mass with no identifiable right colon, no colonic air, or bowel obstruction may be seen. The distal large bowel will be relatively gas free due to hyperperistalsis. This appearance, with the above clinical features, necessitates an emergency contrast enema for diagnosis and, if necessary, reduction before the intussusceptum strangulates and necroses. Absolute contraindications to an enema include intestinal perforation and peritonitis. Positive diagnostic enemas will demonstrate a well-delineated cutoff, usually within the transverse colon. Ultrasound has been used with increasing success. A pseudo kidney appearance or bullseye is often diagnostic.

Three tries with the bag 3 feet above the table is the standard barium setup. If the radiologist chooses a pneumatic approach then appropriate pressure gauges are necessary to guard against perforation from overdistention; 120 mm is the magic number for pressure with the child at rest. The examination is complete when there is visualization of the cecum with reflux into a normal terminal ileum. If the enema fails the patient goes to surgery.

Notes

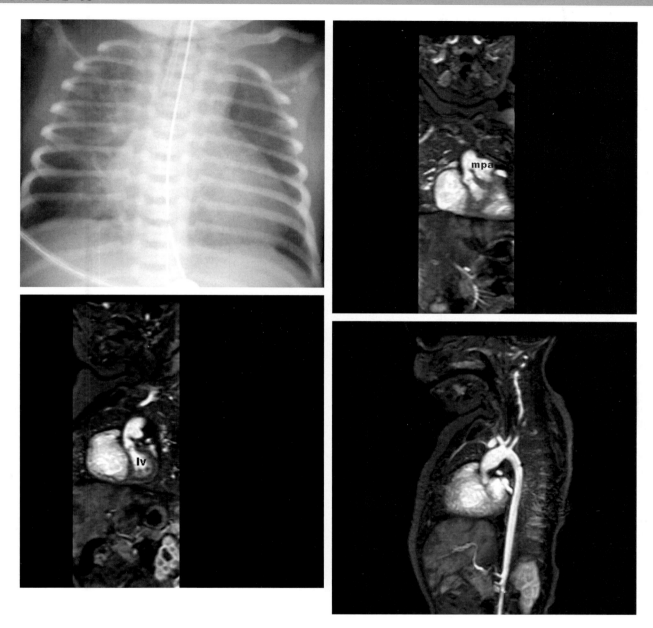

1. What chromosomal anomalies are associated with this entity?

2. What percentage have chromosomal anomalies?

3. What are the findings of prenatal ultrasound?

4. Are these patients cyanotic or acyanotic?

Hypoplastic Left Heart Syndrome

1. Turner syndrome, trisomy 13, 18, 21.

2. 30% have chromosomal anomalies.

3. Prenatal ultrasound at 16–20 weeks demonstrates an enlarged right ventricle and pulmonary artery.

4. Cyanotic.

Reference

Allen HD, Gutgesell HP, Clark EB, et al.: *Moss and Adams Heart Disease in Infants, Children and Adolescents: Including the Fetus and Young Adult,* 6th edn. Baltimore: Lippincott Williams & Wilkins, 2000, pp 1011–1026.

Cross-Reference

Pediatric Radiology: THE REQUISITES, 2nd edn, p 60.

Comment

Hypoplastic left heart syndrome is characterized by hypoplasia or absence of the left ventricle with an atretic aortic and mitral valve. Atretic aortic and mitral valves require a large intra-atrial shunt (left-to-right shunt) and patent ductus arteriosus (right-to-left shunt) to sustain life. The cause is unknown.

Clinically, patients present with cardiovascular collapse and metabolic acidosis at birth as the ductus begins to close cutting off shunted blood from the pulmonary artery. Femoral pulses are diminished and the patients usually have hyperkalemia. If the ductus remains patent, presentation is delayed by a few days.

Radiographically, the heart may show mild cardiomegaly with mild pulmonary edema. The echocardiogram will demonstrate a small left ventricle, small aorta, enlarged right ventricle and enlarged pulmonary artery.

Patients undergo either a transplant or a three-step staged reconstruction of the heart: the Norwood, Glenn, and Fontan procedures.

Notes

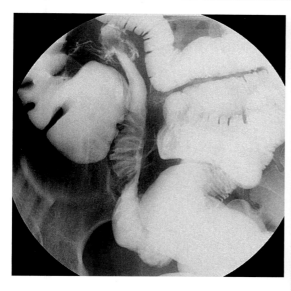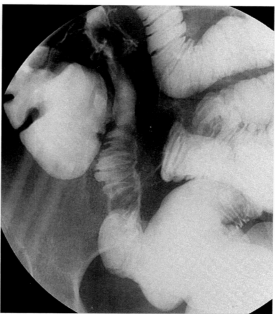

1. Are there skin manifestations?

2. What is the difference between shortened and foreshortened?

3. Is CT indicated?

4. What is the eponym for amyotrophic lateral sclerosis?

Crohn Disease

1. Yes, erythema nodosum.

2. Foreshortening is merely the illusion of shortening, as the barrel of a gun might appear as you are looking end on.

3. Complicated Crohn will develop fistula and abscesses that are easily detected by CT.

4. Lou Gehrig's disease. The apostrophe connotes that the Yankee first baseman of the 1920s had in fact been afflicted with the disease. Alternatively, Crohn had described regional enteritis while personally being free of inflammatory bowel disease, hence the eponym Crohn disease not Crohn's disease.

Reference

Jabra AA, Fishman EK, Taylor GA. Crohn disease in the pediatric patient: CT evaluation. *Radiology* 179: 495–498, 1991.

Cross-Reference

Pediatric Radiology: THE REQUISITES, 2nd edn, p 118.

Comment

Regional enteritis is characterized by segmental, full-thickness, granulomatous involvement of the bowel wall. Presentation includes failure to thrive, recurrent abdominal pain, diarrhea, and rectal bleeding. The peak age is between 20–40 but many cases begin in early adolescence. Crohn is rare in infants and young children. Ten per cent of children may have sacroilitis or large joint arthritis.

Radiographically, plain film may show obstruction or bowel wall thickening. Contrast studies demonstrate fistulae, cobblestoning, or a mass. Thickening of folds is secondary to mucosal edema, while a more nodular pattern indicates an edematous submucosa. The terminal ileum is involved in the majority of cases, appearing nodular, thickened, irregular, and rigid. Alternatively, lymphoid hyperplasia may cause filling defects without the rigidity seen in inflammatory bowel disease, a distinction made at real-time fluoroscopy.

Over time, aphtha (pinpoint mucosal erosions) will develop into deep ulcers and later heal with stricturing (string sign), fistula and/or abscess formation. Discontinuous lesions within different segments of colon and eccentric involvement of the lumen with mesenteric predominance are characteristic. Long-standing disease may produce a featureless shortened bowel.

Crohn may involve the GI tract anywhere between the mouth and anus; therefore surgery is used conservatively as it may actually exacerbate the disease.

Notes

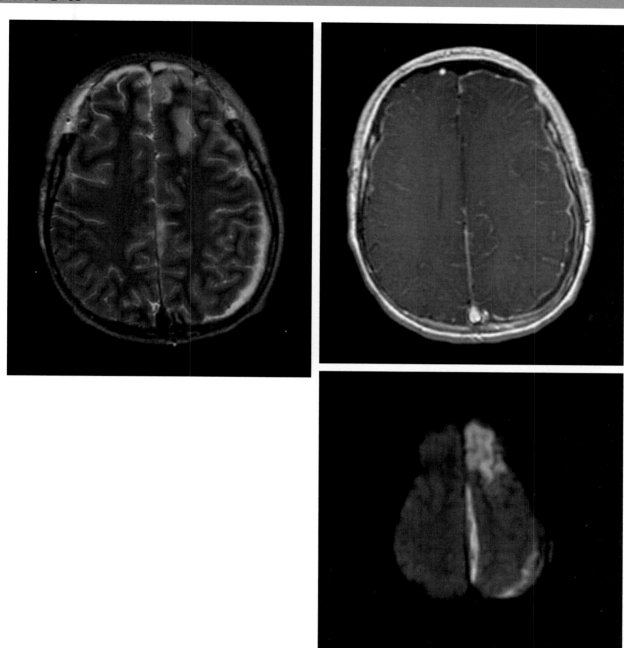

1. What does the Greek prefix lepto mean?
2. What layers compose the leptomeninges?
3. What is the role of imaging in this diagnosis?
4. What are complications of this entity?

Haemophilus influenzae Meningitis

1. Delicate or thin.

2. Leptomeninges refers to the arachnoid and pia. Excluding the durable dura mater.

3. Meningitis is diagnosed by clinical and lumbar puncture lab results. Imaging is reserved for complications in cases with unusual clinical courses.

4. Bacterial meningitis may lead to: hydrocephalus, venous thrombosis, cavernous sinus thrombosis, venous infarction, arterial infarction, effusions, cerebritis and abscess, ventriculitis, and deafness.

Reference

Cockrill HH Jr, Dreisbach J, Lowe B, et al.: Computed tomography in leptomeningeal infections. *Am J Roentgenol* 130(3): 511–515, 1978.

Cross-Reference

Pediatric Radiology: THE REQUISITES, pp 276–278.

Comment

Bacterial meningitis is an infection of the leptomeninges. The bacteria that cause meningitis vary with age. In the neonatal period, *Escherichia coli* and group B streptococci are common. In childhood, *H. influenzae* predominates, while in adolescents and young adults *Neisseria meningitidis* is the culprit. The elderly are prone to *Streptococcus pneumoniae* and *Listeria monocytogenes*. There are five roots of entry to the meninges: (1) direct hematologic spread across the blood–brain barrier, (2) through the choroid plexus, (3) direct extension from a ruptured cortical abscess, (4) penetrating trauma, and (5) direct extension from a superficial structure, i.e. sinusitis. Clinically, patients present with fever, stiff neck, and headache. Other signs include photophobia, diplopia, irritability, nausea, and vomiting. Untreated patients may progress to seizures, coma, and death.

On CT and MR subdural effusions are present due to irritation of the meninges and subsequent weeping of transudative fluid, a characteristic especially common in H flu. The fluid will follow the attenuation and intensity of CSF on CT and MR sequences respectively. Effusions are most commonly located over the frontal and temporal regions and will resolve with the clinical course over several days. Distinguishing sterile effusions from pus containing empyemas is not so simple. Helpful signs include slight hyperintensity to CSF in empyemas on T1- and T2-weighted scans. Loculation of empyema is seen in 50% of patients. Subdural effusions are most often bilateral while subdural empyemas are unilateral. Empyema will enhance on both CT and MR, while subdural effusions will not. Substantial vasogenic edema and cerebritis in underlying parenchyma is associated with empyema but not to the same degree as with subdural effusions. Underlying parenchymal signal abnormalities, including enhancement, may reflect the effect of inflamed meninges on the brain or possible infarction. Other complications are listed above.

Treatment by antibiotics is life saving. Roughly a third of patients have significant neurologic complications.

Notes

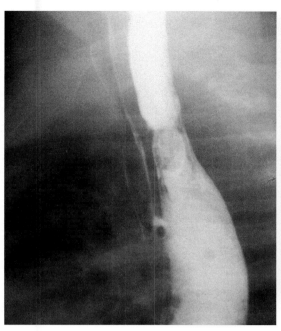 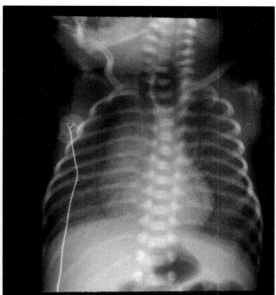

1. What is the incidence?

2. What are the associated abnormalities?

3. What is VACTERL?

4. What are the variations of this disorder?

Esophageal Atresia (EA)/ Tracheoesophageal Fistula (TEF)

1. 1 in 3000 live births.

2. Down, prematurity, VACTERL.

3. **V**ertebral abnormalities, **A**nal atresia, **C**ardiac abnormalities, **T**racheoesophageal fistula and/or **E**sophageal atresia, **R**enal agenesis, and **L**imb defects. Rarely are all findings present.

4. EA and distal fistula (82%), EA and no fistula (9%), H fistula, EA and two fistulas, EA and proximal fistula.

Reference

Berrocal T, Torres I, Gutiérrez J, Prieto C, et al.: Congenital anomalies of the upper gastrointestinal tract. *Radiographics* 19:855–872, 1999.

Cross-Reference

Pediatric Radiology: THE REQUISITES, 2nd edn, pp 92–95.

Comment

Development of the upper airway begins at 4 weeks with budding and eventual separation of the trachea from the esophagus. Failure of the normal process may lead to atresia or, less commonly, tracheoesophageal fistulae. Coughing, choking, and cyanosis are the symptoms with the first feeding on day one.

Radiographically, one may see an air-distended esophageal atretic pouch that may often contain a curled NG tube. Excessive dilatation of the stomach and or small bowel will be seen as a result of the distal fistula communicating between the lungs and the esophagus. A careful confirmatory contrast study may be attempted but is usually not necessary.

Treatment is surgical; reanastomosis with follow-up water-soluble studies to assess integrity. Follow up for evaluation of the associated VACTERL complex. The VACTERL complex refers to a constellation of symptoms that are thought to occur due to a gestational insult during a specific period of development (question 3). The VACTERL complex is seen in a third of EA/TEF cases.

Notes

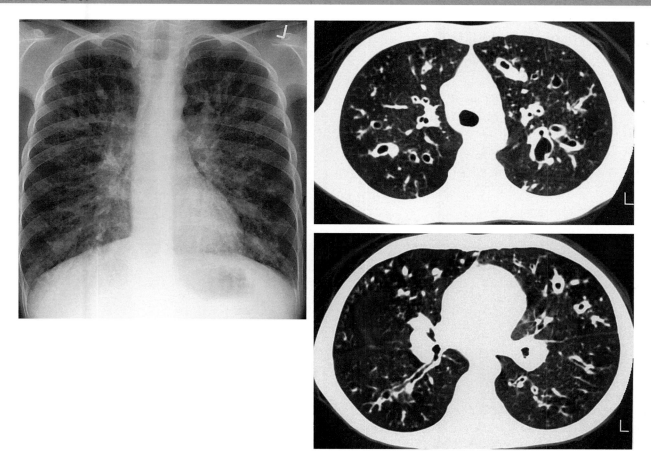

1. What other systems are usually affected?
2. What is the Brassfield Classification?
3. Would you be surprised if this patient had sickle cell as well?
4. What percentage of these patients presented with meconium ileus?

Cystic Fibrosis (CF)

1. Pulmonary, upper respiratory tract, gastrointestinal, and genitourinary.

2. Scoring system used to correlate imaging with clinical picture to guide therapy in cystic fibrosis.

3. Yes, you would! CF: Whites, 1 in 1500; Blacks, 1 in 20,000. Sickle cell: Whites, 1 in 40,000; Blacks, 1 in 500.

4. 20% of CF patients present with meconium ileus.

Reference

Colin AA, Wohl ME: Cystic fibrosis. *Pediatr Rev* 15: 192–200, 1994.

Cross-Reference

Pediatric Radiology: THE REQUISITES, 2nd edn, pp 41–42.

Comment

Cystic fibrosis is an autosomal recessive disease that affects the transport of chloride and water across the cell membrane, a deficit most pronounced in mucus-producing glands. Normal chloride transport across the cell membrane causes water to osmotically leave the cell and hydrate mucus produced by the glands. A dehydrated highly viscous mucus "gunks up" the cilia, preventing the normal clearance of debris and bacteria, leading to chronic infection, bronchitis, and chronic obstructive pulmonary disease (COPD).

Patients may have respiratory symptoms at all ages, although in a small group the earliest symptoms are gastrointestinal, including meconium ileus, malabsorption, fatty liver, and failure to thrive. Respiratory involvement includes bronchiolitis in infants while older children are plagued by recurrent respiratory infection with COPD developing in adolescents.

Findings on chest films run the gamut between normal and bronchiolitis. Hyperinflation due to mucus plugging with subsequent parenchymal damage causes bronchial wall thickening, peribronchial cuffing, and eventually bronchiectasis. The bronchiectasis has an upper lobe predominance. Initially, hilar enlargement is due to reactive nodal hyperplasia from chronic infection, but later results from enlarged pulmonary arteries secondary to pulmonary hypertension.

Pneumothorax from a ruptured bleb is likely to show a limited degree of collapse due to the fibrotic stiffened lung's reduced compliance. An enlarged cardiac silhouette suggests cor pulmonale that develops secondary to pulmonary hypertension caused by hypoxia from poor gas exchange at the mucus and debris-filled alveoli.

Therapy for cystic fibrosis includes mucus-busting enzymatic aerosols and drugs that alter electrolyte transport. Future strategies are aimed at the cellular insertion of genes to repair the defect.

Notes

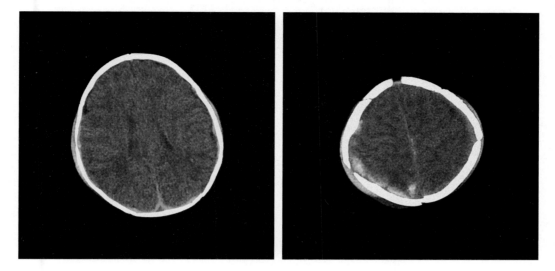

1. What is the appearance of hyperacute hemorrhage on T1 and T2?

2. What is the appearance of acute bleed on T1 and T2?

3. What is the appearance of early subacute (intracellular met hemoglobin) hemorrhage on T1 and T2?

4. What is the appearance of late subacute (extracellular met hemoglobin) hemorrhage on T1 and T2?

5. What is the appearance of chronic hemorrhage on TI and T2?

Subdural Hematoma

1. T1 iso, T2 bright.

2. T1 iso, T2 dark.

3. T1 bright, T2 dark.

4. T1 bright, T2 bright.

5. T1 dark, T2 dark rim.

Reference

Demaerel P, Casteels I, Wilms G: Cranial imaging in child abuse. *Eur Radiol* 12(4):849–857, 2002.

Cross-Reference

Pediatric Radiology: THE REQUISITES, p 280.

Comment

There is a wide range of CNS abnormalities that are caused by child abuse. Strangulation and suffocation may lead to global brain hypoxia and infarction. The shaken baby syndrome, publicized by high-profile court cases, is characterized by subdural hemorrhage, subarachnoid hemorrhage, retinal hemorrhage, cerebral edema, diffuse axonal injury, and small cerebral contusions with minimal evidence of external trauma. A direct blow to the head may produce skull fractures, subdural hematomas and cerebral contra coup contusions.

Clinical presentation includes irritability, blunted affect, episodes of vomiting, cyanosis, weight loss, recurrent encephalopathy, and seizures. Patient histories that do not reflect the severity of injury are also red flags.

In cases involving head injury, recommendations by the ACR suggest head CT in children under 2, as CT is more sensitive to acute subdural and subarachnoid hematomas than MR. MR is indicated in subacute cases in which the blood has an isodense appearance on CT. When reading any head CT it is important to view the scout tomograph or scanogram of the skull, as a skull fracture in the plane of the scan may be difficult to detect.

On CT, subdural hematomas are the most common bleeds in child abuse followed by epidural, subarachnoid, and parenchymal hemorrhage. Anoxia, secondary to suffocation, will appear as diffuse cerebral edema with loss of normal gray-white differentiation and effacement of sulci. Retinal hemorrhages may be apparent on CT as well.

MRI is sensitive (gradient echo) to shear injuries and small cortical contusions undetected by CT. Shear injuries are found in the white matter usually at the corticomedullary junction, centrum semiovale, or corpus callosum. Hemorrhage on MR may be dated by knowledge of hemorrhage evolution. Blood spills out of the vessels in an oxygenated state, oxyhemoglobin, and later, approximately 1–2 days, relinquishes the oxygen to the surrounding cells that have become oxygen hungry due to poor perfusion. Then 2–7 days later the deoxyhemoglobin becomes oxidized forming methemoglobin. Between 1–4 weeks the formation of methemoglobin leads to lysis of the cell and spillage of heme in the extracellular space, which is eventually picked up by macrophages. Months later there is a detectable buildup of hemosiderin due to metabolized heme within the brain parenchyma. See the question section for the appearance of hemorrhage on MR.

One-half of abuse cases lead to permanent sequelae or death.

Notes

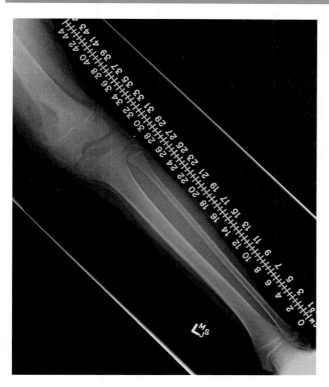

1. What are the two histologic bone tumor types?
2. Which type is this case?
3. Name some examples of each histologic type.
4. Is there any genetic predisposition?

Osteosarcoma

1. Round cell and mesenchymal.

2. Mesenchymal.

3. Mesenchymal, bone and cartilage: enchondromas, osteochondromas, chondroblastomas, and osteosarcoma. Round cell, marrow infiltrative: Ewing sarcoma, lymphoma, and Langerhans cell histiocytosis.

4. Hereditary retinoblastoma patients have an increased risk of osteosarcoma.

Reference

Murphey MD, Robbin MR, McRae GA, et al.: The many faces of osteosarcoma. *Radiographics* 17:1205–1231, 1997.

Cross-Reference

Pediatric Radiology: THE REQUISITES, pp 227–228.

Comment

Osteosarcoma is the most common primary bone sarcoma, affecting the under 30 age group in 80% of cases. Osteosarcoma is thought to be caused by a mutation in mesenchymal cells that leads to destruction and replacement of bone with formation of neoplastic cartilage and bone matrix. The tumor may arise from either the medullary cavity or cortex of the metaphysis. The most common location is about the knee, with the distal femur (40%) twice as common as the proximal tibia (20%). The proximal humerus is third (15%) with flat-bones such as the jaw and maxilla composing the rest. These tumors favor areas of fast growth, hence the above-described distribution. The tumor is divided histologically into either osteoblastic, fibroblastic, or chondroblastic categories. Clinically, osteosarcoma presents between 10 and 20 years with pain, local swelling, and a palpable mass.

Radiographically, osteosarcoma appears as an ill-defined lytic lesion with mineralized osseous matrix in a cloud-like morphology that will often extend beyond the normal contours of the bone. The more aggressive the tumor the more lytic its appearance. A fast-growing osteosarcoma will elevate the periosteum as it destroys cortex. The periosteum will respond by the formation of radial spicules responsible for the often mentioned sunburst spiculation appearance. New bone formation as a result of periosteal elevation will be partially destroyed by the advancing tumor leaving in its wake the Codman triangle, the shortest side representing the tumor margin. Associated soft tissue masses may also be seen in a fair number of cases.

MRI is key for evaluating the extent of tumor involvement. Short tau inversion recovery (STIR) images with their exquisite sensitivity to bone marrow edema will demarcate presumed tumor margin. Dark on T1, bright on T2, MR will allow for detection of physeal, intra-articular, and soft tissue involvement. In the future, gadolinium may have a role in monitoring chemotherapy tumor response.

Fifteen per cent of osteosarcomas present with mets. Metastatic disease commonly travels to the lung, demonstrating multiple dense pulmonary nodules (mineralized osseous matrix) that may cavitate and result in pneumothorax. Osteosarcoma may also metastasize to bone with either skip lesions (normal bone found between the two lesions) or across the joint.

Neoadjuvant therapy to debulk the tumor followed by resection and post-resection chemotherapy in the absence of metastatic disease will yield 5-year survival rates of 80%. Much of the prognosis rests on tumor grade with the less aggressive more differentiated lower grades demonstrating better sensitivity to chemotherapy. Resection of pulmonary mets has demonstrated increased survival.

Notes

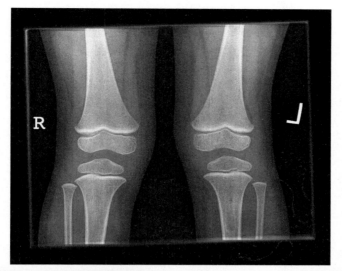

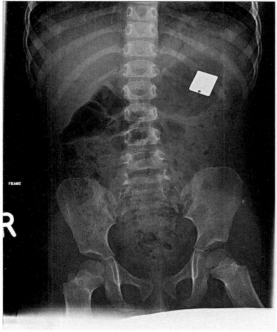

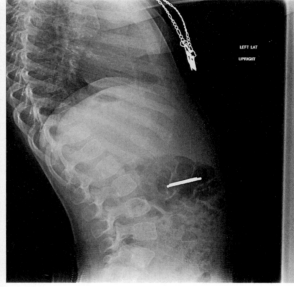

1. What is Wimberger sign?

2. In what disease is Wimberger sign seen?

3. How is this entity treated?

4. How long do these findings persist?

Lead Poisoning

1. Small divots of metaphyseal destruction seen at the proximal medial portion of the tibia.

2. These lucent bands of metaphyseal destruction are seen in congenital syphilis, osteomyelitis, fibromatosis, and hyperparathyroidism.

3. Blood lead levels above 10 μg/dL are treated with chelation therapy.

4. Lead lines will resolve after approximately 4 years.

References

DeLuca SA: Lead poisoning. *Am Fam Physician* 30(1): 179–180, 1984.

Blickman JG, Wilkinson RH, Graef JW: The radiologic "lead band" revisited. *Am J Roentgenol* 146(2): 245–247, 1986.

Cross-Reference

Pediatric Radiology: THE REQUISITES, p 217.

Comment

Ingested lead is a toxic substance that competes with calcium and is readily taken up by bone. Lead clears rapidly from the blood but will have a half-life of 30 years once deposited in bone. Even though 80% of ingested lead finds its way into the bones, the amounts are so minute as to be undetectable by radiography. Lead lines are the result of lead's effect on osteoclastic resorption of the provisional zone of calcification, the mineralized cartilaginous template that is eventually removed and replaced by osteoblast-formed matrix that is later mineralized. In the case of lead poisoning, osteoclasts are unable to resorp the mineralized cartilage, which continues to grow by active osteoblasts. The lines do not disappear with therapy, they merely "migrate" away from the physis as the zone of provisional calcification moves in the direction of the growth plate away from the diaphysis. Eventually with the normal turnover of bone the lines disappear after 4 years. Lead lines do not appear until the blood levels reach between 50–80 μg/dL.

Dense metaphyseal bands do carry a differential diagnosis that includes normal physiologic sclerosis, heavy metal intoxication, radiation injury, hypervitaminosis D, treated hyperthyroidism, and bisphosphonate therapy. The most common, physiologic sclerosis, can be differentiated from lead poisoning by using the proximal fibular metaphysis as a reference. Fast-growing bones are more commonly affected by lead poisoning whereby physiologic sclerosis will show no disparity between the tibia and the slow-growing fibula.

Notes

Fair Game Cases

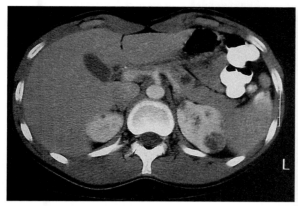
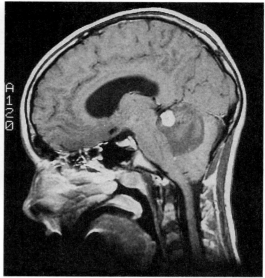

1. What criteria are required for diagnosis?

2. What would account for increased hematocrit levels?

3. What percentage of patients have a single finding?

4. There is an associated 10-fold increased in pheochromocytoma, true or false?

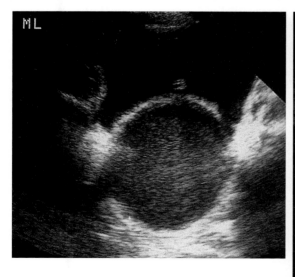
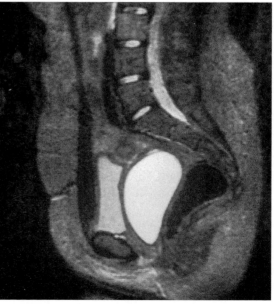

1. If this lesion is seen before puberty, what is the sonographic appearance?

2. If this lesion is seen after puberty, what is the sonographic appearance?

3. What are the congenital etiologies?

4. What are the acquired etiologies?

Von Hippel–Lindau (VHL) Syndrome

1. VHL family history plus CNS hemangioblastoma or one visceral lesion; two or more CNS hemangioblastomas; one hemangioblastoma and one visceral lesion.

2. Hemangioblastomas may secrete erythropoetin-causing polycythemia.

3. 50% will have one manifestation.

4. True, there is a 10-fold increase in pheochromocytoma.

Reference

Smirniotopoulos JG, Murphy FM: The phakomatoses. *Am J Neuroradiol* 13(2):725–746, 1992.

Cross-Reference

Pediatric Radiology: THE REQUISITES, pp 272–273.

Comment

Von Hippel–Lindau is a syndrome caused by a mutation of a tumor suppressor gene, which gives rise to neoplasms in the CNS. Involved organs include the cerebellum, retina, spinal cord, neural crest cell derivatives, kidney, and pancreas. The disease is also known as CNS hemangioblastomatosis due to the preponderance of cerebellar hemangioblastomas. VHL is transmitted as an autosomal dominant trait.

VHL presents as early as the teen years but most commonly in the 20s, with eye symptoms secondary to retinal hemangiomas. Soon after, cerebellar hemangiomas may be detected, while renal cell carcinoma is commonly encountered in older patients. Given the pathophysiology of tumor suppressor mutations, the chances of developing any of these lesions increases over time. Other associated entities include spinal cord hemangioblastomas, pheochromocytoma, liver and kidney angiomas, and cysts of the pancreas, liver, and kidney.

On imaging, 80% of hemangioblastomas appear as mural nodules, that is, a cystic structure with a solid component in contiguity with a wall. The cysts may contain very proteinaceous fluid and appear much like blood on MR. Cysts, relative to CSF, may be hyperintense on T1 while hypointense on T2, reflecting their relative protein content. As this is a vascular neoplasm there is intense contrast enhancement.

Therapy of brain lesions varies from surgery to radiation therapy. Renal cysts are imaged for development of solid components, strong evidence of malignancy. Nephrectomy is not performed but rather the tumors are scooped out of the renal parenchyma as a means of preserving renal function. The killers here are hemangioblastoma (50%) and renal cell carcinoma (30%).

Notes

Hydrometrocolpos

1. If before puberty, the secretions appear anechoic.

2. After puberty, menstruation gives the fluid a hyperechoic appearance.

3. Imperforate hymen, vaginal septum, vaginal atresia, rudimentary horn.

4. Endometrial tumors, cervical tumors, or from post-irradiation fibrosis.

Reference

Nalaboff KM, Pellerito JS, Ben-Levi E: Imaging the endometrium: disease and normal variants. *Radiographics* 21: 1409–1424, 2001.

Cross-Reference

Pediatric Radiology: THE REQUISITES, p 188.

Comment

Hydrometrocolpos is defined as a fluid-filled uterus and vagina secondary to obstruction. Causes include imperforate hymen, vaginal septum, vaginal atresia, or vaginal diaphragm. Hydrometrocolpos may be accompanied by imperforate anus, dysraphic abnormalities of the vertebrae and urinary tract abnormalities, such as solitary kidney or renal ectopia. Most cases of hydrometrocolpos caused by imperforate hymen are not discovered until menarche and may then present as an abdominal or pelvic mass. Infantile hydrometrocolpos presents as an abdominal mass; ultrasound is the screening modality of choice.

On ultrasound there is a marked distention of the vagina and endometrial cavity with fluid. Pre-menarche patients have anechoic collections, while post-menarche patients demonstrate hypoechoic fluid with fluid–fluid levels secondary to retained blood products.

Notes

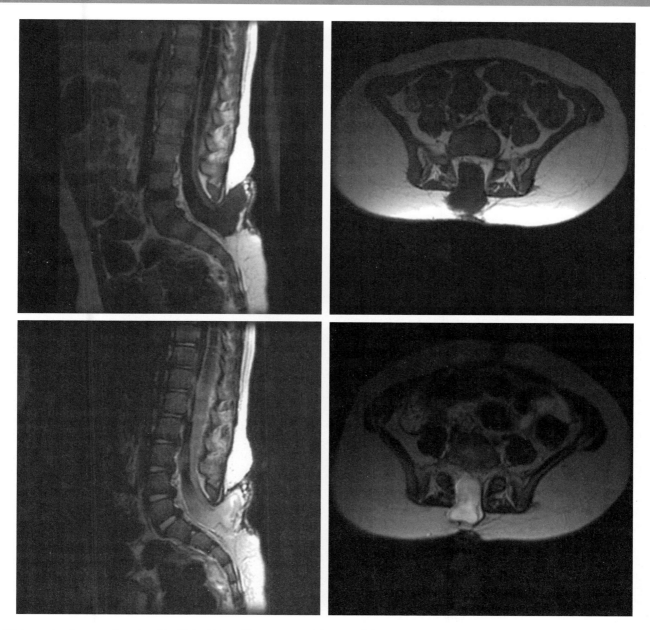

1. This entity is associated with Chiari I malformations. True or false?

2. What nutritional deficiency has been linked to this entity?

3. What is a dorsal dermal sinus?

4. Is this entity more common in males or females?

Myelomeningocele

1. False. Chiari II.

2. Folic acid.

3. Epithelial lined dural tubes that extend from the skin surface to the cord.

4. Females.

Reference

Tortori-Donati P, Rossi A, Biancheri R, et al.: Magnetic resonance imaging of spinal dysraphism. *Top Magn Reson Imaging* 12(6):375–409, 2001.

Cross-Reference

Pediatric Radiology: THE REQUISITES, p 268.

Comment

Neural tube defects are a result of abnormal neurulation, a process by which the neural plate folds, forming a tube and separating from overlying ectoderm (disjunction). As the ectoderm fuses, mesenchymal cells fill the space between the neural tube and future skin, eventually forming the bony posterior spinal arch, paraspinal muscles, and meninges. The mesenchymal cells are normally isolated from the canal formed by the neural tube. If the tube fails to close the mesenchymal cells will be induced to form a lipoma, a common finding in neural tube defects. Failure to completely form the tube or separate from the ectoderm or both will cause a spinal dysraphism ranging from a spina bifida to myelomeningocele.

Myelomeningoceles arise from a failure of neural tube closure leaving an expanded and raised surface of neural elements, the placode, exposed to the exterior. The placode can be thought of as a "splayed" spinal cord exposed to the surface posteriorly with the anterior aspect connected to the dorsal and ventral nerve roots. Vertebral body anomalies are present as the mesenchymal cells are unable to insinuate themselves between the future cord and skin.

Open dysraphisms occur in 0.3% of live births and are more common in females. Elevated alpha-fetoprotein, a protein synthesized in the fetal liver, is present in both the maternal serum and amniotic fluid in open cord defects. Surgery is required as there is 75% mortality associated with open spinal dysraphisms. Imaging is used to follow patients following surgery. Postoperative complications include syringomyelia, tethered cord, arachnoid cysts, cord ischemia, and arachnoiditis.

On plain films there is a widened spinal canal and interpedicular distances. Associated bony abnormalities include hemivertebrae, absent vertebral bodies, fused vertebral bodies, fused pedicles, posterior arch fusions, posterior arch distortions, and scoliosis.

On MR there is widening of the cord due to hydromyelia. A coexistent lipoma may be seen as explained above. There is medial and posterior displacement of the aorta and kidneys (pseudo horseshoe kidney). Chiari II malformation is seen in 99% of myelomeningocele. Hydrocephalus is seen in over 75% of patients. The defect demonstrates a spinal cord that extends through a defect in the posterior arch as it terminates at skin level in the placode. The placode is most often seen in the lower lumbar spine.

Notes

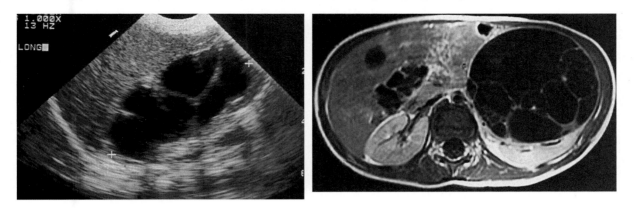

1. 50% of cases occur in boys aged less than 3 years. True or false?

2. These lesions are primarily exophytic. True or false?

3. Hemorrhage is often present. True or false?

4. The lesion is hypervascular in the nephrographic phase. True or false?

Multilocular Cystic Nephroma

1. True.

2. True.

3. False. Rarely is hemorrhage present.

4. False. Avascular or hypovascular.

Reference

Geller E, Smergel EM, Lowry PA: Renal neoplasms of childhood. *Radiol Clin N Am* 35(6):1391–413, 1997.

Lowe LH, Isuani BH, Heller RM, et al.: Pediatric renal masses: Wilms tumor and beyond. *Radiographics* 20(6): 1585–1603, 2000.

Cross-Reference

Pediatric Radiology: THE REQUISITES, pp 171–173.

Comment

Multilocular cystic nephroma (MLCN) is a cystic neoplasm comprising septae containing histologically mature cells. MLCN is seen in young children and young adults with a male predominance in children and a female predominance in adults. It presents as an abdominal mass. The cells of origin are the primitive metanephic blastema.

CT, MRI, and ultrasound show multiple noncommunicating cysts of variable size that tend to be herniated into the renal pelvis. If in Louisville you are shown a mass that extends into the renal pelvis remember to place MLCN into the differential. If you mention it on an intravenous pyelogram with a pelvic filling defect you'll be on your way to the Breast section (Breast follows Pedi at the boards). These tumors rarely hemorrhage and demonstrate little vascularity. It is difficult to differentiate multilocular cystic nephroma from a cystic Wilms tumor or multicystic dysplastic kidney. Consequently nephrectomy provides the definitive diagnosis.

Notes

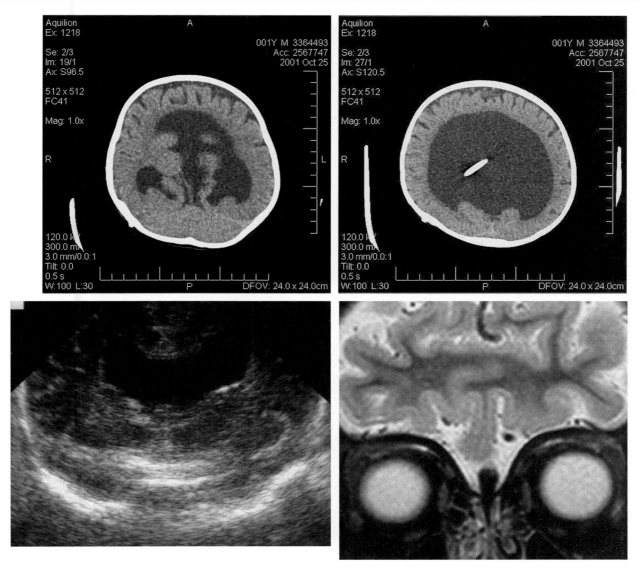

1. Are there associated abnormalities?

2. What is the incidence of this entity?

3. What are the etiologies of this entity?

4. Will the brainstem be affected?

Holoprosencephaly

1. 40% of cases have chromosomal abnormalities. Trisomy 13 is most common.

2. 10:10,000.

3. Sporadic mutations, inherited defects involving chromosomes 7, 13, and 18, diabetes mellitus, TORCH, maternal phenytoin, retinoic acid, and alcohol use.

4. No, the brainstem is spared.

References

Albayram S, Melhem ER, Mori S, et al.: Holoprosencephaly in children: diffusion tensor MR imaging of white matter tracts of the brainstem—initial experience. *Radiology* 223:645–651, 2002.

Filly RA, Chinn DH, Callen PW: Alobar holoprosencephaly: ultrasonographic prenatal diagnosis. *Radiology* 151:455–459, 1984.

Cross-Reference

Pediatric Radiology: THE REQUISITES, pp 261, 263, 269–270.

Comment

Holoprosencephaly is a developmental anomaly in which there is failure of forebrain cleavage into two hemispheres. Holoprosencephaly varies across a spectrum of findings, ranging from near complete segmentation to a single large ventricle and horseshoe brain. I shy away from using the term "fused" as this is a physiologic process of one into two parts, not two fusing to form one. The timing of the disturbance determines the severity of the disorder.

Holoprosencephaly is divided into the groups lobar, semilobar and alobar in order of severity. Corpus callosum abnormalities vary with segmentation severity, ranging from complete absence to partial formation. Unique to holoprosencephaly though is the absence of the head and preservation of the tail. Nonholoprosencephaly agenesis of the corpus callosum usually manifests as absence of the tail, a good clue for distinguishing the two. Facial abnormalities are present as well.

Prenatal imaging will easily show a large ventricle with a rim of brain along the cortex differentiating the finding from hydranencephaly, an ischemic insult to the anterior circulation that will shows no parenchyma laterally. On MR, findings will vary with severity of the developmental disorder. The interhemispheric fissure, and falx cerebri, may be absent or formed or somewhere in between. The septum pellucidum is always absent. The basal ganglia and thalami may demonstrate absence of segmentation.

Prognosis is nearly normal for mild cases of the lobar form, while death is certain with the alobar form.

Notes

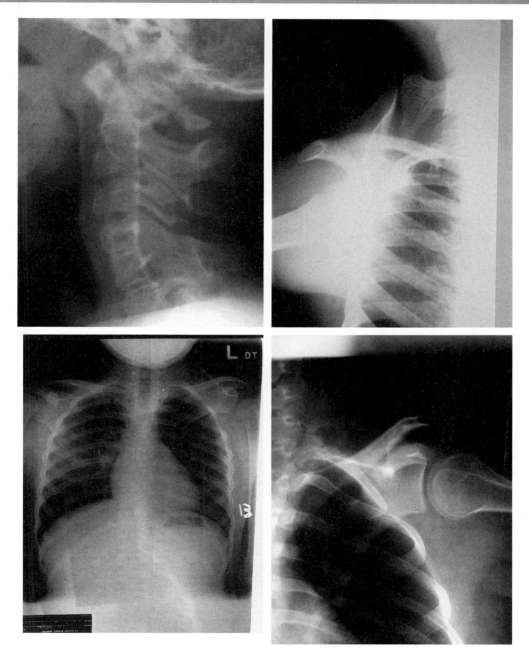

1. How else might you want to image this patient?

2. What are the organ systems involved in this entity?

3. What is the VACTERL complex?

4. In the cervical spine, what distinguishes this entity from juvenile chronic arthritis?

Klippel–Feil Syndrome

1. Ultrasound to look for renal agenesis. MR to examine the spine.

2. Cardiac, skeletal, renal, neuro.

3. **V**ertebral abnormalities, **A**nal atresia, **C**ardiac abnormalities, **T**racheoesophageal fistula and/or **E**sophageal atresia, **R**enal agenesis or dysplasia, and **L**imb defects.

4. Vertebral bodies demonstrate lack of segmentation in Klippel–Feil while there is posterior fusion in juvenile rheumatoid arthritis.

Reference

McBride WZ: Klippel-Feil syndrome. *Am Fam Physician* 45(2):633–635, 1992. Review.

Cross-Reference

Pediatric Radiology: THE REQUISITES, 2nd edn, p 21.

Comment

Did you miss the scapula or spine? Klippel–Feil (K-F) anomaly is a congenital abnormality of failed vertebral segmentation yielding a reduced number of cervical vertebra. One often hears references to congenital fusion, but in fact the spine develops from one column of somites that split or segment sometime between weeks 4 and 8. Alternatively, fusion of the posterior elements is associated with juvenile rheumatoid arthritis. A Sprengel deformity (congenital high-riding scapulae) may be seen in 25% of cases and may be associated with an omovertebral bone. An omovertebral bone is a calcified structure that runs from the vertebrae to the scapula. More commonly a fibrous band extends from the scapula to the lower cervical vertebrae. Clinically, a web-neck coupled with limited range of motion and low posterior hairline suggests the diagnosis of K-F.

Due to the abnormal vertebrae the spine shows hypermobility and instability, features that result in abnormal stress at the joints with subsequent sclerosis and osteophyte formation. Commonly, radiculopathy may result from neural foraminal encroachment or disc herniation.

Associated anomalies include renal agenesis, cardiac abnormalities, extremity deformities, Chiari I formation, and the very rare neurenteric cyst.

Notes

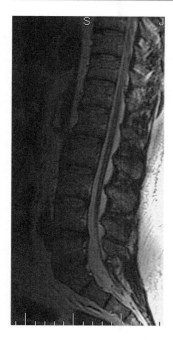

1. Is there an increased incidence of VACTERL syndrome in these patients?
2. When should the conus be at its normal level (T11–L2)?
3. Does a normal positioned conus rule out this entity?
4. What is considered a thickened filum?

Tethered Cord

1. Yes.

2. By 2 months.

3. No, a cord can still be tethered.

4. Over 2 mm.

Reference

Tortori-Donati P, Rossi A, Biancheri R, et al.: Magnetic resonance imaging of spinal dysraphism. *Top Magn Reson Imaging* 12(6):375–409, 2001.

Cross-Reference

Pediatric Radiology: THE REQUISITES, p 293.

Comment

Tethered cord is a syndrome of neurologic symptoms that is due to an abnormal low position within the canal. The tethered cord might be primary or secondary. Primary cord abnormalities include a tight filum terminale and tethered conus. Secondary etiologies include diastematomyelia, internal meningocele, neurenteric cyst, dermoid cyst, and lipomeningocele.

Clinically, patients present with gait disturbance, weakness, muscle atrophy, bowel or bladder dysfunction, urinary incontinence, or recurrent UTIs.

On MR or ultrasound, the conus should normally reside no lower than the body of L2. Tethered cord will demonstrate a low conus with an associated short thick filum terminale. It is thought that the low position may result from multiple etiologies: incomplete differentiation, failure of involution of the caudal neural tube, or from abnormally short filum nerve fibers. Tethered cord will demonstrate a thickened filum measuring greater than 2 mm at the level of L5. There may be a fatty component seen as T2 hyperintensity. Tethered cord is associated with lipomyelomeningocele, dermal sinus, diastematomyelia, lipoma, dermoid, or epidermoid.

Surgery is directed at freeing the conus from adhesions or repairing the associated spinal dysraphism.

Notes

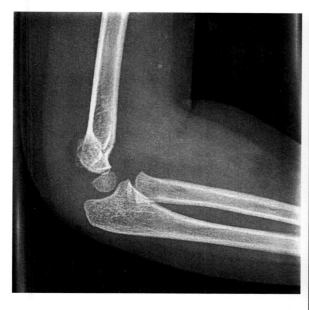 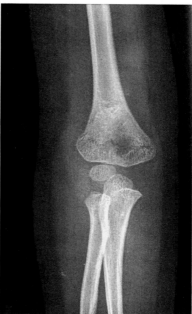

1. What is the classification system for this fracture?

2. How are they treated?

3. The trochlea forms from one ossification center. True or false?

4. The olecranon is formed from multiple ossification centers. True or false?

Supracondylar Fracture

1. Gartland I (nondisplaced), II (incomplete and angulated), III (complete).

2. Type I and stable type II are treated with closed reduction and casting. Unstable type II and type III undergo closed reduction with percutaneous pinning.

3. False. The trochlea forms from multiple ossification centers.

4. True. The olecranon is formed by multiple ossification centers.

Reference

Rogers, LF: *Radiology of Skeletal Trauma,* 3rd edn. New York: Churchill Livingstone, 2002.

Cross-Reference

Pediatric Radiology: THE REQUISITES, p 200.

Comment

The most common elbow fracture in childhood is the supracondylar fracture. Supracondylar fractures commonly occur between the ages of 3 and 10. The fracture is most commonly caused by fall on an outstretched hand.

As childrens' bones are far more plastic than adults' you may easily miss subtle fractures if you rely solely on cortical disruption or trabecullar discontinuity. Several lines are useful. The anterior humeral line is drawn along the anterior cortex bisecting (pass through the middle third) the capitellum. A supracondylar fracture may displace the capitellum a full width posterior to the anterior humeral line and still not demonstrate a fracture line. Normal alignment of the radius and capitellum is confirmed by drawing a line parallel to the radial tuberosity and proximally thought the humerus bisecting the capitellum. The line ought to pass through the capitellum on every projection; if not, then radial head dislocation or capitellar displacment is present. Fall on an outstretched hand may cause varus angulation. The angulation may be measured using the Bauman angle. The Bauman angle is measured by the intersection of the capitellar-humeral metaphysis and the long axis of the humerus and normally measures 75°– 80°. Use the angle to evaluate the post-reduction film.

Another indirect method in detecting fracture is the presence of elevated fat pads. Abnormal joint fluid will insinuate itself in between the fat and bone lifting the pads out of the olecranon and coronoid fossas. Small effusions will elevate the anterior fat pad while larger amounts are required to displace the posterior. If you don't see an anterior fat pad, you most probably don't have an intra-articular fracture. If you have a posterior fat pad you most probably have an intra-articular fracture. The anterior fat pad sign is sensitive while the posterior fat pad sign is specific. In cases where an effusion is detected without identifying a break you must assume an occult fracture and treat accordingly. Additional views, while increasing radiation dose, health care costs, and treatment time, will not change therapy as children with effusions are treated as if fractured.

Notes

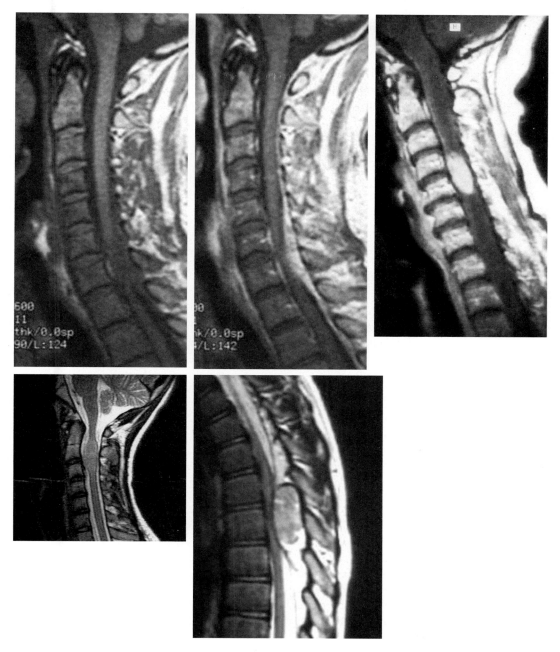

1. Astrocytomas are most commonly found in which part of the spine?

2. Are drop mets more common in children or adults (given the presence of an intracranial tumor)?

3. What tumors are associated with drop mets?

4. What are the CT findings of drop mets?

C A S E 80

Spinal Neoplasms

1. Thoracic, then cervical, and least commonly in the lumbar region.

2. More common in children.

3. Medulloblastoma, ependymoma, anaplastic glioma, germinomas, choroids plexus tumors, pinealcytoma, pineoblastoma.

4. Thickening and nodularity of the thecal sac, nerve root, and spinal cord.

Reference

Schick U, Marquardt G: Pediatric spinal tumors. *Pediatr Neurosurg* 35(3):120–127, 2001.

Cross-Reference

Pediatric Radiology: THE REQUISITES, p 299.

Comment

Spinal tumors in children may arise within the spinal cord (intramedullary), within the dura but outside the spina cord (intradural extramedullary), or outside the dura (extra dural) originating from the bony spine or paraspinal soft tissues.

Cord (intramedullary) lesions are predominantly gliomas, the most common being astrocytomas, ependymomas, and gangliogliomas. Astrocytomas appear on MR as focal or long-segment areas of T1 hypointensity and T2 hyperintensity. Astrocytoma comes in two flavors, the more common pilocytic (well circumscribed) and the fibrillary (infiltrating). The fibrillary form demonstrates fusiform enlargement, syrinx, or cystic changes of the cord. Enhancement is the rule.

Intradural (extramedullary intradural) lesions include nerve sheath tumors, neoplastic seeding and developmental tumors. The most common benign lesions include schwannomas and neurofibromas that may occur sporadically or as part of neuro-fibromatosis. Neoplastic seeding of the subarachnoid space occurs most commonly with medulloblastoma, germ cell tumors, ependymoma, and pineal neoplasm. Gadolinium-enhanced MR is the imaging procedure of choice and shows laminar or nodular enhancement along the cord surfaces and nerve roots.

Epidural (extradural) lesions include abscesses and hematomas. Abscesses will appear as fluid collections that rim enhance and are usually associated with contiguous discitis (80%). On T1 the fluid will appear dark, on T2 the fluid will appear bright, and on post-contrast images the rim enhances. Hematoma occurs secondary to acute trauma, surgery, and disc herniation. The signal characteristics of a hematoma will vary with the age of the bleed.

Notes

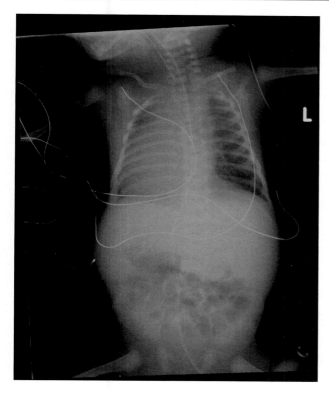

1. What is the definition of dextrocardia?
2. What is the definition of dextroposition?
3. What is the definition of inversion?
4. What is the definition of heterotaxy?

Situs Inversus Totalis/Solitus/Ambiguous

1. Dextrocardia indicates the position of the heart within the thorax, on the right.

2. Dextroposition describes cardiac displacement by an extrinsic phenomenon (e.g., pectus excavatum).

3. Inversion describes an alteration in the location of an asymmetric organ on the contralateral side.

4. Heterotaxy describes organ relationships other than situs solitus or its mirror image situs inversus.

Reference

Applegate KE, Goske MJ, Pierce G, et al.: Situs revisited: imaging of the heterotaxy syndrome. *Radiographics* 19(4):837–852, 1999.

Cross-Reference

Pediatric Radiology: THE REQUISITES, 2nd edn, p 69.

Comment

An in-depth analysis of complex cardiac malformations begins with the determination of situs. Situs can be determined by recognizing asymmetry of the tracheo-bronchial tree and position of the abdominal organs. The right and left atria develop on the same side as the thoracic and abdominal viscera: the right atrium on the right side of the mediastinum, and the left atrium on the left—the "visceral–atrial" rule. This is also referred to as situs solitus; the reverse is situs inversus. In cases of symmetric lungs, situs cannot be determined: situs ambiguous. Next, the orientation of the cardiac apex is evaluated. Its location enables one to determine the presence or absence of cardiac malposition.

Primary dextrocardia implies that the cardiac axis (silhouette) is predominantly "pointed" to the right of the spine and that there is associated inversion of the cardiac chambers (mirror image). Secondary dextrocardia may occur when a normal heart is "pushed" to the right, as occurs with a left sided tension pneumothorax, congenital diaphragmatic hernia, or scoliosis. In primary dextrocardia, the incidence of CHD is considerable; 2% of children with CHD have dextrocardia. Levocardia refers to the cardiac silhouette pointing to the left, with normal chamber orientation. Mesocardia occurs when left or right cannot be determined, and situs solitus or inversus may also be present.

Atrioventricular concordance occurs when the right atrium is appropriately aligned with the right ventricle, and the left atrium is appropriately aligned with the left. Atrioventricular discordance occurs when there is an abnormal relationship between the right atrium and left ventricle and the left atrium and right ventricle. Angiography and MRI can shed further light on whether the ventricles are inverted, whether there is a L- or D-loop rotation, or whether there is transposition of the great vessels. Atrioventricular discordance is often associated with CHD.

In the heterotaxy syndrome, the atrioventricular connection is ambiguous because either two right or two left atria may exist. The heterotaxy syndrome includes developmental complexes that are characterized by a tendency for symmetric development of normally asymmetric organs or organ systems. Thus, these abnormalities should be considered whenever there is a discordance between the cardiac apex and abdominal situs. Although they are rare in and of themselves, the severe CHD that is associated makes identification of these lesions worthwhile as most infants survive the early postnatal period.

Asplenia, a teratogenic insult that occurs at 4 weeks' gestation, is characterized by bilateral trilobed (right side) lungs with short eparterial bronchi (bronchi that are above the pulmonary arteries). Almost all cases are accompanied by severe CHD, an asymmetric liver, and GI tract malformations (microgastria, biliary atresia). The affected children are almost always boys, are cyanotic, and are prone to developing sepsis.

Polysplenia is characterized by bilateral bilobed (left side) lungs with long hyparterial bronchi (bronchi that are below the pulmonary arteries). Some children have associated severe CHD, and there are often renal anomalies. The affected children are almost all girls and have less severe malformations than in asplenia. Bilateral SVCs can occur in both variants: in 55% of asplenia, and in 35% of polysplenia.

Notes

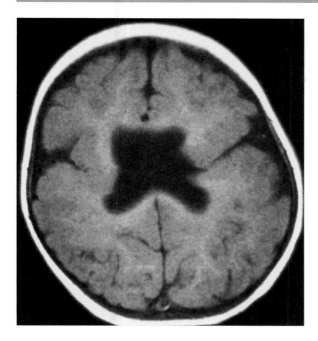

1. What percentage of cases are bilateral?

2. What percentage of these patients have septo-optic dysplasia?

3. Is there a genetic cause?

4. Patients that present with seizures and developmental delay ought to be imaged in how many planes?

Schizencephaly

1. 35%.

2. 25%–50%.

3. Some cases are the result of a mutation of the EMX2 homeobox gene that functions in germinal matrix development.

4. At least two planes, as a mild case of schizencephaly within the plane of the scan may be missed.

Reference

Barkovich AJ, Kuzniecky RI: Neuroimaging of focal malformations of cortical development. *J Clin Neurophysiol* 13(6): 481–494, 1996.

Cross-Reference

Pediatric Radiology: THE REQUISITES, p 273.

Comment

Schizencephaly is a disorder of cortical development thought to occur due to a second trimester localized ischemic event. A competing genetic cause has been suggested with mutation of a gene involved in neuronal migration. Schizencephaly is defined as a CSF-filled cleft extending from the surface of the cortex to the lining of the ventricle. Clefts may either be closed or open lipped, uni- or bilateral. Most clefts are found in the frontal and temporal locations. Clinically, patients with open-lipped schizencephaly present with hydrocephalus and seizures, while the "closed lippers" present with hemiparesis and motor delay.

On MR, the easily seen open-lip defects are filled with CSF usually communicating with a lateral ventricle. Gray matter is seen to line the surface of the cleft. The ipsilateral cerebral hemisphere is smaller than the unaffected contralateral size. The septum pellucidum is absent in the majority of open-lipped cases. The more subtle closed-lipped schizencephaly often manifests as a dimple of the lateral wall of the lateral ventricle.

Treatment is consevative. Prognosis is variable from near normal in closed-lipped cases to severe impairment in bilateral open-lipped schizencephaly.

Notes

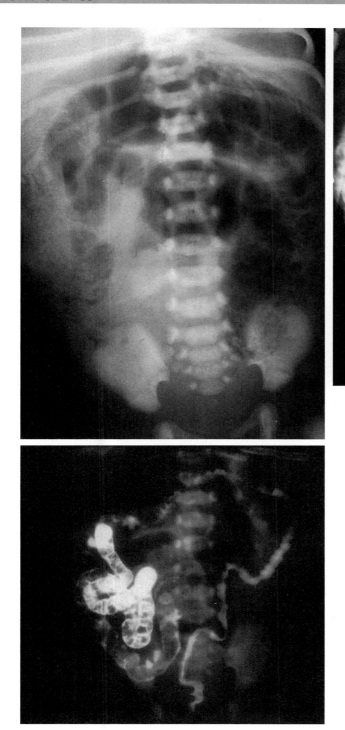

1. What is the significance of calcifications in the scrotum?

2. What is meconium ileus equivalent?

3. Does the infant's first stool smell foul?

4. What is the differential diagnosis?

Meconium Ileus

1. Dystrophic calcification secondary to meconium peritonitis can travel into the scrotum as the processus vaginalis is patent.

2. *Jeopardy:* Stool in the small bowel in teenagers with respiratory symptoms.

3. No, there are no bacteria present in the gut until after birth with feeding.

4. Ileal atresia.

Reference

Agrons GA, Corse WR, Markowitz RI, et al.: Gastrointestinal manifestations of cystic fibrosis: radiologic-pathologic correlation. *Radiographics* 16:871–893, 1996.

Cross-Reference

Pediatric Radiology: THE REQUISITES, 2nd edn, pp 112–113.

Comment

Meconium is the first bowel movement; bacteria free and consisting of succus entericus—bile salts, bile acids, and intestinal mucosal debris. Meconium is usually passed within the first 6 hours of birth but owing to perinatal stress may be evacuated in utero presumably due to vagal response.

Meconium ileus occurs when meconium inspissates, becoming thick like molasses and obstructs the distal ileum in patients with cystic fibrosis. Twenty per cent of patients with cystic fibrosis present with ileus. Normal infants will present with distention and vomiting within hours of birth. One quarter of all bowel obstructions in this age group are caused by meconium ileus. It is the leading cause of neonatal bowel obstruction presenting as abdominal distention. Meconium ileus may be complicated by volvulus, perforation, and peritonitis.

Radiographically, the ileus appears as multiple dilated loops of differing calibers with a paucity of air. A differential consideration, ileal atresia, will demonstrate abundant bowel gas with multiple air fluid levels. The soap bubble appearance (Neuhauser sign) is seen in the right lower quadrant. Differential considerations include Hirschsprung disease, ileal atresia, and meconium plug syndrome/small left colon.

A contrast study is diagnostic and often therapeutic as a microcolon is demonstrated.

Notes

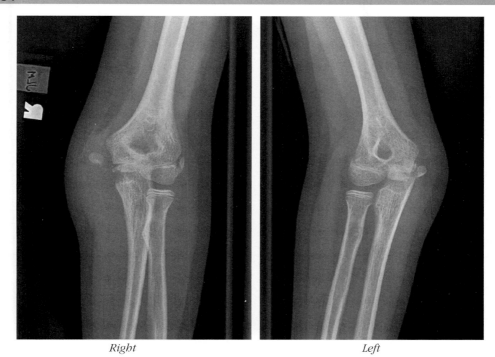

Right   *Left*

1. At what age does the trochlear ossification center appear on radiographs?
2. What is the stabilizer in valgus strain in the adult?
3. What is the valgus stabilizer in children?
4. What is the "weakest link" in the skeletally immature elbow?

C A S E 84

Little League Elbow: Medial Elbow Apophysitis

1. The trochlea should begin to ossify at 9 years in girls and 10 years in boys.

2. The medial collateral ligament consisting of the anterior, posterior, and transverse band.

3. The common flexor–pronator tendon.

4. The apophyses are weakest, leading to avulsions in children as opposed to ligamentous disruption in adults.

Reference

Donnelly LF, Bisset GS, Helms CA, et al.: Chronic avulsive injuries of childhood. *Skeletal Radiol* 28(3): 138–144, 1999.

Cross-Reference

Pediatric Radiology: THE REQUISITES, p 239.

Comment

Little league elbow refers to a range of clinical entities that occur from repetitive valgus stress on the skeletally immature elbow. Little league elbow does not refer to a specific entity but rather the effect of either chronic tensile stress on the medial elbow (apophysistis) and/or compressive forces on the lateral elbow (osteochondritis dissecans, OCD). Entities under the little leaguer's elbow designation include medial epicondylitis, fragmentation, delayed or accelerated apophyseal growth of the medial condyle, delayed closure of the medial epicondyle growth plate, OCD of the capitellum, osteochondritis of the radial head, hypertrophy of the ulna, and olecranon apophysitis. In adults, the majority of the articular strength and stability comes from ligamentous support. Children's ligaments, however, are normally lax until late adolescence, joints thereby gain their strength from tendinous insertions. At the elbow the main stablizer against valgus strain is the common flexor–pronator tendon. In adults, severe valgus stress leads to sprain or rupture of the medial collateral ligament, whereas in children this ligament complex is lax, transferring the force to the tendon. The nonfused medial ephicondyle apophysis is far weaker than the tendon and leads to either apophysitis or avulsion in the pediatric age group.

Radiographically, an acute sudden avulsion will demonstrate soft tissue swelling and visible separation of the medial epicondyle. A contralateral view is recommended for comparison in more subtle cases. A more chronic repetitive type injury will demonstrate fragmentation on radiographs. In addition to throwing injuries, medial epicondyle avulsion may occur due to fall on an outstretched hand or posterior dislocation. Both may lead to an entrapped epicondyle that may easily be confused for a trochlear ossification center. Know the age of the patient and know the time of trochlear ossification! Trapped fragments will lead to disabling degenerative arthritis.

Epicondylitis on MR will demonstrate low T1 and high T2 signal consistent with edema of the epicondyle. Alternatively, MR may prove useful in evaluation of an avulsed medial or lateral epicondyle in cases where the medial (under 7 years) and lateral (under 11 years) have yet to ossify. Posterior dislocations may lead to displacement of the ulnar nerve, an important finding easily detected on MRI.

Treatment of epicondylitis is conservative with rest. Treatment of epicondyle avulsions ranges from conservative to surgery depending on the degree of displacement as well as the individual's athletic demands. Ulnar neuropathy may develop in cases of conservatively treated avulsions.

Notes

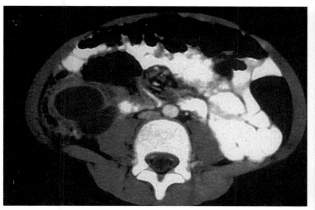
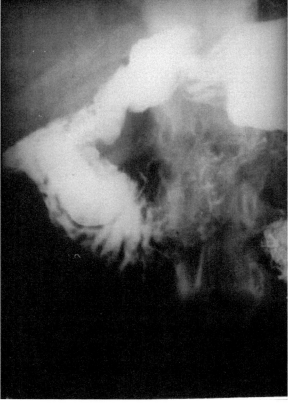

1. Where is the most common location for this entity?
2. Where is the second most common location for this entity?
3. What terms are used to describe the extraluminal aspects of the bowel?
4. What is the differential diagnosis?

Duplication Cyst

1. Distal ileum, 35%.

2. Distal esophagus, 20%.

3. Mesenteric and antimesenteric.

4. Omental cyst, choledochal cyst, mesenteric cyst, giant Meckel diverticulum, ovarian cysts.

References

Macpherson RI. Gastrointestinal tract duplications: clinical, pathologic, etiologic, and radiologic considerations. *Radiographics* 13:1063–1080, 1993.

Berrocal T, Torres I, Gutiérrez J, et al.: Congenital anomalies of the upper gastrointestinal tract. *Radiographics* 19:855–872, 1999.

Cross-Reference

Pediatric Radiology: THE REQUISITES, 2nd edn, p 111.

Comment

The normal fetal gut begins as a tube, fills in, and then hollows out (recanalization) at 8–10 weeks gestation. One abnormality of recanalization is enteric duplication. Tubular or spherical enteric mucosal-lined cystic structures are located on the mesenteric side of the small bowel. They rarely communicate with the true lumen. Duplications may present as obstruction and/or abdominal mass, but are usually asymptomatic. Obstruction may be due to compression or intussusception. Duplications may also grow over time and hemorrhage.

While fluoro studies will generally show compression and dilatation of the bowel, ultrasound may directly establish a diagnosis. If you see a cystic mass with an inner echogenic layer (mucosa) and an outer hypoechoic layer (muscle), you've nailed the diagnosis.

Notes

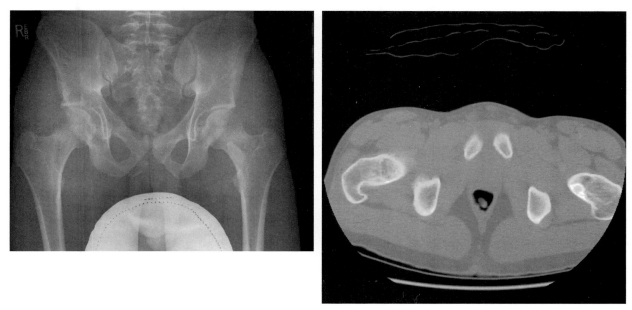

Patient Reported No Hip Pain

1–5. When you spot a bone lesion on conventional radiography you ought to think of five things. What are they?

Fibrous Dysplasia

1. Where is the lesion? Diaphyseal, metaphyseal, epiphyseal? Does it abut the articular surface?

2. Is it lytic or blastic?

3. What is the matrix? Chondroid, osseus, fibrous?

4. Is the zone of transition wide or narrow?

5. Is there periosteal new bone formation and/or cortical destruction?

Reference

Kransdorf MJ, Moser RP, Jr, et al.: Fibrous dysplasia. *Radiographics* 10:519–537, 1990.

Cross-Reference

Pediatric Radiology: THE REQUISITES, pp 220–221.

Comment

Fibrous dysplasia is a nonheritable skeletal developmental anomaly in which fibroblasts proliferate and produce fibrous tissue that combines with immature woven bone trabeculae. The lesion is commonly found in the marrow space but may extend to the cortex. The abnormal trabeculae give the characteristic ground glass appearance on conventional radiograph. A relative dearth of trabeculae will impart a lucent lesion. A reactive thick rind of dense sclerosis is seen encircling the ground glass lucency as the osteoblasts attempt to wall off the fibrous lesion. However, absence of a sclerotic border does not exclude fibrous dysplasia. Base of skull lesions are often sclerotic. Nuclear bone scan demonstrates hot lesions. Bowing deformity (shepherd's crook deformity) may be present as the fibrous woven bone does not contain the same level of strength found in lamellar bone. Either fracture or leg length discrepancy is a common presentation.

Fibrous dysplasia may affect one bone (monostotic) or multiple bones (polystotic). The great majority of cases involve one bone in patients between 5 and 20 years of age. Bones most often affected include the femur, tibia, and ribs. The skull is also often affected with the facial bones commonly involved (frontal bossing), a "differential distinguisher" from histiocytosis X, which prefers the calvaria. Differential diagnostic considerations include enchondroma, aneurysmal bone cysts, and histiocystosis X. Sarcomatous transformation is exceedingly rare. Management is conservative.

Notes

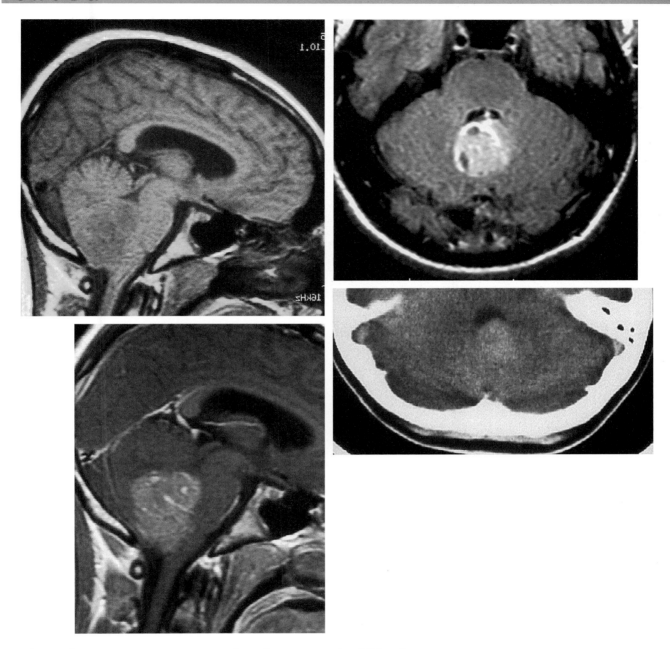

1. What is the most common posterior fossa brain tumor in children?

2. What is the second most common poterior fossa brain tumor in children?

3. Is there a gender predominance?

4. A drop met is in what space?

Medulloblastoma

1. Cerebellar astrocytoma.

2. Medulloblastoma.

3. M:F = 4:1 for medulloblastoma.

4. Extramedullary, intradural.

Reference

Blaser SI, Harwood-Nash DC: Neuroradiology of pediatric posterior fossa medulloblastoma. *J Neurooncol* 29(1): 23–34, 1996.

Cross-Reference

Pediatric Radiology: THE REQUISITES, pp 288–289.

Comment

Medulloblastoma is a highly malignant primitive neuroectodermal round cell tumor with a misleading name; there is no such thing as a medulloblast. So where do they come from? They are thought to arise from neuroepithelial cells on the roof of the fourth ventricle. In adulthood these cells migrate into the cerebellar parenchyma. They are the second most common posterior fossa tumor in children (40%) and account for 15% of all childhood brain tumors. Seventy-five per cent of cases are seen within the first year. Clinically, patients present with increasing head size or vomiting from obstructing hydrocephalus.

On CT, medulloblastoma appears as a well-defined, hyperdense mass of the cerebellar vermis or hemisphere. These cells are packed with nuclear material, giving them a much denser precontrast appearance compared with the similar appearing astrocytoma. There may be calcific or cystic components to the mass. Midline lesions are typical in children, while adolescents and adults will usually demonstrate hemisphere involvement. Enhancement is typically homogeneous.

On MR, the lesion appears nonspecific, shifting the emphasis on to patient age and tumor location for diagnosis. Most often medulloblastoma is hypointense on T1 and hypo-isointense on T2. There is heterogeneity on T2 thought to be a result of cystic components. There is homogenous enhancement of moderate intensity. The tumor may spread through the CSF to the cisterns, ventricles or the spinal cord. Drop mets are best evaluated with contrast scans as they enhance brightly.

Surgery, radiation, and chemo are used in concert, although 5-year survival is approximately 50%.

Notes

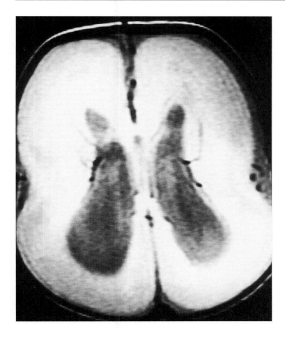

1. How many layers of cortex form in this entity?

2. There is often hypoplasia of the corpus callosum. True or false?

3. There are often associated pulmonary abnormalities. True or false?

4. There has been an association between this entity and congenital cytomegalovirus (CMV). True or false?

Lissencephaly

1. Four instead of six layers.

2. True. There is corpus callosum hypoplasia.

3. False. There are cardiac not pulmonary abnormalities.

4. True. CMV has been associated with lissencephaly.

Reference

Barkovich AJ, Gressens P, Evrard P: Formation, maturation, and disorders of brain neocortex. *Am J Neuroradiol* 13(2):423–446, 1992.

Cross-Reference

Pediatric Radiology: THE REQUISITES, p 274.

Comment

Lissencephaly means smooth brain and is thought to occur due to deletions of chromosome 17 and the X chromosome. The gene is hypothesized to encode a protein involved in neuronal cell migration. The brain appears smooth as there are few gyri or sulci present. There are two types of lissencephaly: Type 1, or classical lyssencephaly, and Type II, cobblestone lissencephaly. Type 1 is characterized by a thickened cortex seen laterally and absence of gray–white interdigitations. Type II is primarily an abnormality at the gray–white interface and is associated with muscular dystrophy. Clinically, mental retardation and seizures reflect the abnormal histologic architecture present in neuronal migration abnormalities.

On imaging the "hourglass" or "figure-of-eight" configuration are the Louisville buzzwords that describe the shape of the brain on axial section. There is failed opercularization of the sylvian fissures (absence of the normal temporal lobes lateral to the sylvian fissures). On MR there is a global reduction in the number of gyri and sulci with thinning of the cortex and smoothing of the gray–white matter interface and ventriculomegaly. High signal abnormality due to cortical laminar necrosis has been described.

Seizure meds are the limit of treatment. Patients usually die in childhood or in their teens due to pneumonia, presumably from aspiration.

Notes

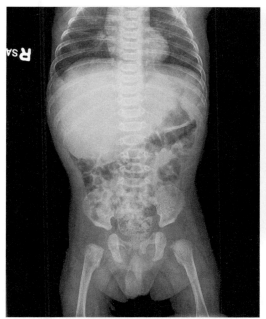

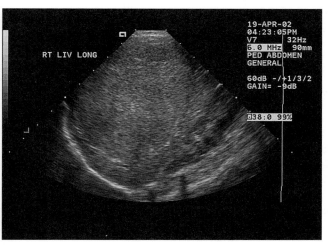

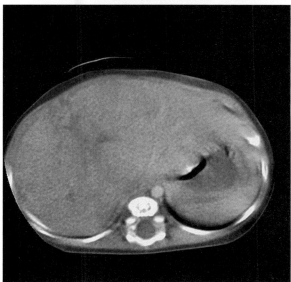

1. Is cirrhosis a risk factor?

2. Are there elevated alpha-fetoprotein levels?

3. Are most of these tumors hyper or hypoechoic?

4. What is the classic pimp sign on angiography?

Hepatoblastoma

1. No, cirrhosis is *not* a risk factor.

2. Yes, malignant epithelial tumors produce alpha-fetoprotein.

3. Most of these tumors are hyperechoic.

4. A spoke-wheel pattern.

Reference

Siegel MJ. Pediatric liver imaging. *Semin Liver Dis* 21(2):251–269, 2001.

Cross-Reference

Pediatric Radiology: THE REQUISITES, 2nd edn, p 137.

Comment

Hepatoblastoma is the most common hepatic tumor in children. Patients present with an right upper quadrant mass and are under 5 years, usually less than 2 years of age. Males are affected twice as often as females. The tumor is rapidly progressive and metastases to the lung. Associated findings include Beckwith–Wiedemann, hemihypertrophy, precocious puberty, Gardener syndrome, trisomy 18, fetal alcohol syndrome, maternal use of gonadotropins, maternal exposure to metals or petroleum products, and siblings with hepatoblastomas. Cirrhosis is not a risk factor. Pathologically, the mass is large and usually solitary, affecting the right lobe more frequently. There are two histologic types: (1) epithelial, which is a solid mass with homogenous appearance and is considered to be favorable histologically; (2) mixed epithelial and mesenchymal (less favorable), composed of cysts, necrosis, and hemorrhage with thick fibrotic septae and vascular invasion. The latter type contains osteoid, which may calcify.

The ultrasound appearance of hepatoblastoma is variable, often showing a heterogeneous, echogenic mass with poorly defined margins. Tumor invasion of the vessels may be detected with the use of color Doppler. Precontrast CT will demonstrate a low attenuated mass with areas of inhomogeneity related to hemorrhage or necrosis. Stippled or coarse calcification is common. Enhancement is less than normal liver parenchyma.

Complete surgical resection is needed for long-term survival. This can only be attempted in the absence of mets, IVC, aorta, or main portal vein invasion, and three or fewer lobes involved. Aggressive chemotherapy is given to decrease tumor bulk preoperatively. Only 50–70% are resectable at presentation.

Notes

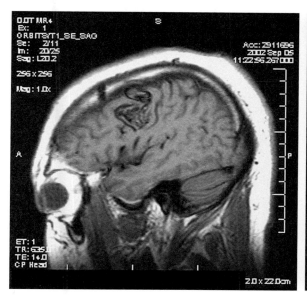
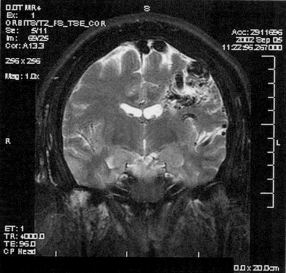

1. What did Spetzler and Martin classify?

2. What is the most common cause of intracranial spontaneous bleed in children less than 15?

3. What functions are ascribed to eloquent regions of brain?

4. What regions of the brain are eloquent?

Arteriovenous Malformation

1. Arteriovenous malformations.

2. Arteriovenous malformations.

3. Eloquent refers to those areas which control speech, motor functions, and senses.

4. Primary motor cortex, primary sensory cortex, speech, auditory, visual, thalamus, internal capsule, and brainstem.

Reference

Wright LB, James CA, Glasier CM: Congenital cerebral and cerebrovascular anomalies: magnetic resonance imaging. *Top Magn Reson Imaging* 12(6):361–374, 2001.

Cross-Reference

Pediatric Radiology: THE REQUISITES, p 265.

Comment

Arteriovenous malformations (AVMs) are congenital lesions in which there is absence of a capillary bed and direct connection between arterioles and venules. AVMs are thought to arise from the persistence of primitive connections between arterioles and venules. Connections between arterioles and venules without intervening capillaries creates a low-resistance shunt that steals blood away from other perfused regions and causes progressive enlargement of the involved arteries and veins. AVMs are found within brain parenchyma located above the tentorium in 85% of cases. By far the biggest concern of AVMs is their propensity to bleed, which is estimated at 2–3% per year.

Clinically, AVMs typically present between 20 and 40 years of age with hemorrhage, seizures, headaches, or progressive neurologic defects. Twenty per cent of patients are under 20. AVM is responsible for 40% of spontaneous bleeds in children. Seizures are seen in 70% of cases. Headaches are thought to occur as a result of hypertrophic dural vessels. Progressive neurologic effects have been attributed to vascular steal or venous hypertension.

On contrast-enhanced CT you will see densely dilated veins and an abnormal tangle of vessels. Hematoma and calcification are common. MR will demonstrate a tightly packed nidus with flow voids seen in the tangled malformation. Parenchymal loss and hemosiderin staining indicate previous hemorrhage. On angiography a tightly packed tangled collection of arteries with early draining enlarged veins is seen.

Treatment is directed at removing the AVM via surgical excision, radiosurgery, or embolization. The grading system devised by Spetzler and Martin aids in prognosis. The Spetzler–Martin system grades on the basis of size (<3 cm or >6), location (eloquent location vs. noneloquent), and venous drainage (deep or superficial).

Notes

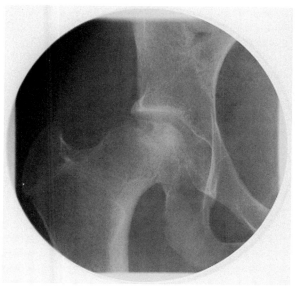 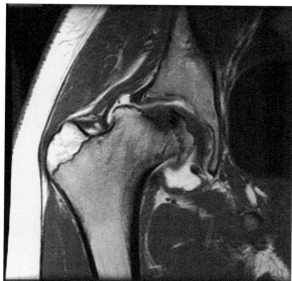

1. Why are the epiphyses of unequal size?

2. What is the differential diagnosis?

3. Does the abnormal widened joint space resolve during adulthood?

4. Name risk factors for this disease.

Legg–Calve–Perthes Disease

1. There has been growth arrest of the cartilage due to ischemia.

2. Hypothyroidism, sickle cell, Gaucher, Meyer dysplasia.

3. No, the widened joint space persists into adulthood.

4. Sickle cell disease, steroid therapy, bone marrow transplant, malignancy, autoimmune disease.

Reference

Donaldson JS, Feinstein KA: Imaging of developmental dysplasia of the hip. *Pediatr Clin N Am* 44(3): 591–614, 1997.

Cross-Reference

Pediatric Radiology: THE REQUISITES, p 246.

Comment

Legg–Calve–Perthes disease is a long acronym for pediatric osteonecrosis. It does, however, differ from adult avascular necrosis as there is healing and remodeling of the necrotic femoral heads. The disease commonly presents between 5 and 8 years and is usually asymmetric (80%). The M:F ratio is 5:1. A definitive etiology for L-C-P has yet to be worked out but some form of epiphyseal ischemia or raised intra-articular pressure from transient synovitis appears to play a role. The four stages are devascularization, collapse and fragmentation, reossification, and remodeling. The growth plate and epiphysis arrest, while the synovial-fed articular cartilage continues to grow. Fragmentation occurs as blood supply is reestablished at various sites from independent collaterals, reactivating the previously arrested ossification process at multiple sites. The result is a fragmented appearance on radiograph. Collapse is caused by subchondral resorption and leads to pain, limping, and possible premature physis closure.

The approach to L-C-P is to intervene before collapse and its relentless progression to osteoarthritis. The femoral head requires the acetabulum and the acetabulum requires the femoral head for normal morphologic development. As deformity of the femoral head occurs with subchondral collapse and remodeling, the head migrates laterally, often times yielding a hinge joint. Reapposition of the head and the femur is crucial for proper healing. An adequate look at the unossified head to assess shape requires arthrography, although recent studies have suggested the use of MR.

Radiographically, numerous abnormalities have been described: soft tissue fullness on the lateral joint aspect secondary to effusion, small laterally displaced femoral epiphysis, flattening of the epiphysis, and intra-epiphyseal gas. Metaphyseal cyst of uncertain etiology and widening and shortening of the femoral neck due to abnormal physeal growth are common.

The MR findings of osteonecrosis in young children vary greatly from the appearance seen in adults or adolescents. The epiphysis may demonstrate either increased or normal T2 signal. Frank necrosis will appear dark on both T1 and T2. Studies have suggested that perfusion imaging greatly increases sensitivity, as quantitative subtraction methods will demonstrate areas of nonenhancement adjacent to regions of intense enhancement. The enhancement represents areas of recanalization and is associated with a good prognosis. MR has also been shown useful in evaluating the degree of femoral head flattening a predictor for early degenerative arthritis.

Therapy ranges from non-weight-bearing via casting to femoral varus osteotomy or shelf acetabuloplasty. Surgery is aimed at reducing the likelihood of early degenerative arthritis.

Notes

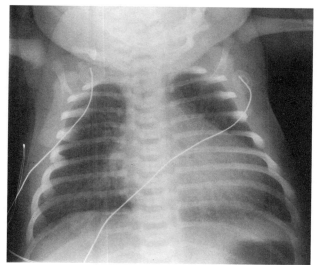

Cyanotic patient.

1. Is there increased or decreased pulmonary vascularity?
2. If the vascularity was decreased what is your differential?
3. If the vascularity was increased what is your differential?
4. What is the classic sign describing the appearance of the heart in this case?

Transposition of the Great Vessels/Arteries (TGA)

1. Increased pulmonary vascularity.

2. Cyanotic with decreased vascularity: tetralogy of Fallot (normal heart size), Ebstein anomaly, pulmonic atresia, and tricuspid atresia (the latter three with enlarged heart).

3. Cyanotic with increased vascularity: TGA, truncus, total anomalous pulmonary venous return, and single ventricle.

4. The "egg-on-a-string" sign.

Reference

Allen HD, Gutgesell HP, Clark EB, et al.: *Moss and Adams Heart Disease in Infants, Children and Adolescents: Including the Fetus and Young Adult,* 6th edn. Baltimore: Lippincott Williams & Wilkins, 2000, pp 1027–1084.

Cross-Reference

Pediatric Radiology: THE REQUISITES, 2nd edn, pp 60–61.

Comment

In transposition of the great vessels or transposition of the great arteries there is switching of the relative positions of the pulmonary artery and the aorta. The aorta is connected to the right ventricle, while the pulmonary artery is connected to the left ventricle. Without a patent ductus arteriosus (PDA) or atrial or ventricular septal defect the circulations are entirely separate. Blood leaves the LV through the PA and then back to the LA through the normal pulmonary veins. This condition is rapidly fatal. Bidirectional shunting is necessary to sustain life. Increased pressure in the right atrium from systemic back pressure causes the foramen ovale to remain open, allowing the life-sustaining communication between the separate circulations. Clinically, patients present with cyanosis on the first day of life.

Radiographically, films rarely show increased blood flow as surgical intervention is performed early. For Kentucky purposes though, the findings include: narrowing of the superior mediastinum due to a hypoplastic thymus, poorly seen aortic arch and loss of the pulmonary artery trunk, the right PA is higher and larger than the left as the LV outflow tract is "pointed" to the right. There is a right-sided aortic arch in 5% of cases. The "egg-on-a-string" sign appearance is the applicable buzzword and reflects the right atrial and ventricular enlargement coupled with a hypoplastic thymus. On ultrasound d-TGA demonstrates the aorta anterior to the pulmonary artery, 11 o'clock and 5 o'clock respectively.

The normal relationship includes an aorta at 8 o'clock and the anterior PA at 2 o'clock.

Prostaglandins are administered to prevent PDA closure. Patients are treated surgically with balloon septostomy, whereupon a balloon is stuck through the atrial septum and inflated, enlarging the hole for improved mixing. The Mustard procedure attempts to leave the anomaly as is and redirect the normal pulmonary veins and IVC, creating a systemic right side and a pulmonary left side. Unfortunately, this commonly leads to RV failure over time. Preferably, the aorta and PA are interposed via the Jatene arterial switch procedure.

Notes

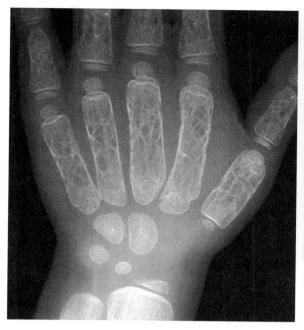
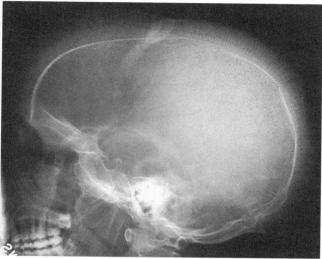

1. What are the findings of hemophilic pseudotumor?

2. What is the differential diagnosis for Erlenmeyer flask deformity?

3. What percentage of adult marrow is devoted to hematopoiesis?

4. What are rodent facies?

Thalassemia

1. Soft tissue mass, periosteal elevation, buttressing, and bony destruction.

2. Anemia, storage disease (Gaucher), mucopolysaccharidosis, osteopetrosis, and Pyle disease.

3. 50%.

4. Rodent facies are caused by forward displacement of the incisors and are pathognomonic of thalassemia.

Reference

Tunaci M, Tunaci A, Engin G, et al.: Imaging features of thalassemia. *Eur Radiol* 9(9):1804–1809, 1999.

Cross-Reference

Pediatric Radiology: THE REQUISITES, p 218.

Comment

Thalassemia is a genetically transmitted disease manifested by a defect in the globin portion of hemoglobin. There is a homozygous form, thalassemia major and a heterozygous form, thalassemia minor. An understanding of marrow pathophysiology is helpful in interpreting the imaging findings.

Marrow is composed of red cell, white cell, and platelet progenitors. In addition, fat comprises a percentage of the make-up, depending on the age and metabolic state of the bone. Marrow is divided into two forms, red and yellow. Red marrow is the hematopoietically active fat-poor state, while yellow marrow is the resting, fat-rich state. Infants are born with red marrow as the need for growth and demand for hematopoiesis is high. Beginning at birth there is a predictable and programmed conversion to yellow marrow with a distal to proximal direction. Eventually, red marrow resides only in the spine, ribs, clavicles, scapulae, skull, and long bone metaphyses. On MR the fatty yellow marrow is bright on T1 and T2, while red marrow is relatively dark. At times when the body demands increased hematopoiesis the yellow marrow will reconvert to red marrow in just the reverse order, proximal to distal.

In cases of severe chronic anemia, marrow reconversion will take place. Other diseases such as plasma cell myeloma, myelofibrosis, leukemia, lymphoma, skeletal mets, and various anemias such as sickle cell and thalassemia will cause marrow expansion as the continued demand for normal blood products fails to be met. Radiographically, the marrow hyperplasia will cause widened medullary cavities with coarsened trabeculae and squaring of the bones. During adolescence the most severe manifestations shift from the appendicular skeleton to the axial skeleton. The calvaria demonstrates widening, hair-on-end appearance, and obliteration of the diploic space. The axial skeleton demineralizes as hydroxyapatite and osteoid are replaced by marrow-forming elements. The Erlenmeyer flask deformity is seen as the metaphyses get packed and expanded by hematopoietic cells intent on churning out new red blood cells. Extramedullary hematopoiesis refers to extraosseous blood cell production as in the liver, spleen, and lymph nodes. The large paraspinal soft tissue masses that may compress the spinal canal are in fact extraosseous extensions of medullary tissue derived from vertebral bodies and ribs.

Notes

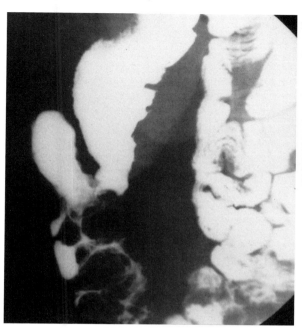

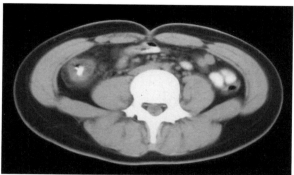

1. What is Rovsig's sign?

2. What are the etiologic agents for the above entity?

3. Can foreign body perforation yield this appearance?

4. What is splinting and who loves it?

Typhlitis

1. Pain from appendicitis mirroring McBurney's point on the left.

2. *Candida*, *Pseudomonas*, and cytomegalovirus.

3. Most certainly yes, focal thickening of bowel should always trigger thoughts of a foreign body perforation.

4. Splinting is an acute curvature of the lumbar spine secondary to an ipsilateral inflammatory process (such as appendicitis) aimed at relieving tension on the inflamed peritoneum. Board examiners love it, so look for it!

Reference

McNamara MJ, Chalmers AG, Morgan M, et al.: Typhlitis in acute childhood leukaemia: radiological features. *Clin Radiol* 37(1):83–86, 1986.

Cross-Reference

Pediatric Radiology: THE REQUISITES, 2nd edn, pp 121–123.

Comment

Typhlitis is a necrotizing colitis that affects the right colon and ileum in neutropenic patients. The neutropenia is often secondary to leukemia, lymphoma, aplastic anemia, cyclic neutropenia, AIDS, or transplantation. Current theory suggests direct bacterial invasion of the "chemotherapy weakened" bowel wall. Presentation is characterized by distention, right lower quadrant pain, bloody stools, and vomiting.

Radiographically, small bowel obstruction, ileus, paucity of right lower quadrant air, thickened right colon, and pneumatosis may be seen on plain film. The striking CT appearance of massively thickened colon limited to the ascending segment of large bowel in the appropriate clinical setting is pathognomonic. Ultrasound of the right lower quadrant will demonstrate a target sign representing the thickened bowel with an echogenic mucosa.

Therapy is supportive and conservative with antibiotics. Perforation and peritonitis buy a trip to the OR.

Notes

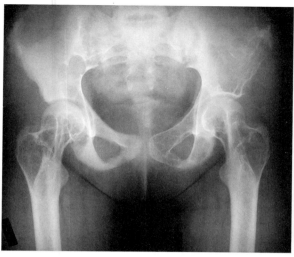 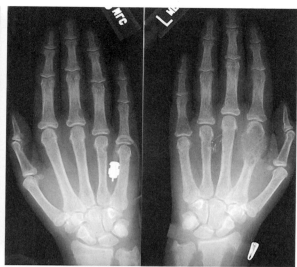

1. What is the cause of osteitis fibrosa cystica?
2. Which bone cell secretes alkaline phosphatase?
3. Has chondrocalcinosis been reported with this disorder?
4. Is chronic renal disease associated with these findings?

Hyperparathyroidism

1. Hyperparathyroidism.

2. Osteoblasts. Elevated levels are seen in hyperparathyroidism as osteoblasts attempt to catch up with high parathormone driven osteoclast activity.

3. Yes.

4. Yes, renal disease leads to vitamin D deficiency, hypocalcemia, and compensatory secondary hyperparathyroidism.

Reference

States LJ: Imaging of metabolic bone disease and marrow disorders in children. *Radiol Clin N Am* 39(4): 749–772, 2001.

Cross-Reference

Pediatric Radiology: THE REQUISITES, pp 214–216.

Comment

Primary hyperparathyroidism, an adult disorder, can be caused by an adenoma, hyperplasia, or the rare parathyroid carcinoma. Increased parathormone levels recruit osteoclasts to resorb calcium and phosphate from the bones while simultaneously increasing excretion of phosphate in the urine and resorption of calcium in the renal collecting tubules. The net effect is serum calcium up and phosphate down. Skeletal changes include resorption of subperiosteal bone with decreased mineralization, coarsened trabeculae and erosive changes at the insertion of muscles, i.e., the lumbricals inserting at the radial aspects of the phalanges. Aggregates of osteoclasts, cellular debris, and hemorrhage come together to form solitary expansile lucent lesions known as brown tumors. Brown tumors are more commonly associated with primary versus secondary hyperparathyroidism.

Secondary hyperparathyroidism is caused by any condition that causes sustained decreased serum calcium levels. Remember that low calcium increases parathyroid hormone levels. The most common cause of decreased serum calcium levels is renal disease. Vitamin D is integral at maintaining calcium levels by increasing intestinal and renal resorption. The nonfunctioning kidney cannot convert vitamin D to its active form, thus rendering the patient functionally vitamin D deficient. Low vitamin D leads to low calcium, while phosphate levels climb due to loss of normal renal function. This combination drives parathyroid levels abnormally high. So called renal osteodystrophy develops with widening of growth plates, frayed metastases, coarsening of the trabecular pattern, demineralization and cortical thinning. Slipped capital femoral epiphysis is commonly seen.

Tertiary hyperparathyroidism refers to unlucky patients with long-standing renal osteodystrophy who develop autonomous parathyroid adenomas that will not respond to vitamin D therapy. Surgery is required.

Notes

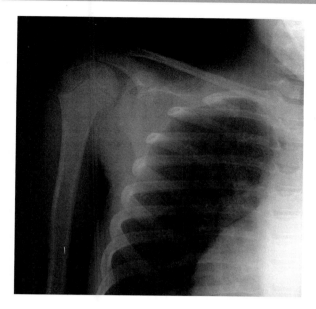

1. Name several epiphyseal equivalents.

2. What is the differential diagnosis?

3. If this lesion was centered in the metaphysis you might include what rare lesion in your differential?

4. Where is this lesion most commonly found?

Chondroblastoma

1. Talus, anterior vertebral bodies.

2. Epiphyseal only: subchondral cyst, osteomyelitis, or Langerhans cell histiocytosis. Epiphysis extending into metaphysis: enchondroma, osteoblastoma, and aneurysmal bone cyst.

3. Chondromyxoid fibroma, metaphyseal based, and appearing similar to chondroblastoma.

4. Distal femur, proximal tibia, proximal humerus, and proximal femur.

Reference

Ecklund K, Jaramillo D, Buonomo C: Pediatric case of the day. Chondroblastoma. *Radiographics* 16:979–982, 1996.

Cross-Reference

Pediatric Radiology: THE REQUISITES, pp 233–234.

Comment

Chondroblastoma is a rare benign tumor of hyaline-cartilage-producing origin residing within the epiphysis or hypophysis. The tumor occurs in adolescents with a 2:1 predominance in males. Clinically, chondroblastomas are painful and usually produce an effusion or reduced joint mobility as they are commonly intra-articular. Treatment is curettage and bone grafting.

Radiographically, these lesions appear as eccentrically located rounded lucencies in the epiphyses. Well-defined margins with a narrow zone of transition and thin rim of sclerosis are characteristic of chondroblastoma. The lesion may extend into the metaphysis and/or expand the cortex. Stippled calcification of chondroid matrix is seen in a large number of cases. A periosteal reaction may be seen in those tumors with periosteal contiguity.

MR of chondroblastoma demonstrates a lobular appearance with a heterogeneity on T2 imaging. Of note is the substantial peritumoral bone marrow edema on short tau inversion recovery (STIR) and T2 fat sat images that falsely projects a more aggressive nature to this tumor. Do not get sucked into diagnosing tumors on MR; conventional radiographs will hold the diagnosis in the vast majority of cases. Rather, use MR to stage, detect tumor recurrence, or problem solve in narrowed diagnostic scenarios.

Notes

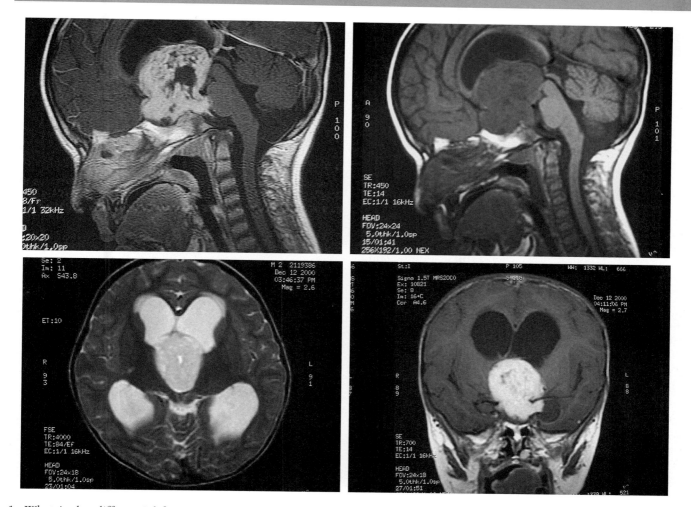

1. What is the differential for a suprasellar mass?

2. Which form of this mass is seen in children, adamintinomatous or papillary?

3. Which suprasellar masses are cystic?

4. What percentage of these cases are calcified and cystic?

Craniopharyngioma

1. SATCHMO: **S**ellar lesion with superior extension, **A**neurysm, **T**eratoid lesions, **C**raniopharyngioma, **H**ypothalamic glioma, **M**etastases, **O**ptic nerve glioma.

2. Adamantinomatous occurs in children, while papillary is seen in adult craniopharyngioma.

3. Rathke's cleft cyst, large pituitary adenoma, glioma, mets, and aneurysm.

4. 90% of these cases are calcified and cystic in the childhood form.

Reference

Johnsen DE, Woodruff WW, Allen IS, et al.: MR imaging of the sellar and juxtasellar regions. *Radiographics* 11:727–758, 1991.

Cross-Reference

Pediatric Radiology: THE REQUISITES, p 287.

Comment

Craniopharyngioma is a tumor thought to arise from either the remnant of the craniopharyngeal duct or squamous epithelial cells in the pars tuberalis of the adenohypophysis. The tumor is most commonly found in children and adolescents. Craniopharyngioma commonly grows in a suprasellar location, although you may find them entirely within the sella. Two varieties exist, a childhood form with a calcified cystic predominance that presents between 11–14 years and an adult form seen in the 50s that appears less cystic. The childhood form carries with it a poor prognosis. The sella and surrounding area is a pretty tight space, so clinically mass effect is responsible for headache, visual deficits, hydrocephalus, pituitary dysfunction, and frontal lobe behavior changes.

On CT a large heterogenous suprasellar mass is seen with linear and peripheral calcifications. Look for lobulated cysts, bony erosion, and expansion of the dorsum sella. On MR, T1-weighted images of these cysts may appear dark, intermediate, or bright, depending on their protein content. The lesions may appear homo or heterogenous. On MR these cysts will appear bright on T2. Ninety per cent of childhood craniopharyngiomas are both cystic and calcified. These suprasellar masses will often extend inferiorly into the sella. If you give gadolinium, expect some enhancement of the solid components. And don't forget to give the sella a quick look on lateral c-spine.

Craniopharyngioma is treated with surgery and radiotherapy. Prognosis is variable.

Notes

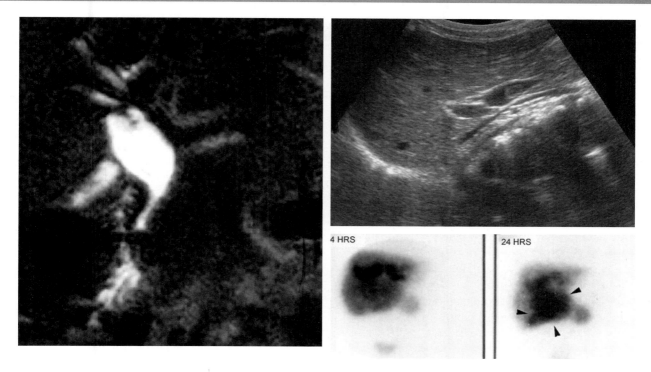

1. Is there an association with medullary sponge kidney?
2. What finding will be apparent on upper GI?
3. Is there a role for magnetic resonance cholangiopancreatography?
4. This entity is lined by gastric mucosa, true or false?

Choledochal Cyst

1. 80% of patients with Caroli disease have medullary sponge kidney.

2. Widening of the duodenal C loop.

3. Ultrasound is usually adequate.

4. False, they are lined by duodenal mucosa.

Reference

Kim OH, Chung HJ, Choi BG: Imaging of the chole-dochal cyst. *Radiographics* 15(1):69–88, 1995.

Cross-Reference

Pediatric Radiology: THE REQUISITES, 2nd edn, pp 128–129.

Comment

Choledochal cysts are localized dilatations or aneurysms of the biliary tree. The etiology ranges from congenital weakness in neonates to reflux biliopathy with second-ary dilatation. There are four types based on locations and size of the dilated segments: Type I, cystic fusiform dilitation of the common bile duct (CBD) with an anom-alous junction of the pancreatobiliary ductal system; Type II, a diverticulum protruding from the wall of the CBD; Type III, a diverticulum of the CBD; Type IV is considered by some synonymous with Caroli disease, diffuse fusiform intrahepatic dilatations without evidence of obstruction.

Presentation includes abdominal pain (50%), fever, obstructive jaundice (80%) and a mass (50%). The clas-sic triad of episodic abdominal pain, jaundice and a right upper quadrant mass on the right side presents in 20% of cases.

Conventional radiographs may show a right upper quadrant mass with displaced bowel loops. Ultrasound will yield much morphologic information about the cysts. A cystic mass in the porta hepatis that can be shown to connect to the CBD, cystic duct, or hepatic duct will nail the diagnosis. Endoscopic retrograde cholangiopancreatography and HIDA scans will confirm a communication between the cysts and biliary tree.

Treatment is excision with enteric drainage of the bil-iary tree. A delay in treatment may lead to cirrhosis, portal hypertension, cholangitis or pancreatitis. Increased risk of biliary tract carcinoma is 20 times that of the normal population.

Notes

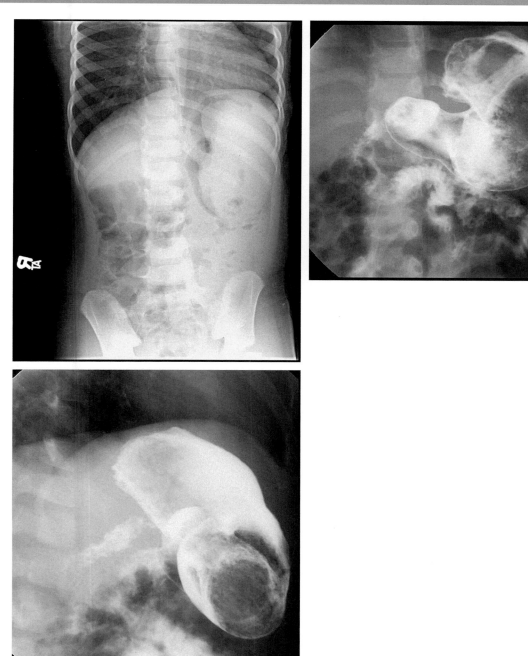

1. Does hairstyle matter in this entity?

2. Is proctitis related to this entity?

3. Is this entity more common in breast-fed infants?

4. What are the three most common etiologic agents in this entity?

Bezoar

1. Braids are commonly seen in trichobezoar.

2. Yes.

3. No, lactobezoar are more common with formula.

4. Milk, pits, and hair.

References

Sinzig M, Umschaden HW, Haselbach H, et al.: Gastric trichobezoar with gastric ulcer: MR findings. *Pediatr Radiol* 28(5):296, 1998.

Bhattacharyya NC, Goswami A: Phytobezoars in infants. *Indian Pediatr* 30(9):1146–1149, 1993. Review.

Cross-Reference

Pediatric Radiology: THE REQUISITES, 2nd edn, p 105.

Comment

Do not forget to include bezoars and foreign bodies as they are not rare but merely uncommon. Bezoars are indigestible organic materials that form a collection in the stomach. Specific names describe the contents, trichobezoar (hair), phytobezoar (indigestible plant or vegetable material), and milk curd (the dreaded lactobezoar). Radiographically, the bezoar is seen on fluoroscopy as a mobile mass that fails to exit the stomach. Presentation varies from abdominal mass to halitosis often in emotionally troubled children or adolescents. Anorexia and weight loss are usually associated symptoms.

Notes

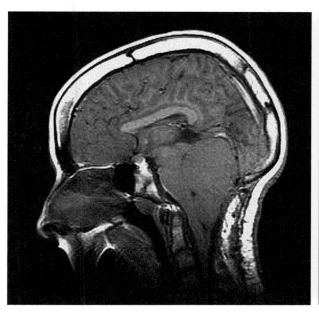 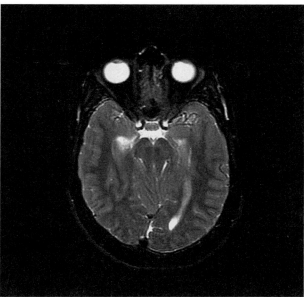

1. What percentage of these patients have a myelomeningocele?

2. What is an encephalocele?

3. What is a meningocele?

4. What is a myelomeningocele?

Chiari II (Arnold–Chiari)

1. Greater than 95%.

2. Encephalocele: meninges and brain extending through skull defect.

3. Herniation of meninges through defect in the posterior spine, most often the lumbosacral region.

4. Herniation of meninges and neural elements through defect in the posterior spine, most often the lumbosacral region.

Reference

Rauzzino M, Oakes WJ: Chiari II malformation and syringomyelia. *Neurosurg Clin N Am* 6(2):293–309, 1995.

Cross-Reference

Pediatric Radiology: THE REQUISITES, pp 268–269.

Comment

Type II of the four types of Chiari malformations also goes by the name Arnold–Chiari and refers to a group of abnormalities, including inferior displacement of the cerebellum, brain stem, and fourth ventricle, narrowed fourth ventricle, small posterior fossa, and a lumbar myelomeningocele. It appears that an abnormality in ventricular growth inhibits normal development of the posterior fossa. The small posterior fossa produces the Chiari type II abnormalities due to posterior fossa crowding.

Clinically, these patients present at birth with myelomeningocele requiring immediate surgery. Hindbrain herniation will manifest as lower cranial nerve dysfunction, upper extremity weakness, opisthotonus, and spasticity.

On CT findings include hydrocephalus, an enlarged foramen magnum, Lückenschädel sign (lacunar skull or skeletal dysplasia), and scalloping of the clivus. On MR sagittal sections will clearly show a small posterior fossa with inferior displacement of the brainstem and inferior cerebellum in addition to upward migration of the superior cerebellum. The corpus callosum will demonstrate some form of dysgenesis. Tectal beaking with fusion of the colliculi may be easily seen on the sagittal midline with the cerebellum wrapping itself around the brainstem. Syringomyelia and hydrocephalus are present as well as gray matter heterotopias and aqueductal stenosis.

Treatment is directed toward repair of the myelomeningocele as well as VP shunt placement for hydrocephalus.

Notes

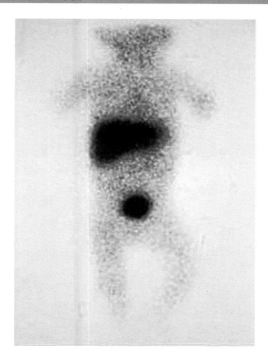

1. What is Caroli disease?

2. Is there an increased risk of cancer with Caroli?

3. What is the normal common bile duct measurement in infants?

4. What is the differential diagnosis of neonatal ascites?

Biliary Atresia

1. Multiple choledochoceles.

2. Yes, cholangiocarcinoma.

3. Up to 3 mm.

4. Free urine secondary to rupture calyx (posterior urethral valve), hydrops fetalis, chylous, and perinatally ruptured thoracic duct.

Reference

Gubernick JA, Rosenberg HK, Ilaslan H, et al.: US approach to jaundice in infants and children. *Radiographics* 20(1):173–195, 2000.

Cross-Reference

Pediatric Radiology: THE REQUISITES, 2nd edn, pp 127–128.

Comment

The causes of neonatal jaundice are infectious hepatitis, biliary atresia intravascular hemolysis, extravascular hemolysis, resorption local hemorrhage, alpha-1-antitrypsin deficiency, and biliary obstruction. Jaundice persisting beyond 4 weeks is either due to neonatal hepatitis or biliary atresia. Some have suggested that biliary atresia is secondary to sclerosing cholangitis from neonatal hepatitis. Associated abnormalities include polysplenia, preduodenal portal vein, and malrotation. Imaging plays a central role in distinguishing these two entities.

Imaging is directed toward demonstrating a normal morphologic and functional biliary system. Ultrasound will effectively rule out either extrahepatic biliary dilatation or choledochal cysts. Visualization of the gallbladder is suggestive of hepatitis, while nonvisualization, in the absence of morphologic abnormality, indicates atresia. A normal-sized gallbladder is present in 10–20% of patients with biliary atresia. Ultrasound is nonspecific and a HIDA scan must be used to differentiate hepatitis from atresia. Atresia is amenable to surgery with best results prior to 2 months of age.

HIDA is 99mTc-labeled IDA, which is injected intravenously and extracted by hepatocytes leading to excretion into the biliary system and duodenum. There are three patterns: normal uptake with excretion in GI tract (neonatal hepatitis), normal uptake with no excretion into the GI tract (atresia), and poor uptake with little or no excretion (severe hepatitis, atresia can not be ruled out). An intraoperative cholangiogram is performed for definitive diagnosis as well as evaluation for surgical correction. Most often a Kasai procedure is performed wherein a loop of jejunum is brought up to a dissected porta hepatis for drainage of bile. If Kasai fails, transplantation is considered.

Notes

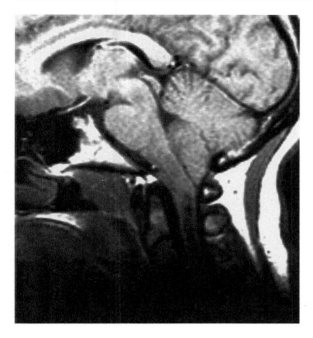

1. What is thought to be the cause of the syrinx in this entity?

2. What is the incidence of hydrocephalus in these patients?

3. Why have VP shunts been implicated as a cause of this entity?

4. Define basilar invagination.

C A S E 102

Chiari I

1. Abnormal CSF flow dynamics are thought to contribute to flow abnormalities leading to hydrosyringomyelia.

2. 25%.

3. The VP shunt lowers the intracranial pressure necessary to keep the sutures open, allowing for growth.

4. An upward displacement of the odontoid process through the foramen magnum.

Reference

Barkovich AJ, Wippold FJ, Sherman JL, et al.: Significance of cerebellar tonsillar position on MR. *Am J Neuroradiol* 7(5):795–799, 1986.

Cross-Reference

Pediatric Radiology: THE REQUISITES, p 268.

Comment

There are four types of Chiari malformations. Type I malformation is defined by a low position of the cerebellar tonsils, inferior vermis, or cervicomedullary junction below the foramen magnum. The foramen magnum is defined by a line drawn from the basion to the opisthion. The number to remember here is 5 mm. The tonsils may extend no more than 5 mm below the line to be considered normal, greater than 5 mm and symptoms are invariably present. The cause of Chiari I malformation is thought to be a dysplastic occipital bone that causes crowding of the cerebellum and squeezing of the tonsils through the foramen magnum. An alternative etiology in some patients suggests a transient hydrocephalus that herniates the posterior fossa contents inferiorly where they remain permanently. Clinically, young adults will complain of headache, neck pain, weakness, dizziness, and nystagmus.

On imaging the tonsils will be seen to extend beyond 5 mm of the foramen magnum. Syringomyelia is a commonly associated finding within the cervical cord. Treatment is dependent upon the clinical picture and involves decompression of the foramen magnum and cervical laminectomy.

Notes

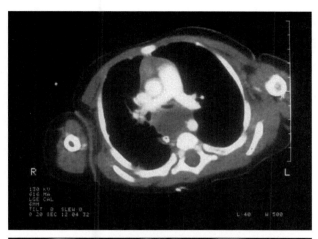

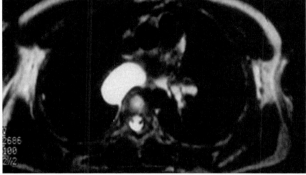

1. At what thoracic level is this abnormality most commonly found?

2. What is the differential diagnosis?

3. What accounts for the density?

4. Is it more common on the right or left?

Bronchogenic Cyst

1. T4–5, tracheal bifurcation.

2. Bronchogenic, enteric cyst.

3. Serous or mucoid fluid fills the cysts.

4. Right.

Reference
Moore KL, Persaud TVN: *The Developing Human: Clinically Oriented Embryology,* 5th edn, Philadelphia: W.B. Saunders Company, 1993.

Cross-Reference
Pediatric Radiology: THE REQUISITES, 2nd edn, p 29.

Comment
Lung development begins at the fourth week with division of the bronchial buds from the laryngotracheal tube. The laryngotracheal tube differentiates into bronchi, bronchioles, and then finally alveoli. Abnormal separation of tracheal buds from the tracheal tree lead to fluid-filled respiratory epithelial-lined cysts. Sequestrations have similar origins, although their peripheral location may induce further differentiation due to their close proximity to pulmonary mesenchyme.

On imaging, bronchogenic cysts appear as well circumscribed, rounded, uniform, often solitary water densities. Cross-sectional imaging is useful, especially prior to biopsy, to exclude vascular abnormalities. Histologic identity is determined by the presence of respiratory epithelium. Bronchogenic cysts are most commonly found in the middle mediastinum at the level of tracheal bifurcation, they will not enhance unless infected. On MR, T2WI will yield bright signal as they are often fluid filled.

Other foregut malformations include enteric cysts and neurenteric cysts. Enteric cysts are often larger and located more commonly in the posterior than in the middle mediastinum. Esophageal duplications are lined with either esophageal or gastric mucosa and have been associated with vertebral anomalies and esophageal atresia. Cysts containing gastric mucosa will rupture from acid secretions, causing hemoptysis.

Neurenteric cysts are found in the posterior mediastinum and are associated with vertebral anomalies.

Notes

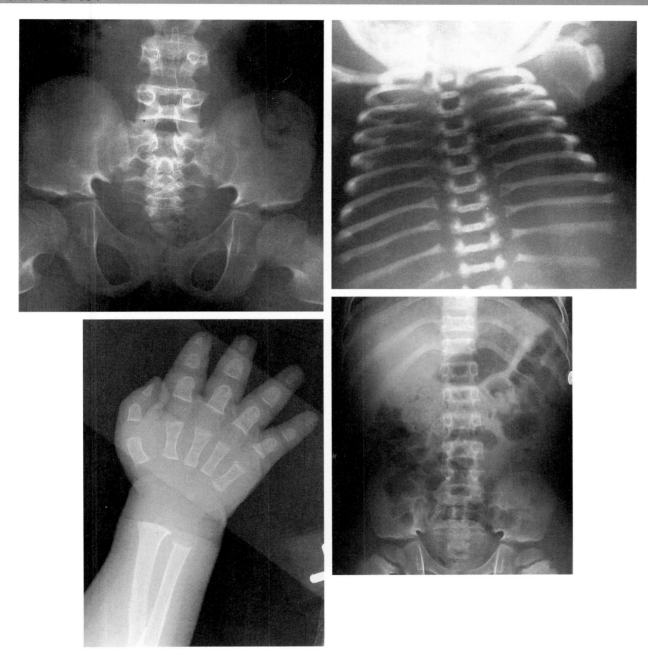

1. What is the genetic inheritence?

2. Name three causes of dural ectasia resulting in scalloping.

3. Name three causes of anterior scalloping.

4. Can syringomyelia cause posterior scalloping?

C A S E 104

Achondroplasia (Rhizomelic Dwarfism)

1. Autosomal dominant, although most cases are sporadic.

2. Neurofibromatosis, Marfan syndrome, Ehlers–Danlos syndrome, ependymoma, communicating hydrocephalus.

3. Lymphoma/leukemia, and lymphadenopathy, aortic aneurysm.

4. Yes, syringomyelia can cause posterior scalloping.

Reference

Silverman FN: Radiologic features of achondroplasia. *Basic Life Sci* 48:31–44, 1988.

Cross-Reference

Pediatric Radiology: THE REQUISITES, p 198.

Comment

Short stature can be symmetric or asymmetric. Asymmetric forms include short-limb, short-trunk, and proportional dwarfism. Short-limbed dwarfs are subdivided on the basis of distribution: rhizomelic, mesomelic, and acromelic. Rhizomelic involves the proximal appendicular skeleton (humeri and femura), mesomelic the middle skeleton (radius–ulna and tibia–fibula), and acromelic the distal skeleton (metacarpals, metatarsals, and phalanges).

Achondroplasia is an autosomally dominant disorder caused by a spontaneous mutation linked to advanced paternal age. The gene affected codes for a fibroblast receptor. The vast majority of cases are heterozygous and demonstrate less severe manifestations than homozygotes. The incidence is 1:26,000. It is the most common form of dwarfism and the result of a defect in enchondral bone formation. Intramembranous flat bone formation is relatively normal and responsible for the normal truncal appearance relative to the shortened limbs. As enchondral formation is responsible for bone lengthening, this entity leads to shortened limbs. Normal long-bone growth proceeds by both enchondral formation and periosteal cortical formation. Periosteal growth is normal in achondroplasia, yielding normal diameter bones with grossly shortened lengths due to enchondral formation dysfunction.

Radiographically, long bones are shortened and flared. Brachycephaly, frontal bossing, and small facial bones are caused by a composite of intramembranous bone outgrowing and compensating for dysplastic enchondral formation (skull base). The spinal interpedicular distances normally increase caudally, while in achondroplasia they decrease. Pedicles are shortened and lead to spinal stenosis, a common condition in adulthood. There is posterior scalloping of the vertebral bodies in addition to anterior beaking. The pelvis may demonstrate flared iliac wings and sacral dysplasia yielding a champagne or margarita glass appearance.

On fetal ultrasound heterozygous acondroplasia has been identified as early as the second trimester. Upper limb shortening, macrocranium, frontal bossing, depressed nasal bridge, midface hypoplasia and brachydactyly are identified in utero. The femur length will fall behind the biparietal diameter as early as 21 weeks and as late at 27 weeks gestation. Chorionic villous sampling at 10–12 weeks in achondroplastic parents will allow for detection of the genetic defect that has been mapped to chromosome 4.

Notes

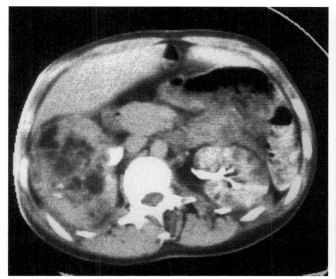

Patient 1

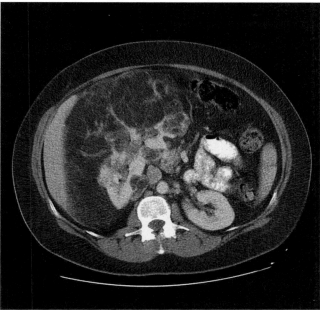

Patient 2

1. How might this condition present?

2. Would you expect this lesion to be hyperechoic on US?

3. Who was Hounsfield?

4. Is the presence of fat diagnostic?

Angiomyolipoma

1. Flank pain.

2. Yes.

3. British electrical engineer, born in 1919 and awarded the 1979 Nobel Prize in Physiology or Medicine for building the prototype CT scanner in 1972.

4. Yes, fat is diagnostic. Few cases of fat containing renal cell carcinomas have been reported.

References

Lowe LH, Isuani BH, Heller RM, et al.: Pediatric renal masses: Wilms tumor and beyond. *Radiographics* 20(6):1585–1603, 2000.

Wagner BJ, Wong-You-Cheong JJ, Davis CJ, Jr: Adult renal hamartomas. *Radiographics* 17:155–169, 1997.

Cross-Reference

Pediatric Radiology: THE REQUISITES, pp 173–174.

Comment

Angiomyolipoma is a hamartomatous benign tumor that contains elements of muscle, fat, and vasculature. Eighty per cent of children with angiomyolipoma will have tuberous sclerosis (TS), while only 50% of pediatric patients with tuberous sclerosis will have angiomyolipoma. Translation: find an angiolipoma on a CT and the patient will have an 80% chance of having tuberous sclerosis. Find a tuberous sclerosis patient on your CT table and you will have a 50% chance of finding an angiomyolipoma. Angiomyolipomas in patients without tuberous sclerosis are unilateral and are seen in middle-aged women.

Clinically the TS angiomyolipomas are relatively silent compared with non-TS-associated angiomyolipomas. These hypervascular lesions tend to develop small aneurysms that bleed, potentially causing life-threatening hemorrhage. Therapy is directed toward removing tumors more likely to bleed (greater than 4 cm). Again, bleeding and partial nephrectomy are more common in the middle-aged female group than in the pediatric group.

Radiologists love angiomyolipomas, as histology can be inferred by imaging studies without deferring to pathologists. The presence of fat is the clincher. On CT, small, multiple, well circumscribed, bilateral areas or low attenuation mixed with soft tissue attenuation are seen. The presence of fat distinguishes angiomyolipoma from renal cell carcinoma; however, isolated reports of fat-containing RCC have been reported.

Notes

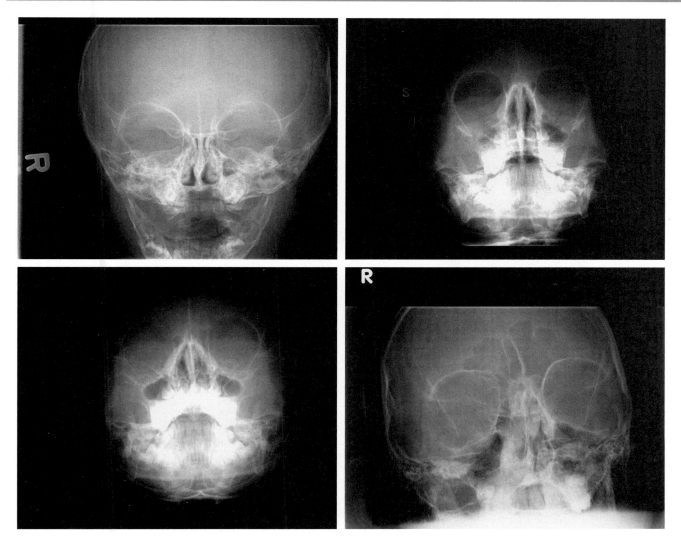

1. What is the differential diagnosis of sinus wall destruction?
2. What is the most common sinus mass?
3. What is the most common benign soft tissue tumor of the sinuses?
4. What is the most common malignant soft tissue tumor of the sinuses?

Sinus Development

1. Rhabdosarcoma, lymphoma, leukemia, hemangioma, lymphangioma, ondontogenic tumors, mucoceles (cystic fibrosis), Wegener granulomatosis, histiocytosis X, infection, and most commonly trauma.

2. Mucus retention cyst.

3. Juvenile nasopharyngeal angiofibroma.

4. Rhabdomyosarcoma.

Reference

Zeifer B: Pediatric sinonasal imaging: normal anatomy and inflammatory disease. *Neuroimaging Clin N Am* 10(1): 137–159, ix, 2000.

Cross-Reference

Pediatric Radiology: THE REQUISITES, p 264.

Comment

Only the paranasal sinuses are present in rudimentary form at birth. The maxillary, ethmoidal, frontal, and sphenoidal air cells develop sequentially. The maxillary antra and ethmoid air cells begin pneumatization before the age of 6 months and are fully pneumatized by approximately 10 years. By 7 years, variable pneumatization of the frontal sinuses should be evident. The sphenoid sinus pneumatizes from anterior to posterior by 10 years. The size and shape of the pneumatized sinuses vary from individual to individual and with age. There is wide variation in the appearance of soft tissues within the sinuses. In asymptomatic infants less than 2 years opacification is common and thought to be due to redundant mucosa and normal fatty changes that precede pneumatization. For this reason, sinus radiographs in infants less than 2 years of age are often not reliable for assessing sinusitis.

Inflammatory reaction to foreign material often causes bilateral thickening of the mucosal membranes. However, a sinus air–fluid level in the absence of trauma suggests an acute bacterial infection. Chronic inflammatory changes of the mucosa may result in retention cysts, polyps, or mucoceles. Polyps are associated most often with cystic fibrosis and allergies. Intracranial and intraorbital extension are well illustrated by computer tomography. CT sets the standard for evaluating inflammation of the nasosinus structures.

Notes

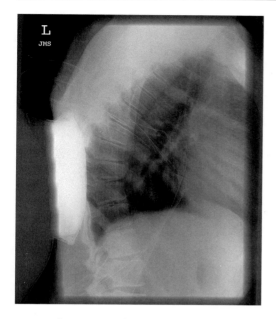

1. At what age is the vertebral column fully ossified?
2. What is limbus vertebrae?
3. What segment of the spine is most commonly affected?
4. What is a Schmorl's node?

Scheuermann Disease

1. The vertebral column is completely ossified at 25 years.

2. Limbus vertebrae results from a small herniation of disc material between the cartilaginous growth plate and underlying bone yielding a small isolated segment of bone.

3. The lower thoracic and upper lumbar segments are most commonly affected.

4. A Schmorl's node is protrusion of the nucleus pulposis into the vertebral body endplate.

Reference

Afshani E, Kuhn JP: Common causes of low back pain in children. *Radiographics* 11:269–291, 1991.

Cross-Reference

Pediatric Radiology: THE REQUISITES, p 291.

Comment

Five secondary ossification centers appear in the vertebrae following puberty. These ossification centers are located at the tips of the spinous and transverse processes as well as the inferior and superior endplates (annular epiphyses). The nonossified cartilaginous endplates are thought to be susceptible to damage by increased forces from manual labor or athletics. Scheuermann disease primarily affects males from ages 13–17 who present with back pain.

Radiographically, findings may range from irregularity of the endplates to wedging and loss of height of the vertebral bodies and disc spaces. The endplates lose their sharp, smooth outline and develop a sclerotic appearance. Anterior wedging or central depression of the endplates yields kyphosis or scoliosis which may develop depending upon the location of the defects. Scheuermann varies from three vertebral levels with at least 5° of wedging to entire spinal involvement. Approximately half of patients have associated spondylolysis. Three-quarters of cases affect the thoracic spine, while the remaining 25% involve the thoracolumbar regions. Healing may lead to fusion of adjoining endplates and permanent progressive kyphotic deformity. The abnormal forces on the endplates often lead to further herniation of the disc material into the vertebral body, imparting a biconcave appearance. Abnormal forces on the disc have also been hypothesized to produce discal calcification. One Scheuermann variant, juvenile lumbar osteochondrosis, demonstrates only lumbar involvement. Radiographically, affected vertebral bodies are widened with similar endplate changes noted in Scheuermann disease.

Patients are observed if the kyphosis is less than 50°. A brace is recommended for curvatures less than 75°, provided the patient is still growing. Braces have demonstrated 50% improvements in kyphotic deformity. Rods and fusion are recommended in skeletally immature patients at 75°, while adults undergo surgery at 60°. Surgery leads to approximately a 50% improvement equally efficacious to the brace in less severely affected patients.

Notes

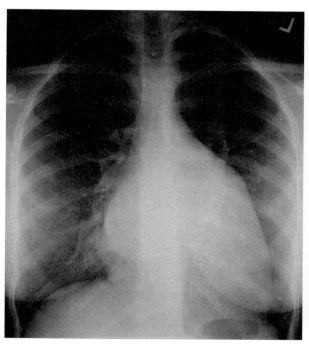 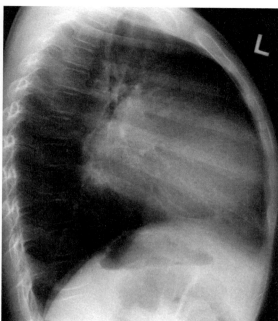

1. What is the etiologic agent?

2. What is the characteristic histologic feature?

3. What is the order of valvular involvement?

4. Do these patients require antibiotic prophylaxis?

Rheumatic Heart Disease

1. Group A beta hemolytic *Streptococcus*.

2. Myocardial Aschoff nodules.

3. Mitral, aortic, tricuspid, and pulmonic.

4. Yes, for 5–10 years after their initial episode.

Reference

Allen HD, Gutgesell HP, Clark EB, et al.: *Moss and Adams Heart Disease in Infants, Children and Adolescents: Including the Fetus and Young Adult,* 6th edn. Baltimore: Lippincott Williams & Wilkins, 2000, pp 1226–1241.

Cross-Reference

Pediatric Radiology: THE REQUISITES, 2nd edn, p 71.

Comment

Rheumatic fever is the most common cause of acquired heart disease in both children and adults. Rheumatic fever is an autoimmune process in which an initial streptococcal infection induces antibody production that cross-reacts with various tissue of the body including heart, joints, brain, and skin. Myocarditis is seen in 50% of cases and represents the most serious complication of acute rheumatic fever. Left-sided valve involvement is typical with inflammation and later scarring, fibrosis, and fusion of the mitral leaflets. These changes lead to the hallmarks of rheumatic fever; mitral insufficiency and mitral stenosis. Aortic insufficiency occurs in 20% of cases. The left atrium enlarges due to the mitral stenosis. The left ventricle may enlarge as well if aortic insufficiency and stenosis are present.

Clinically, patients are usually between 5 and 15 years who have a history of streptococcal pharyngitis 1–3 weeks prior to clinical manifestations of rheumatic fever. Rheumatic fever may cause a pancarditis that may manifest as heart failure, pericarditis, polyarthritis, chorea, erythema marginatum, and subcutaneous nodules. Patients will present with dyspnea and failure.

Radiographically, the chest film demonstrates a normal heart size with a prominent left atrial appendage. On the lateral, left atrial enlargement will cause posterior displacement of the left mainstem bronchus and esophagus. In older children a double wall or density is seen on the PA just medial to the left heart border, as well as splaying of the trachea and elevation of the left mainstem bronchus. Pulmonary venous hypertension will manifest as Kerley B lines, pleural effusion, and indistinct vasculature. If aortic stenosis and/or regurgitation is/are present (20% of cases) LV enlargement and post-stenotic dilatation of the ascending aorta are commonly seen. Left ventricular enlargement appears as a drooping cardiac apex and increased convexity of the superior left cardiac border. The lateral will demonstrate the posterior cardiac border to project beyond (posteriorly) the IVC at the level of the diaphragm.

Patients are initially treated with antibiotics to combat the streptococcal infection. Acute pancarditis is treated conservatively with aspirin or steroids. There is often complete resolution of valvular disease.

Notes

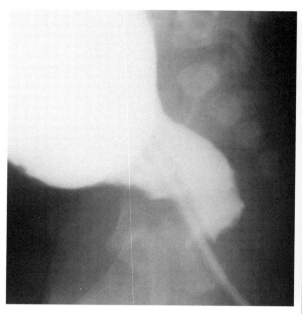 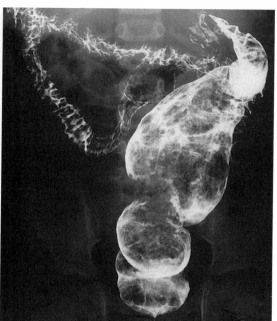

1. What is the incidence?
2. What is the differential diagnosis?
3. Why are delayed films important?
4. Are there associated anomalies?

Hirschsprung Disease

1. 4500:1.

2. Imperforate anus, colonic atresia, meconium plug syndrome, ileal atresia, meconium ileus.

3. Delayed films may be illustrative of poor transit time.

4. Yes, 20% of patients may have Down, cardiac, GI, and GU anomalies.

Reference

Das Narla L, Hingsbergen EA: Case 22: Total colonic aganglionosis-long-segment Hirschsprung disease. *Radiology* 215:391–394, 2000.

Cross-Reference

Pediatric Radiology: THE REQUISITES, 2nd edn, pp 114–116.

Comment

Aganglionosis of the distal sigmoid or rectum prevents relaxation of the denervated bowel, causing a functional obstruction with proximal dilatation. Presentation is often within the first month of life and includes failure to pass meconium in the first 24 hours, abdominal distention, water stools, fever, and shock.

Radiographically, plain films demonstrate dilated bowel to the transition zone. The dilated bowel is histologically normal, while the narrowed bowel is denervated. The transition zone is most commonly located in the rectum (70%), the left colon (15%), transverse (5%), right colon (5%), and ileocecal valve (5%). Contrast examination is performed to identify a transition point, a diagnostic marker. Transition points can be either abrupt or gradual. A normal rectum is always wider than the sigmoid; a rectum/sigmoid ratio > 1 excludes the diagnosis at that location. If the imaging is inconclusive the patient goes on to rectal manometry and suction biopsy. A full-thickness biopsy is the test of last resort. Therapy entails resection with pull-through.

Notes

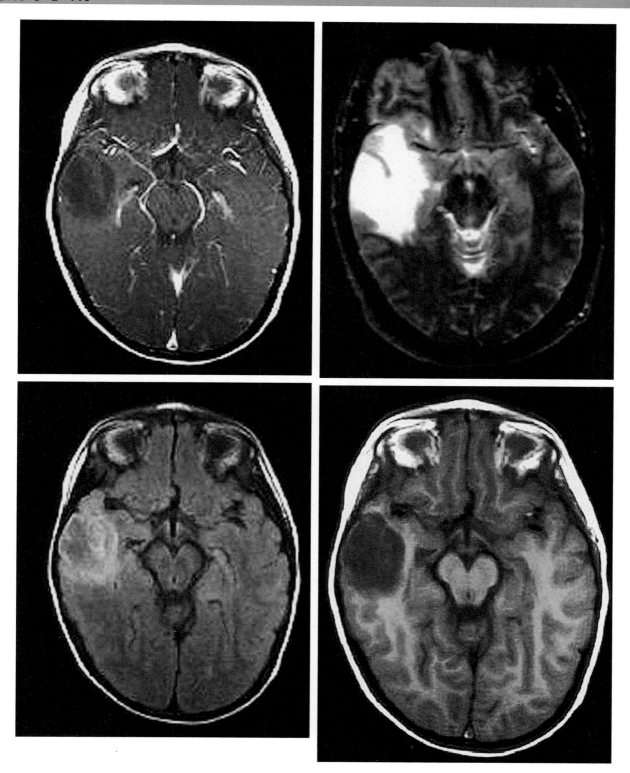

1. Is this entity more commonly unilateral or bilateral?

2. What is the etiologic agent?

3. What is the classic distribution?

4. Would you expect involvment of the basal ganglia?

Herpes Simplex Encephalitis

1. Bilateral but asymmetric.

2. HSV I.

3. Temporal lobes.

4. No, the basal ganglia are usually spared.

Reference

Enzmann DR, Ranson B, Norman D, et al.: Computed tomography of herpes simplex encephalitis. *Radiology* 129:419–425, 1978.

Cross-Reference

Pediatric Radiology: THE REQUISITES, p 278.

Comment

Herpes encephalitis affects the pediatric population in a third of cases. The infection is caused by HSV1 rather than HSV2, which is responsible for neonatal herpes. HSV1, commonly associated with oral cold sores, is thought to penetrate the oral mucosa and infiltrate the gasserian ganglion, remaining latent until reactivation. The virus then spreads toward the limbic structures in the frontal and temporal lobes through the trigeminal branches that innervate the meninges in the anterior and middle cranial fossa.

Herpes encephalitis infection is one of those rare instances in which current medical science can intervene successfully instances and hence it is of utmost importance that the diagnosis be made and timely treatment administered. Patients present with a prodrome of fever and malaise in a majority of patients that within several days develops into altered consciousness, fever, vomiting, seizures, cranial nerve palsies, and hemiparesis.

If clinically suspicious, MR is the modality of choice as early changes are easily detected. Hyperintense signal in the mesial temporal lobes is an early sign best seen on fluid attenuated inversion recovery (FLAIR). Later, the insula, inferior frontal lobes, and cingulate gyrus will demonstrate a bilateral asymmetric abnormally high T2 signal. The basal ganglia are spared. Enhancement is present in the areas of cortical involvement. Late changes demonstrate atrophy and dystrophic calcifications.

Treatment is antiviral meds. Prognosis is variable depending on promptness of therapy. Mortality is 25–75%.

Notes

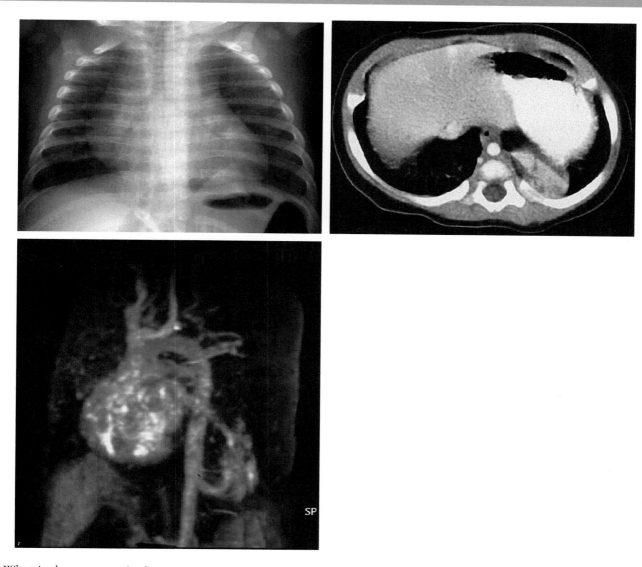

1. What is the presentation?

2. What lobes are affected most commonly?

3. What is a common name for a Turkish sword?

4. Can this lesion be detected prenatally?

Intralobar vs. Extralobar Sequestration

1. Recurrent infection, lung abscess, bronchiectasis, and hemoptysis.

2. Lower lobes, commonly the posteromedial segments.

3. Scimitar.

4. No, as it is fluid filled and cannot be distinguished from the fluid-filled lung.

Reference

Frazier AA, Rosado de Christenson ML, Stocker JT, et al.: Intralobar sequestration: radiologic-pathologic correlation. *Radiographics* 17(3):725–745, 1997.

Rosado de Christenson ML, Frazier AA, Stocker JT, et al.: From the archives of the AFIP. Extralobar sequestration: radiologic-pathologic correlation. *Radiographics* 13(2):425–441, 1993.

Cross-Reference

Pediatric Radiology: THE REQUISITES, 2nd edn, p. 26.

Comment

A sequestration is simply lung tissue that is not connected to either bronchial tree or pulmonary arteries. Commonly, vascular supply is through persistent fetal vessels (an anomalous artery via the aorta) with variable venous drainage. The terms intralobar and extralobar refer to the drainage pattern of the anomaly. Intralobar drainage is through the left atrium via the pulmonary veins (normal). Extralobar drainage is through the inferior vena cava or azygous vein. Most sequestrations are intralobar with left-sided involvement greater than right.

Patients present with recurrent pneumonia. Intralobar sequestrations are seen in older children and adults, while extralobar sequestration is present in the neonatal period. Extralobar sequestration has a stronger association with congenital defects as two-thirds of patients will have abnormalities including diaphragmatic defects, pulmonary hypoplasia, bronchogenic cysts, or cardiac anomalies.

Conventional radiographs may be normal or show a recurrent lower lobe consolidation or lucency. Intralobar may either contain air or fluid density, while extralobar appear airless. Further work-up with MRA and ultrasound may demonstrate the vascular abnormality. Patients most often present with recurrent pneumonia. Therapy for symptomatic patients involves surgical removal of infected sequestration.

Notes

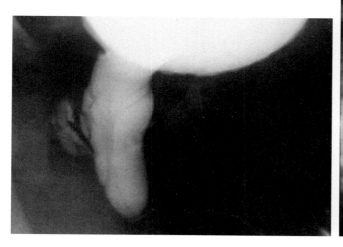
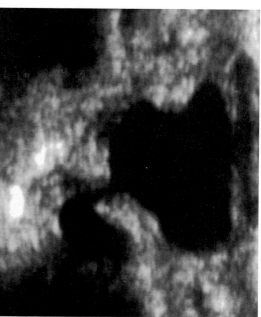

1. Name the segments of the male urethra.
2. In-utero complications of this entity include what?
3. "Hooked" or J-shaped ureters are indicative of what?
4. How often is UTI involved in the presentation of this entity?

Posterior Urethral Valve

1. Penile, prostatic, membranous.

2. Oligohydramnios, urinoma, urine ascites, hydronephrosis, and prune belly.

3. Long-standing obstruction.

4. One-third of cases present with UTI.

Reference

Macpherson RI, Leithiser RE, Gordon L, et al.: Posterior urethral valves: an update and review, *Radiographics* 6:753–791, 1986.

Cross-Reference

Pediatric Radiology: THE REQUISITES, p 162.

Comment

More nomenclature to trip us up. A posterior valve isn't a valve at all, but rather an abnormal fusion of normal mucosal folds within the urethra that obstructs urine. Presentation includes difficulty voiding, bladder distention, UTIs, or hydronephrosis on prenatal ultrasound. Presentation is usually within the first 3 months of life.

A voiding cystourethrogram is the test of choice in ruling out posterior urethral valve. Findings include dilatation and elongation of the posterior urethra. Transverse filling defects are noted indicating the "valve," at the end of the veromontanum (true mountain), with proximal dilatation of the prostatic urethra. Thickened bladder trabeculae are noted as the bladder wall hypertrophies to overcome the increased pressure produced by the urethral obstruction. Reflux may be seen in 30% of cases. Reflux in the setting of high pressure will stunt the normal development of the kidney in utero and destroy renal function. On ultrasound, the posterior urethral valve can be differentiated from reflux by a trabeculated bladder. In addition the kidney may appear small and echogenic with a poorly defined corticomedullary junction. If obstruction is severe, a neonate may present with pulmonary hypoplasia secondary to oligohydramnios.

Treatment is fulguration (electrodesiccation).

Notes

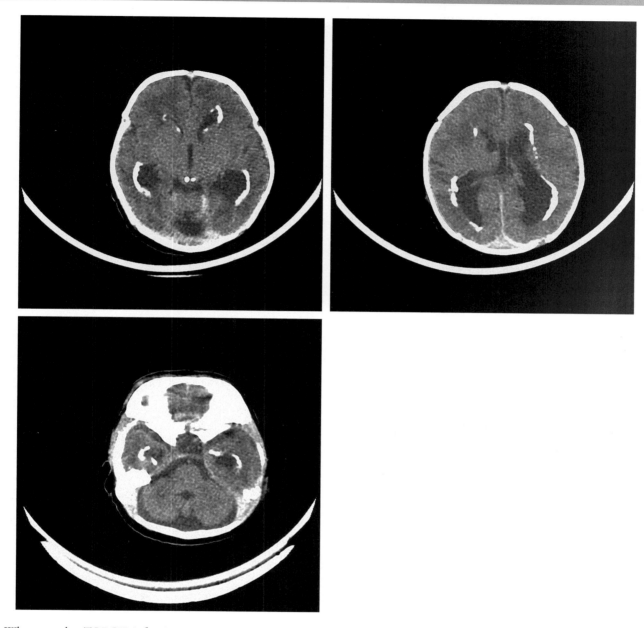

1. What are the TORCH infections?

2. What are the typical four MR findings?

3. Is the basal ganglia spared?

4. Which is the most common TORCH infection?

Cytomegalovirus (CMV) Infection

1. **T**oxoplasmosis, **O**ther, **R**ubella, **C**MV, **H**erpes simplex type 2.

2. Periventricular calcification, cortical malformations, myelination delay, and cerebellar hypoplasia.

3. No, the basal ganglia is commonly involved.

4. CMV occurs in 1% of all births.

Reference
Kapilivsky A, Garfinkle WB, Rosenberg HK, et al.: US case of the day. Congenital cytomegalovirus (CMV) brain infection. *Radiographics* 15:239–242, 1995.

Cross-Reference
Pediatric Radiology: THE REQUISITES, p 278.

Comment
CMV is one of the TORCH infections that is passed transplacentally from the infected mother to the fetus. The etiology is not fully understood with some suggesting that the virus targets the rapidly growing germinal matrix while others claim that the virus attacks the cerebral vasculature with resultant ischemia and infarction. Infection during the first and second trimester will yield developmental abnormalities such as lissencephaly. Third-trimester infections yield focal developmental abnormalities and destructive lesions.

Clinically, 10% of infected infants are symptomatic at birth, while another 10% become symptomatic within the first year. Symptoms include seizures, retardation, sensorineural hearing loss, chorioretinitis, optic neuritis, microcephaly, intrauterine growth retardation, jaundice, hepatosplenomegaly, hemolytic anemia, and pneumonitis.

On imaging, findings vary depending on the stage of the disease. Ultrasound demonstrates branching curvilinear hyperechogenicity in the basal ganglia, referred to as lenticulostriate vasculopathy. There is ventricular enlargement due to encephalomalacia. Additionally, disorganized sulci and gyri may be present. On CT a periventricular pattern of calcification with subependymal cysts and lenticulostriate calcifications is present. MR will demonstrate areas of polymicrogyria or lissencephaly, cerebellar hypogenesis, and abnormal myelination.

Antiviral drugs will arrest further deterioration. Prognosis depends on timeliness of treatment.

Notes

Patient 1

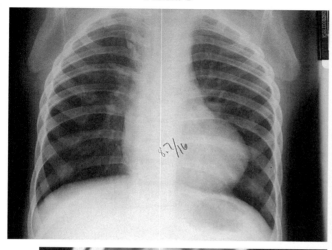

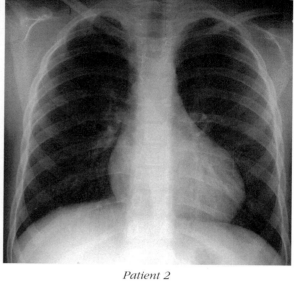

Patient 2

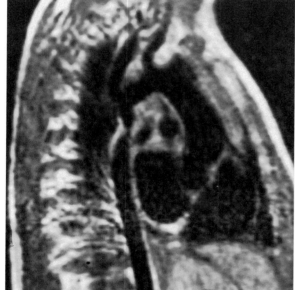

Noncyanotic patient

Patient 3

1. Is there increased or normal pulmonary vascularity?

2. If the vascularity was normal what is your differential?

3. If the vascularity was increased what is your differential?

4. What is the classic sign used to describe the finding in this case?

Coarctation of the Aorta

1. Normal, the LV is enlarged.

2. Acyanotic with normal vascularity: aortic stenosis, pulmonic stenosis, coarctation, and interrupted aortic arch.

3. Endocardial cushion defect, atrial septal defect, patent ductus arteriosus (enlarged LA and enlarged aorta), and ventricular septal defect (enlarged LA and normal aorta).

4. The "reverse 3" describes the appearance of the hypoplastic aortic knob with a dilated postenotic segment.

Reference

Allen HD, Gutgesell HP, Clark EB, et al.: *Moss and Adams Heart Disease in Infants, Children and Adolescents: Including the Fetus and Young Adult,* 6th edn. Baltimore: Lippincott Williams & Wilkins, 2000, pp 988–1010.

Cross-Reference

Pediatric Radiology: THE REQUISITES, 2nd edn, p 66.

Comment

Coarctation of the aorta is a congenital narrowing that can either be focal or diffuse. The focal type is acquired and most commonly seen in adults. The focal type is located at the ductal ligament and thought to occur due to inflammatory conditions including rubella and neurofibromatosis. The diffuse type is seen in children and involves the preductal segment that spans from the innominate to the ductus arteriosus. The diffuse type is thought to occur due to a fusion anomaly of the paired primitive dorsal aorta. Clinically, patients with the diffuse type present early with intracardiac shunts and congestive heart failure. Bounding pulses and nonpalpable leg pulses characterize the physical exam.

Radiographically, the left ventricle is large due to hypertrophy/dilitation. The LV comprises the lower half of the posterior cardiac border on the lateral view. The posterior border ought to cross the IVC 2 cm above the diaphragm. An intersection below this point suggests LV enlargement. The ascending aorta is enlarged and a notch may be seen in the focal type of coarct. The sign is referred to as a "number 3" with the "waist" of the 3 representing the narrowed segment. Rib notching may present after 10 years due to engorged intercostal arteries that erode the rib undersurfaces. The blood is shunted through the subclavian arteries to the intercostals and internal mammaries, inferior epigastrics, iliacs, and back to the abdominal aorta. The first three ribs are supplied by the thyrocervical trunk and are spared from notching. Detailed anatomic information may be gained from relatively noninvasive enhanced MR.

Coarctation is either balloon angioplastied or surgically repaired with excellent outcomes, although complications including aneurysm and restenosis are not uncommon.

Notes

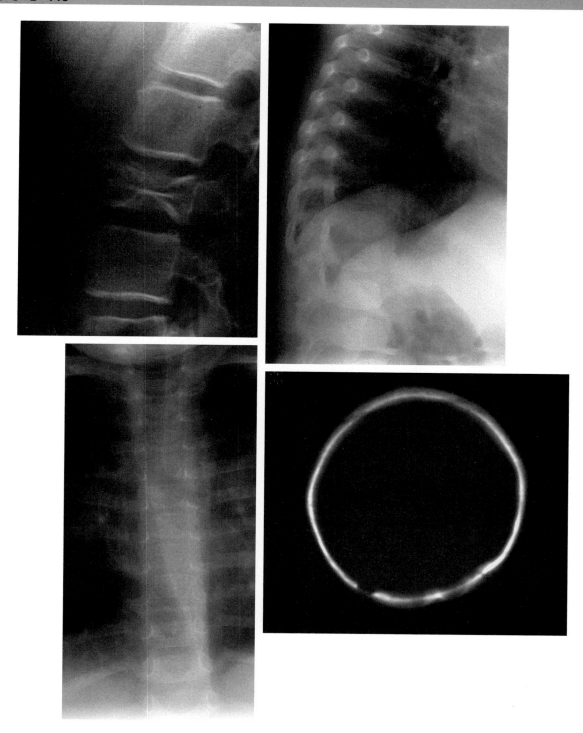

1. What is the differential diagnosis?
2. What is the characteristic skull appearance?
3. What is the characteristic vertebral appearance?
4. How does this entity appear on nuclear bone scan?

Langerhans Cell Histiocytosis (the entity formerly known as eosinophilic granuloma)

1. Osteomyelitis, Ewing sarcoma, and lymphoma (long bones).

2. The lytic skull lesion will appear beveled.

3. A uniformly flattened vertebral body—vertebral plana.

4. From hot to cold; scintigraphy is of limited use in eosinophillic granuloma.

Reference

Williams PH, Fairhurst JJ: Sonographic and radiographic appearance of lesions in an infant with Langerhans' cell histiocytosis. *Pediatr Radiol* 25(5):401, 1995.

Cross-Reference

Pediatric Radiology: THE REQUISITES, p 221.

Comment

Probably the most confusing aspect of eosinophilic granuloma is the nomenclature. Histiocytosis is a term that describes a group of disorders with abnormal proliferation of histiocytes better known as macrophages. An immunoregulatory defect has been proposed as an etiology but the details are currently unknown. There are a number of different histiocytoses, one of which is Langerhans cell histiocytosis (LCH), a disease characterized by clonal proliferation of a Langerhans cell, a special kind of macrophage. In the past, LCH was termed histiocytosis X and was subdivided into Letter–Siwe disease, Hand–Schüller–Christiansen disease, and eosinophilic granuloma. Today, these diseases are considered different expressions of the same entity.

Most often the lesion is seen in the skull (25%), ribs (14%), femur (14%), pelvis (10%), spine (8%), mandible (8%), and humerus (8%). Eosinophilic granuloma prefer flat bones (70%) to long bones (30%). On radiography, the lesions within the skull and flat bones have a lytic well-defined appearance, although sclerosis is variable. Button sequestrum, a little "island" of remaining calvaria surrounded by a "moat" of macrophages, is typical. A beveled appearance to the skull is also common. Long-bone involvement is characterized by radiolucent areas with endosteal erosion and periosteal new bone formation. Vertebral body involvement is typified by loss of height due to flattening—vertebral plana.

MR appearance of EG mimics an aggressive lesion with high signal on T2 fat sat or short tau inversion recovery (STIR) images consistent with bone marrow and soft tissue edema. These nonspecific findings may suggest osteomyelitis or Ewing sarcoma.

Notes

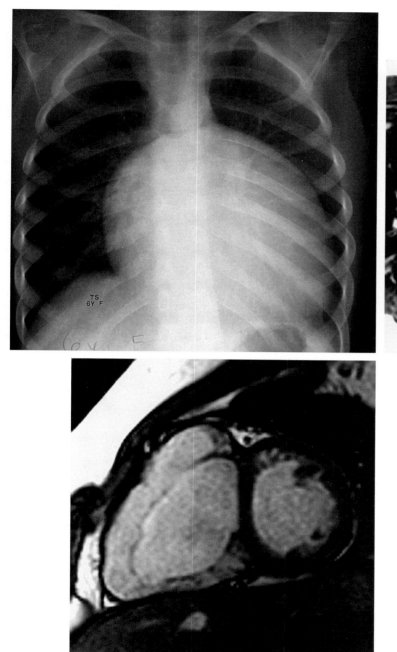

Cyanotic patient

1. Is there increased or decreased pulmonary vascularity?

2. If the vascularity was decreased what is your differential?

3. If the vascularity was increased what is your differential?

4. This entity is associated with maternal use of what drug?

Ebstein Anomaly

1. Decreased pulmonary vascularity.

2. Cyanotic with decreased vascularity: tetralogy of Fallot (normal heart size), Ebstein anomaly, pulmonic atresia, and tricuspid atresia (the latter three with enlarged heart).

3. Cyanotic with increased vascularity: transposition of the great arteries, truncus, total anomalous pulmonary venous return, and single ventricle.

4. Lithium.

Reference

Allen HD, Gutgesell HP, Clark EB, et al.: *Moss and Adams Heart Disease in Infants, Children and Adolescents: Including the Fetus and Young Adult,* 6th edn. Baltimore: Lippincott Williams & Wilkins, 2000, pp 636–651.

Cross-Reference

Pediatric Radiology: THE REQUISITES, 2nd edn, p 65.

Comment

Ebstein anomaly is described as partial atrialization of the right ventricle with tricuspid valve redundancy. Translation: large RA, small RV and tricuspid valve. There is always an associated patent foramen ovale (PFO) or atrial septal defect (ASD). Blood entering the small poorly contracting ventricle exits either through the pulmonary artery or back through the insufficient tricuspid valve. Blood begins to shunt though the PFO or ASD, causing cyanosis.

Clinically, the cyanosis is variable depending upon the volume of shunted blood and tricuspid regurgitation. Cyanosis will present with severe obstruction. EKG findings indicate right bundle branch block and Wolff–Parkinson–White syndrome (lengthening P-Q interval).

Radiographically, severely cyanotic infants may have decreased pulmonary vascularity with massive cardiomegaly from right atrial enlargement. If a substantial amount of right ventricle remains then patients will have normal vascularity with late RV hypertrophy characterized by a box-like configuration on chest films.

Prognosis varies as some patients need no intervention, while others require surgical reconstruction.

Notes

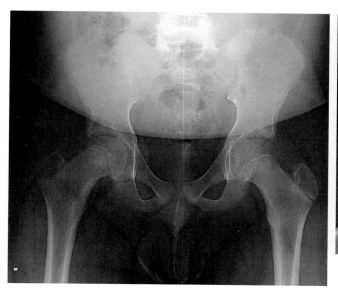 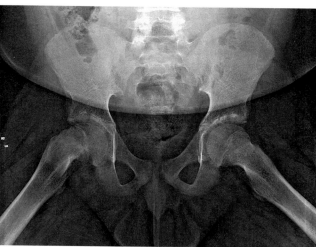

1. Is there a gender predominance?

2. Is this a Salter–Harris fracture?

3. At what age are boys affected?

4. What is the name of the osteonecrosis staging system on conventional radiograph osteonecrosis?

C A S E 117

Slipped Capital Femoral Epiphysis (SCFE)

1. Yes, 3:1 boys:girls.

2. SCFE is not a true Salter–Harris I; it is a fracture through the proliferative and hypertrophic zones, not the hypertrophic and provisional zones (SH I).

3. Boys at 14, girls at 11.

4. Ficat.

Reference

Boles CA, el-Khoury GY: Slipped capital femoral epiphysis. *Radiographics* 17:809–823, 1997.

Cross-Reference

Pediatric Radiology: THE REQUISITES, pp 243–244.

Comment

Slipped capital femoral epiphysis is displacement at the growth plate of the femoral epiphysis relative to the femoral neck. The femoral epiphysis or **H**ead displaces (relative to the the neck) **I**nferiorly and **P**osteriorly (HIP), conversely the femoral neck displaces superiorly and anteriorly. Slippage occurs just prior to closure of the growth plates (3:1 boys:girls) with presentation at 14 years for boys and 11 years for girls. The etiology is thought to be either an underlying metabolic disorder or abnormal biomechanics. The disorder is bilateral in half the cases. Presentation involves hip pain, limp, and decreased range of motion.

Radiographically, the big number to remember is one-sixth as that is the normal fraction of epiphysis that ought to extend laterally when a line is drawn over the lateral aspect of the femoral neck. Less than one-sixth is indicative of SCFE. Two views are used to evaluate the hip, the AP pelvis and the frog leg lateral. The frog leg lateral is more sensitive in demonstrating the slippage. Widened growth plates and metaphyseal irregularity are characteristic of SCFE. In chronic or long-standing cases bony spurring and remodeling may be seen.

Treatment options range from traction to surgical pinning aimed at achieving closure of the growth plate. Surgical manipulation or repositioning of the epiphysis relative to the metaphysis have shown poor results. Avascular necrosis is a long-term complication.

Notes

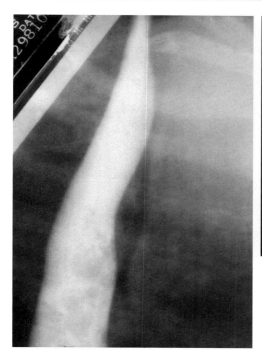
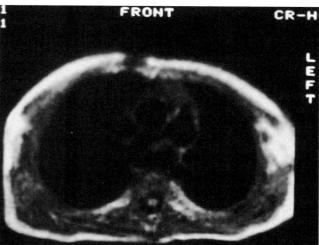

1. Which vascular slings are usually symptomatic?
2. Which vascular slings are normally asymptomatic?
3. What are the symptoms in this entity?
4. An aortic diverticulum causes what GI manifestation?

C A S E 118

Pulmonary Artery Sling

1. Double aortic arch, right arch with aberrant left subclavian and patent ductus arteriosus, and anomalous take-off of the right pulmonary artery.

2. Anomalous innominate artery, anomalous left common carotid, left arch with aberrant right subclavian artery, right arch with aberrant left subclavian artery.

3. Stridor, tachypnea, and respiratory distress.

4. Dysphagia lusoria.

Reference

Allen HD, Gutgesell HP, Clark EB, et al.: *Moss and Adams Heart Disease in Infants, Children and Adolescents: Including the Fetus and Young Adult,* 6th edn. Baltimore: Lippincott Williams & Wilkins, 2000, pp 636–651.

Cross-Reference

Pediatric Radiology: THE REQUISITES, 2nd edn, p 16.

Comment

Pulmonary sling is an abnormal development of the left pulmonary artery, in which it arises from the right pulmonary artery at the level of the carina and swings around behind the trachea passing to the anterior esophagus. On a conventional radiograph there may be an impression on the trachea or right mainstem bronchus. The impression may cause partial obstruction of the lung with asymmetric hyperlucency, a depressed left hilum, or anterior bowing of the trachea or mainstem bronchus. On a lateral view there is an anterior impression of the barium-filled esophagus. Anomalous origin of the left pulmonary artery is the only vascular malformation that will give a posterior tracheal impression and an anterior esophageal impression. Tracheal stenosis may develop in 50% of cases from either the extrinsic compression or an associated complete cartilaginous tracheal ring.

Anterior impressions on the trachea are caused by a high-riding innominate artery or carotid artery. Anterior impressions on the trachea with posterior impressions on the esophagus are caused by a double aortic arch or right aortic arch with an aberrant left sublclavian artery, aortic diverticulum, and left ligamentum arteriosum. Double aortic arch may also give a bilateral impression on the esophagus as the two aortic arches hug the esophagus and trachea before joining to form the descending aorta.

A posterior esophageal impression is due to either a left-sided arch with an aberrant right subclavian or a right aortic arch with an aberrant left subclavian artery.

Normally the vessels arising from the aorta from right to left are: innominate (bifurcating into the right subclavian and right common carotid), left common carotid, and left subclavian. An aberrant right subclavian does not arise from the innominate but rather distal to the subclavian. Aberrant right subclavian is the most common of the aortic arch anomalies and occurs with a frequency of 1 in 200. Alternatively, a right aortic arch with an aberrant left subclavian is a mirror image of the left subclavian with the exception of the variable ductus that when present will form a ring. Right aortic arch is associated with tetralogy, ventricular septal defect, and atrial septal defect, and coarctation.

Notes

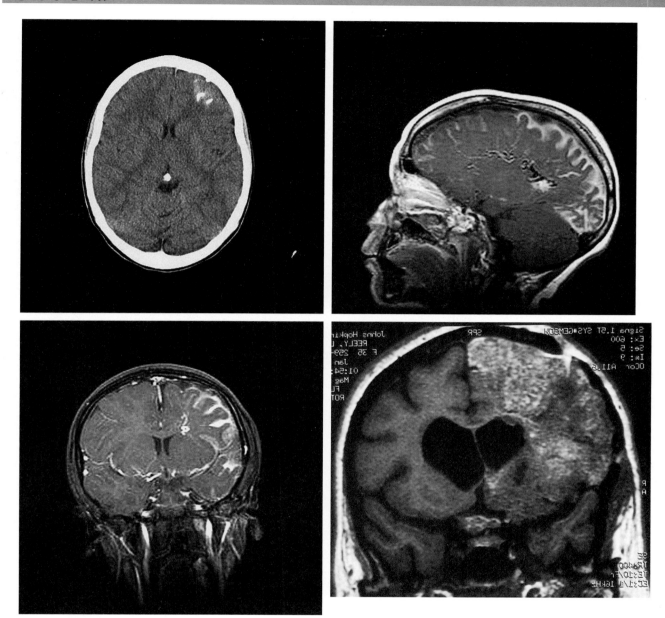

1. What is Dyke–Davidoff–Masson syndrome?

2. What is the significance of tram tracking?

3. What is platybasia?

4. At what age does tram tracking develop?

Sturge-Weber

1. Nonspecific hemicalvarial thickening due to cortical hemiatrophy.

2. Tram tracking may be seen on conventional radiographs of the skull and CT and represents cortical calcification due to cell death in different apposing gyri.

3. It is flattening of the skull base defined by a skull base angle greater than 143°.

4. Between 5 and 15 years.

Reference

Smirniotopoulos JG, Murphy FM: The phakomatoses. *Am J Neuroradiol* 13(2):725–746, 1992.

Cross-Reference

Pediatric Radiology: THE REQUISITES, p 272.

Comment

Sturge-Weber or encephalotrigeminal angiomatosis is a rare neurocutaneous disorder that features cutaneous vascular malformations manifesting as a facial port wine stain capillary, mental retardation, and seizures. Presumably between the fourth and eighth week of gestation there is a regional failure of differentiation involving the ectoderm and mesoderm overlying the face and brain, which leads to abnormal development of the vasculature affecting subsequent skin, leptomeningeal, and brain involvement. Others have suggested that the disorder lies in abnormal vein formation with poor outflow and subsequent persistence of primitive vascular plexus as collateral drainage. Either of these mechanisms leads to poor venous drainage of the cortex with progressive ischemia and functional loss. Clinically patients initially present with intractable seizures within the first year in addition to hemiparesis.

CT findings include "tram-track" cortical calcifications due to ischemia and necrosis with calcification in apposing gyri. Ischemia leads to cortical atrophy. The vacuum created by cortical atrophy is partially filled in by calvarial thickening, enlarging diploic space, elevation of petrous ridge, and increased pneumatization of the mastoid air cells, known as the Dyke–Davidoff–Masson syndrome.

MR will show similar atrophy as seen on CT. There will be intense enhancement in the areas of leptomeningeal angiomatosis. There is white matter hypointensity on T2 secondary to ischemia as well as calcification following the neonatal period. The deep venous structures will dilate secondary to the abnormal venous outflow.

Seizures are managed medically, although hemispherectomy is sometimes used to treat intractable epilepsy. Prognosis is poor.

Notes

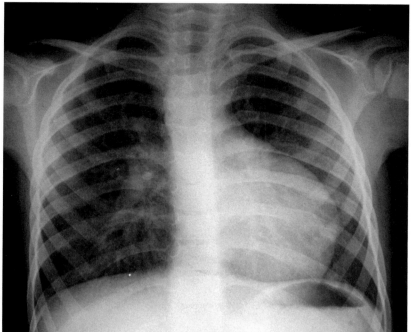

Cyanotic patient

1. Is there increased or decreased pulmonary vascularity?

2. If the vascularity was decreased what is your differential?

3. If the vascularity was increased what is your differential?

4. What percentage of patients with this entity will have transposition of the great vessels?

Tricuspid Atresia

1. Decreased pulmonary vascularity.

2. Cyanotic with decreased vascularity: tetralogy of Fallot (normal heart size), Ebstein anomaly, pulmonic atresia, and tricuspid atresia (the latter three with enlarged heart).

3. Cyanotic with increased vascularity: transposition of the great arteries, truncus, total anomalous pulmonary venous return, and single ventricle.

4. One-third with tricuspid atresia will have transposition.

Reference
Allen HD, Gutgesell HP, Clark EB, et al.: *Moss and Adams Heart Disease in Infants, Children and Adolescents: Including the Fetus and Young Adult,* 6th edn. Baltimore: Lippincott Williams & Wilkins, 2000, pp 636–651.

Cross-Reference
Pediatric Radiology: THE REQUISITES, 2nd edn, p 65.

Comment
Tricuspid atresia is complete absence of the tricuspid valve with no direct connection from the right atrium to the right ventricle. In order to sustain life a patent foramen ovale or atrial septal defect with either a ventricular septal defect (VSD) or patent ductus arteriosus (PDA) must be present. A right-to-left shunt will occur with blood traveling RA, LA, LV through VSD and RV or RA, LA, LV, Ao, PDA, and finally PA. Transposition is associated with tricuspid atresia in a third of cases.

Clinically, half of patients present with cyanosis on the first day. EKG results suggest LV hypertrophy, a finding that in the context of cyanosis is indicative of tricuspid atresia.

Radiographically, a normal or small heart and decreased pulmonary vascularity are noted. The left heart border demonstrates convexity and enlargement consistent with LV hypertrophy. The pulmonary artery trunk is not seen due to low flow and a concavity is seen at the mediastinal–cardiac junction.

Surgical repair ultimately involves the Fontan procedure following early temporizing interventions. The usually successful Fontan procedure is a direct anastomosis or bridging of the RA to the PA and has been linked to numerous complications, including elevated systemic pressure, pulmonary artery thrombosis, and arteriovenous malformations.

Notes

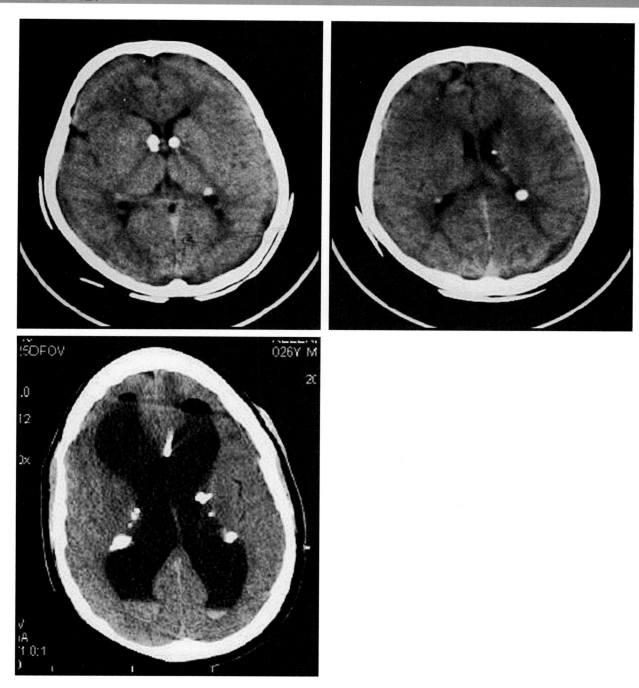

1. What is the Vogt triad?
2. What is Bourneville disease?
3. What is Pringle disease?
4. Is this an autosomal dominant or autosomal recessive inherited entity?

Tuberous Sclerosis

1. Adenoma sebaceum, mental retardation, and seizures.

2. Another name for tuberous sclerosis.

3. Another name for tuberous sclerosis.

4. Autosomal dominant.

Reference

Evans JC, Curtis J: The radiological appearances of tuberous sclerosis. *Br J Radiol* 73(865):91–98, 2000.

Cross-Reference

Pediatric Radiology: THE REQUISITES, p 272.

Comment

Tuberous sclerosis (TS) is a neurocutaneous disorder characterized by multiple hamartomas of the brain, eye, skin, and kidneys. Two genes on separate chromosomes (9 and 16) have been implicated. The gene on chromosome 16 encodes a protein named tuberin that appears to be homologous to GTPase-activating protein, an important cell proliferation regulator. Sixty per cent of new cases are from spontaneous mutations; the remainder is familial transmission through an autosomal dominant pattern of inheritance. Criteria have been devised to establish this clinical diagnosis.

Dysplasia of cortical stem cells produces abnormal masses of disorganized cells, hamartomas. These hamartomas may grow within the cortex, white matter, and subependymal region. On gross examination these hamartomas are firm and smooth and have been likened to potatoes by pathologists. These cortical tubers often cal-cify and may be found anywhere in the cortex. Hamartomas located in the subependymal region are nearly universal. In addition, subependymal giant cell astrocytomas are encountered as well. Hamartomas appear elsewhere in the body and include renal angiomyolipomas, retinal glial hamartomas, and pulmonary and cardiac myomas. Cysts may be found in the liver, kidneys, and pancreas. Cutaneous angiofibromas, shagreen patches, hypopigmentation, and pathognomonic subungal fibromas characterize TS skin involvement.

Clinically, mental retardation and seizures are seen in a majority of patients. Skin manifestations include adenoma sebaceum, which is neither an adenoma or of sebaceous origin. The reddish macules are in fact angiofibromas, a form of dermal hamartoma. Hamartomas are normal histologic components in an abnormal arrangement. Complete Vogt triad is seldom seen as expression of the disease is variable. The most common cause of death appears to be renal complications including bleeding angiomyolipoma, renal failure, and renal cell carcinoma.

On imaging the stage of myelination will play a central role in the intensity of the lesions. Subependymal nodules and cortical tubers will appear hyperintense on T1 and hypointense on T2 before myelination. Following myelination there is T1 isointensity and T2 hypointensity. Seventy-five percent of subependymal tubers calcify and may be detected using a sequence sensitive to susceptibility and blooming as in gradient echo. Cortical lesions are hyperintense on T1 and hypointense on T2 pre-myelination, while post-myelination the pattern inverts; T1 hypo and T2 hyper. White matter demonstrates pre-myelination a T2 hypointense signal and post-myelination a T2 hyperintense signal. Giant cell astrocytomas are located adjacent to the foramen of Monro and enhance intensely.

Notes

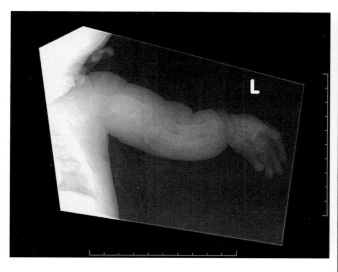
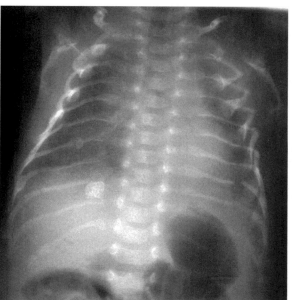

1. What are Wormian bones?

2. What is the differential diagnosis?

3. What is the incidence?

4. Scant callous formation is often encountered in this entity, true or false?

Osteogenesis Imperfecta

1. Wormian bones are prominent intersutural bones that arise from secondary ossification centers.

2. Nonaccidental trauma, congenital insensitivity to pain, hypophosphatasia, juvenile osteoporosis.

3. 20,000–60,000:1.

4. False. Excessive callous formation is characteristic.

Reference
Munoz C, Filly RA, Golbus MS: Osteogenesis imperfecta type II: prenatal sonographic diagnosis. *Radiology* 174:181–185, 1990.

Cross-Reference
Pediatric Radiology: THE REQUISITES, pp 206–208.

Comment
Bone is a type of connective tissue that holds the rare distinction of mineralization in the normal state. This mineralization makes up 65% of bone, while the remaining 35% is organic matrix that houses osteocytes, osteoclasts, and osteoblasts. The organic matrix is held together by collagen protein that acts as the backbone. The collagen is produced by osteoblasts that spin it into a triple helical structure. Osteogenesis imperfecta (OI) is a collagen synthesis disease that is characterized by osteoporosis and skeletal fragility. In fact, OI is a spectrum of disorders that involve different mutations in the genes that code for collagen. Many other tissues are made of collagen and demonstrate manifestations of the disease; blue sclera, deafness, poor dentition, ligamentous laxity, and easy bruising.

The disease is characterized into four types: two congenital and two latent.

Type 1 (AD): Previously known as the tarda form, thin, brittle bones that fracture with exuberant callus formation are characteristic. Skeletal bowing and epiphyseal enlargement are the bony sequelae. Inheritance is autosomal dominant with variable penetrance. Presentation is during the late teenage years with blue sclerae (90%) and occasional (20%) deafness secondary to otosclerosis.

Type 2 (AR): The congenital form is lethal and can be detected in utero by multiple fractures, demineralized calvaria, and a femur length more than three standard deviations bellow the mean. Blue sclerae are always present. Inheritance is autosomal recessive.

Type 3 (AR): Fractures with excessive callus are seen at birth. Normal sclerae and hearing are present.

Type 4 (AD): Osteoporosis, occasional fractures, and discolored teeth are normal. Normal sclerae are present.

Therapy is directed at preventing fractures and straightening long bones via the use of intramedullary rods.

Notes

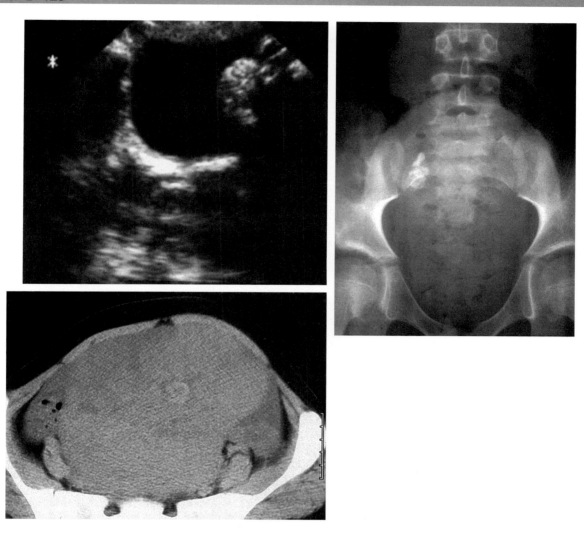

1. What percentage of these lesions are bilateral?

2. Is there a potential for malignant transformation?

3. 66% of ovarian tumors in girls up to age 15 are of what type?

4. These lesions place the patient at an increase risk for ovarian torsion, true or false?

Ovarian Teratoma

1. 15% are bilateral.

2. Yes, 1–2% may transform to squamous cell carcinoma.

3. Mature cystic teratoma.

4. True. Any adnexal mass places the patient at increase risk for ovarian torsion.

Reference

Outwater EK, Siegelman ES, Hunt JL: Ovarian teratomas: tumor types and imaging characteristics. *Radiographics* 21:475–490, 2001.

Cross-Reference

Pediatric Radiology: THE REQUISITES, p 191.

Comment

The benign cystic ovarian teratoma accounts for two-thirds of pediatric ovarian tumors. Teratomas are germ cell tumors derived from the three germ layers, ectoderm, mesoderm, and endoderm. Other germ cell tumors include the malignant dysgerminomas and endodermal sinus tumors. Cystic teratomas are also known as dermoids due to their predominantly ectodermal make up—remember that teeth, skin, hair, and oil (sebum) from sebaceous glands are all ectodermal in origin.

The tumor often presents at 6–10 years as a mass and/or abdominal pain. Plain films demonstrate calcifications in half the cases. Ultrasound shows cystic components with hyperechoic fat and calcified components. A mural nodule, the dermoid plug, is characteristic and occurs in two-thirds of cases. The "tip-of-the-iceberg" sign refers to the echogenic calcium and hair that prevents transmission of sound waves, obscuring the posterior wall of the lesion. Fat–fluid levels may also be noted. CT will further demonstrate the soft tissue, calcium, and fat in the teratoma.

Benign cystic teratomas are treated by cystectomy or wedge resection if bilateral involvement is present.

Notes

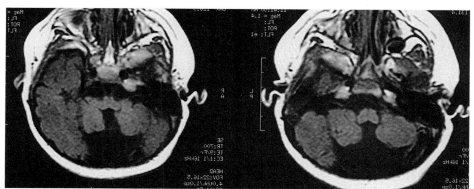

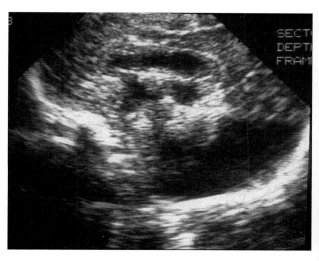

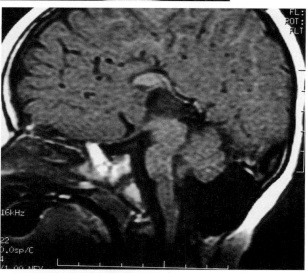

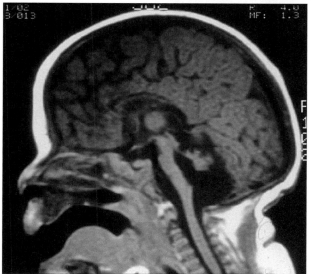

1. What is the PHACE syndrome?

2. What genetic associations are seen with this entity?

3. What CNS associations are there with this entity?

4. What is Joubert syndrome?

Dandy–Walker Malformation

1. **P**osterior fossa malformations, **H**emangiomas, **A**rterial anomalies, **C**oarctation of the aorta, **C**ardiac defects, and **E**ye abnormalities.

2. PHACE, Meckel–Gruber syndrome, Warburg syndrome, Aicardi syndrome, and neurocutaneous melanosis.

3. Agenesis of the corpus callosum, gray matter heterotopia, polymicrogyria, agyria, and schizencephaly.

4. Autosomal dominant disorder with vermian hypoplasia but no cystic component as seen in Dandy–Walker malformation.

References

Pilu G, Visentin A, Valeri B: The Dandy-Walker complex and fetal sonography. *Ultrasound Obstet Gynecol* 16(2):115–117, 2000.

Barkovich AJ, Maroldo TV: Magnetic resonance imaging of normal and abnormal brain development. *Top Magn Reson Imaging* 5(2):96–122, 1993.

Cross-Reference

Pediatric Radiology: THE REQUISITES, pp 268–271.

Comment

Dandy–Walker malformation is defined as partial or complete agenesis of the cerebellar vermis, cystic dilatation of the fourth ventricle, enlargement of the posterior fossa with upward displacement of the transverse sinuses. Dandy–Walker malformation occurs due to migrational abnormality of Purkinje cells from the germinal matrix in the roof of the fourth ventricle. An ischemic event to the fourth ventricle is thought to prevent proper development of the foramina of Luschka and Magendie. Partial or total CSF outflow obstruction follows. A large fourth ventricle cyst splays the developing cerebellum, preventing fusion and vermis formation.

Clinically, there is some combination of macrocephaly, seizures, and developmental delay. Hydrocephalus (75%) leads to headaches, a common presentation.

On MR there is enlargement of the posterior fossa and elevation of the tentorium. The classic torcular–lambdoid inversion is common. Normally, the lambdoid suture confluence is higher than the torcular, while in Dandy–Walker malformation the relationship is inverted with the torcular residing more superiorly. The vermis is small if not totally absent. An enlarged posterior fossa will be filled with a large cyst.

Symptomatic patients with hydrocephalus are VP shunted.

Notes

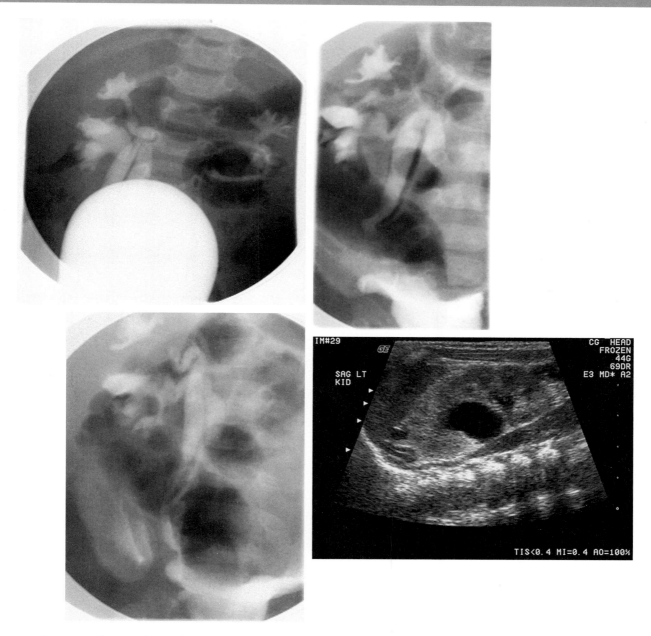

1. Does this entity have a familial incidence?

2. What is the significance of the "drooping lily" sign?

3. What is the most common neonatal abdominal mass?

4. Is power Doppler more or less sensitive to flow than color Doppler?

Duplex Collecting System

1. Yes, duplications are familial.

2. The drooping lily sign signifies the presence of an obstructed (nonfunctioning) upper pole of a duplex system.

3. Hydronephrosis.

4. Power Doppler is more sensitive to flow.

Reference

Fernbach SK, Feinstein KA, Spencer K, et al.: Ureteral duplication and its complications. *Radiographics* 17:109–127, 1997.

Cross-Reference

Pediatric Radiology: THE REQUISITES, pp 157–160.

Comment

A duplex kidney refers to a kidney that is drained by two ureters; perhaps a more accurate description would be duplex ureters. Duplication occurs as a broad spectrum ranging from a bifid pelvis to complete duplication of the ureters. The cause is thought to arise from premature splitting of the ureteric buds. Normally ureteric buds migrate to meet the blastema, inducing differentiation of the normal kidney.

No residency is complete without getting pimped on the Weigert–Meyer rule. The ureter draining the lower pole inserts in its normal trigonal position (orthotopic). The upper pole ureter inserts within the bladder ectopically (abnormal position), medially, and inferiorly. In extreme cases the ureter may insert into the uterus, vagina, or urethra, locations that will present with incontinence. The further the distance from the expected location the more likely a dysplastic kidney. The upper pole is often obstructed and associated with a ureterocele. The incidence of reflux is actually the same as in the general population. Refluxing upper pole ureters tend to be more common on the left, especially in girls.

Radiographic features include mass effect from a hydronephrotic upper pole, abnormal axis of the collecting system, fewer calyces with a drooping lily sign, renal and ureteric lateral displacement, spiral course of the ureter, bladder filling defects.

Notes

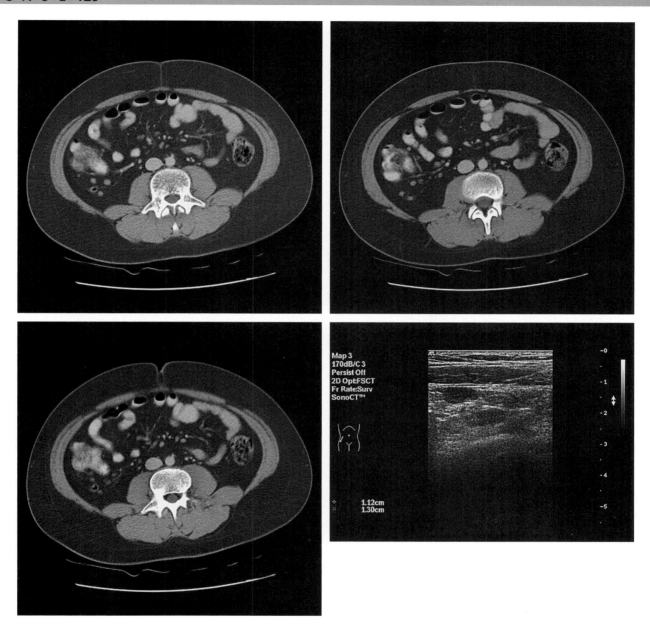

1. What are the differential considerations in the pediatric age group for right lower quadrant pain?

2. What have been considered the most likely etiologic agents?

3. What is the treatment?

4. Is a normal-appearing appendix on CT necessary to make this diagnosis?

Mesenteric Adenitis

1. Appendicitis, constipation, diabetic ketoacidosis, intussusception, pneumonia, urinary tract infection, mesenteric adenitis, ectopic pregnancy, ovarian cyst, testicular and ovarian torsion, and renal calculi.

2. The most likely etiologic agents are *Yersinia enterocolitica*, *Helicobacter jejuni*, *Campylobacter jejuni*, and *Salmonella* or *Shigella*.

3. The treatment is conservative.

4. Yes, a normal-appearing appendix is necessary to make the diagnosis of mesenteric adenitis by CT.

Reference

Rao PM, Rhea JT, Novelline RA: CT diagnosis of mesenteric adenitis. *Radiology* 202(1):145–149, 1997.

Comment

Mesenteric adenitis describes a condition in which enlarged mesenteric lymph nodes are associated with abdominal pathology (secondary form) or as an isolated (primary form) finding. Primary mesenteric adenitis is defined as right-sided adenopathy in the absence of an acute inflammatory process. Secondary mesenteric adenopathy is associated with celiac disease, appendicitis, inflammatory bowel disease. The primary form is considered more common in children than adults. Some have suggested that the primary form reflects nodal enlargement secondary to a low-grade bowel inflammatory process. Clinically, patients present with abdominal pain, fever, leukocyosis, nausea, vomiting, diarrhea, and diffuse or right lower quadrant pain and tenderness. These nonspecific findings lead to a broad differential including, potentially, appendicitis. In fact, in many clinical cases, it is difficult to distinguish mesenteric adenitis from appendicitis. The therapy for mesenteric adentitis is conservative and therefore its detection by CT may save a patient from a trip to the OR.

On CT, primary mesenteric adenitis is defined as three or more enlarged nodes (>0.5 cm on short axis) in the right lower quadrant with absence of other local pathology, i.e., appendicitis. The nodes are usually larger and more widely distributed in mesenteric adenitis than in appendicitis. Be careful not to mistake unopacified small bowel for an enlarged node; oral contrast is key in differentiating the two. Ultrasound will demonstrate a cluster of nodes that will appear rounded and increasingly hypoechoic with tenderness on transduce palpation. Remember: the eye doesn't see what the mind doesn't know, so include it in your rule out appendicitis hunt.

Notes

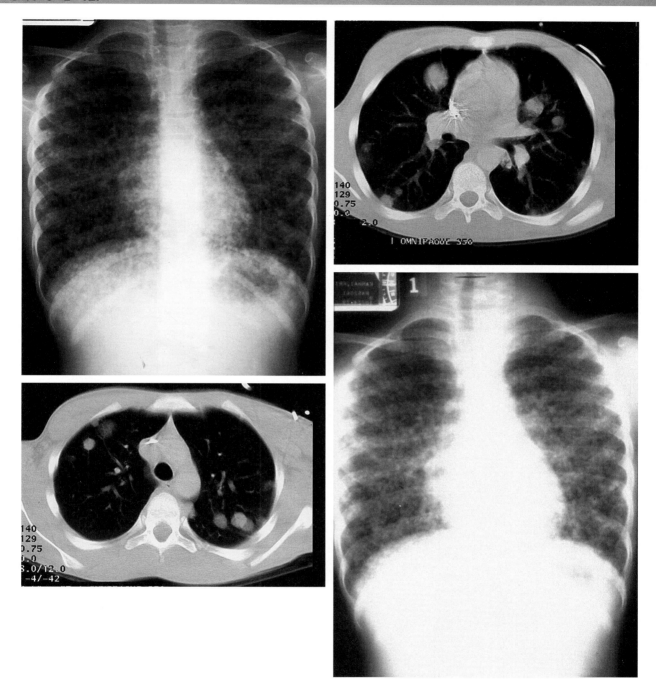

1. Multiple granulomas are more commonly fungal or tuberculous in etiology?

2. What are the most common primarily pulmonary malignancies in children?

3. Are pulmonary metastases usually calcified?

4. What lung metastases are associated with pneumothorax?

C A S E 127

Pediatric Pulmonary Nodules

1. Multiple granulomas are more commonly fungal than tuberculous.

2. Bronchogenic carcinoma, leiomyosarcoma, rhabdomyosarcoma, hemangiopericytoma, and Askin tumor represent the most common primary pulmonary malignancies in children.

3. No, pulmonary mets are usually noncalcified with the exception of thyroid carcinoma. Osteosarcoma metastasis will ossify in the lung and may give a calcified appearance.

4. Osteosarcoma and Wilms are associated with pneumothorax.

Reference
Eggli KD, Newman B: Nodules, masses, and pseudo-masses in the pediatric lung. *Radiol Clin N Am* 31(3):651–666, 1993.

Cross-Reference
Pediatric Radiology: THE REQUISITES, p 40.

Comment
On identifying a pulmonary nodule in the pediatric chest, it is important to decide whether it is solitary or one of many. A small solitary pulmonary nodule in a child is most likely of infectious origin; healed primary tuberculosis. Alternatively, a larger solitary nodule may represent an early focal round pneumonia, sequestration, or possible abscess. Multiple small nodules may represent inflammatory granulomata, pulmonary metastasis as in this case, varicella, lymphangiectasia, lymphocytic interstitial pneumonitis (LIP), laryngeal papillomatosis, or septic emboli. Multiple large nodules are primarily of metastatic origin: Wilms tumor, Ewing sarcoma, and osteosarcoma.

Metastatic lung disease is far more common than primary lung neoplasm in children. Spread to the lungs is usually hematogenous; however, tumors may spread via the lymphatics, airspaces, or pleural space. Wilms tumor, the most common metastatic lung neoplasm, spreads through the venous system. Wilms metastasis characteristically appears as large multiple ovoid masses ranging in size from small to large. Thyroid mets, by contrast, have a milliary appearance with multiple small nodules that range between 2 and 3 mm. The thyroid metastatic nodules are characteristically calcified. Differential diagnositic considerations for small, calcified nodules include healed varicella pneumonia, and histoplasmosis.

In summary, most pulmonary masses in childhood are nonmalignant. Nodular disease is overwhelmingly a result of prior granulomatous infection. Pulmonary mets are caused by Wilms, osteosarcoma, and Ewing sarcoma. Primary malignant neoplasm is exceedingly rare in the pediatric age group.

	Large	**Small**
Multiple	Osteosarcoma	Varicella
	Wilms tumor	Thyroid mets
	Ewing sarcoma	Granulomata
	Septic emboli	Laryngeal
		Papillomatosis
		LIP
		Lymphangiectasia
Solitary	Round pneumonia	Hamartoma
	Abscess (bacterial, fungal)	Granuloma
	Plasma cell granuloma	AV malformation or
	CCAM	varix
	Sequestration	

Notes

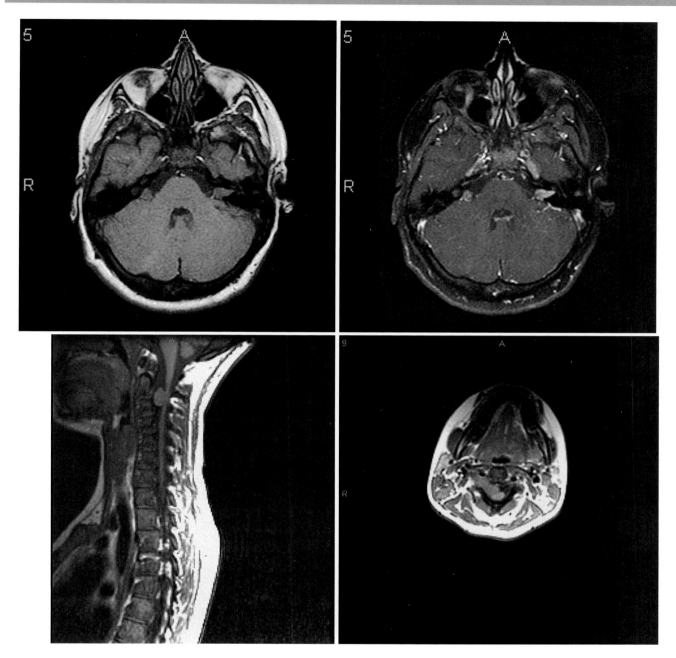

1. How many letters in von Recklinghausen?
2. What is the significance of the above question?
3. How many alphanumerics are in neurofibromatosis type 2?
4. What is the significance of the above question?

Neurofibromatosis Type 2

1. 17.

2. von Recklinghausen or NF-1 is found on the 17th chromosome.

3. 22.

4. NF-2 is found on the 22nd chromosome.

Reference

Smirniotopoulos JG, Murphy FM: The phakomatoses. *Am J Neuroradiol* 13(2):725–746, 1992.

Cross-Reference

Pediatric Radiology: THE REQUISITES, p 272.

Comment

Neurofibromatosis type 2 is a neurocutaneous disorder of one of the phakomatoses that is entirely unrelated to neurofibromatosis type 1. NF-2 is one-tenth as common as NF-1. The NF-2 chromosomal abnormality is located on the 22nd chromosome and codes for a tumor suppressor protein named schwannomin. NF-2 consists of multiple cranial nerve schwannomas (including the pathognomonic bilateral vestibular schwannomas), multiple meningiomas, spinal ependymomas, and nerve sheath schwannomas. Specific diagnostic criteria were revised in 1997 from the consensus conference held in 1987 that laid down specifics for both NF-1 and NF-2.

Clinically, neurofibromas are not a feature of NF-2, prompting Smirniotopolus and Murphy to suggest a term that actually describes the condition, MISME syndrome (Multiple Inherited Schwannomas, Meningiomas, and Ependymomas). Hearing loss occurs between the second and fourth decade.

On MR schwannomas appear as round extra-axial masses that are dark on T1 and bright on T2. Enhancement is intense and homogeneous unless hemorrhage in present. The schwannomas are most commonly found in the cerebellopontine angle where they involve the vestibular branch of the 8th nerve and may compress the 7th and cochlear branch (leading to facial paralysis and tinnitus). The 5th, 9th, and 10th, in order of frequency, may also be involved. Meningiomas appear isodense on T1 and T2 and light up intensely on enhanced scans. Meningiomas are dural based and will often demonstrate the characteristic dural tail. Spinal involvement may include both schwannomas and meningiomas. Schwannomas may present as nerve sheath tumors extending out of the neural foramen in a dumbbell configuration or as intramedullary masses. Ependymomas are intramedullary and often involve the conus or filum.

Treatment options range from observation to radiosurgery in qualifying cases. Prognosis varies with expression of the disease.

Notes

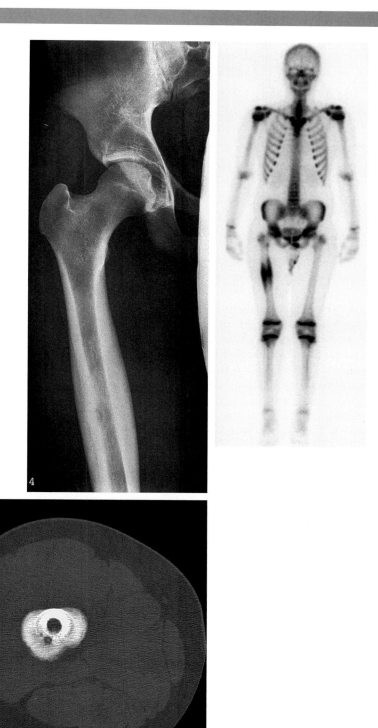

4

1. What is the history?

2. What is the differential diagnosis?

3. What is the therapy?

4. Scintigraphy demonstrates a cold lesion. True or false?

Osteoid Osteoma

1. Dull aching pain most pronounced at night and responds to aspirin.

2. Brodie's abscess, stress fracture.

3. Radiofrequency ablation.

4. False. These lesions are hot on bone scan.

Reference

Kransdorf MJ, Stull MA, Gilkey FW, et al.: Osteoid osteoma. *Radiographics* 11:671–696, 1991.

Cross-Reference

Pediatric Radiology: THE REQUISITES, p 223.

Comment

An osteoid osteoma is a highly vascularized, benign, matrix-producing tumor measuring less than 2 cm. Lesions greater than 2 cm are classified as osteoblastomas. Osteoblastoma is histologically identical but differs in size, symptomatology, and location.

The nidus is a term describing the central radiolucent lesion that often contains a mineralized center. The lytic-appearing portion is nonmineralized osteoid intermixed with fibrovascular connective tissue and surrounded by reactive sclerotic bone. The tumor produces prostaglandins that account for "pain out of proportion to the lesion size." These patients present with night-time pain responsive to aspirin. Seventy-five per cent of patients are between 5 and 35 years, with males composing 65% of those affected.

Radiographically, the lesion appears as a small radiolucent lesion with surrounding reactive sclerosis depending upon the osteoma's location. Osteoid osteomas usually arise in the cortex but may originate in cancellous bone. The femur, tibia, and humerus are most commonly affected. Spine involvement may lead to scoliosis. CT is the modality of choice in detecting the nidus.

Therapy ranges from conservative treatment of analgesics to surgical excision. A successful alternative to surgery is image-guided radiofrequency ablation performed by musculoskeletal radiologists.

Notes

Patient 1

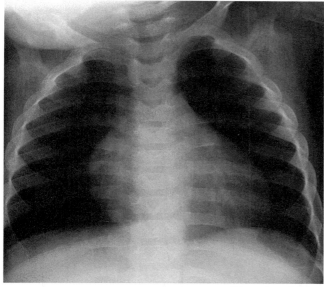

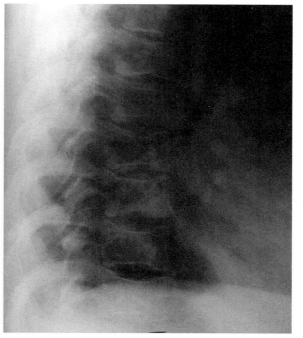

Patient 1

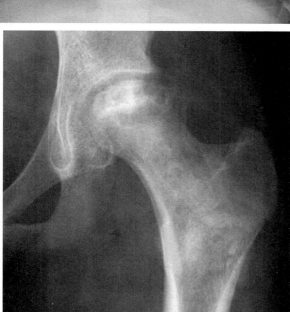

Patient 2

1. When does this disease begin to manifest?

2. What is dactylitis?

3. Avascular necrosis of the humeral epiphysis is seen in which variant of this entity?

4. Would you expect to see inner table widening?

Sickle Cell Disease

1. Fetal hemoglobin persists for 6 months. HbSS will dominate after this period and lead to the clinical disease.

2. The first clinical signs of sickle cell in which small tubular bone infarction of the hands and feet leads to fever, pallor, and swelling of the hands and feet.

3. Sickle C hemoglobinopathy.

4. No, although there is diploic space widening due to increased hematopoiesis; the outer, not the inner table, is affected. This is due to the physics of a pressure within two parallel curved surfaces. The force is exerted only on the outer surface.

Reference

Lonergan GJ, Cline DB, Abbondanzo SL: Sickle cell anemia. *Radiographics* 21:971–994, 2001.

Cross-Reference

Pediatric Radiology: THE REQUISITES, pp 217–218.

Comment

Sickle cell anemia is a heritable defect in the composition of hemoglobin that leads to deformity and loss of function of red blood cells. The disease manifests as an anemia with infarctions present in multiple organ systems. The spleen grows in size as it sequesters the sickled red blood cells packing the sinuses and splenic cords until stasis produces thrombosis and infarction. A new theory of small-vessel ischemia or microinfarction of bone and other tissue appears to be related to the increased expression of adhesion molecules on the membranes of nonsickled cells, in contrast to the previous sickled sludging hypothesis. With autosplenectomy by early adolescence a vital defense against blood-borne microorganisms is lost. Coupled with defects in the complement system, encapsulated organisms can thrive in the chronically immune-weakened anoxic tissues found in sicklers.

Marrow hyperplasia, infarction, and infection all demonstrate characteristic radiographic abnormalities. Marrow hyperplasia manifests on conventional radiographs as widening of long-bone metaphyses, widening of trabeculae, thinning of the cortex, and osteo-penia. Widening of the diploic space in the skull is associated with outer table thinning. Bone infarction is most commonly seen in the proximal femur, proximal humerus, distal femur, or proximal tibia. Infarction will appear as patchy lucency and sclerosis of medullary bone. Cortical bone infarction leads to periosteal reaction with new bone formation. H-shaped vertebrae develop due to infarction of the relatively hypovascular central portion of the vertebral body.

Osteomyelitis is common in these patients. One theory suggests a bacteremia caused by loss of intestinal wall integrity due to infarction. *Staphylococcus* and *Salmonella* are common bugs. Radiographically, osteomyelitis will appear as erosions, lysis, or periosteal reaction. As infection is under pressure the pus will bore through the cortex producing an involucrum.

Notes

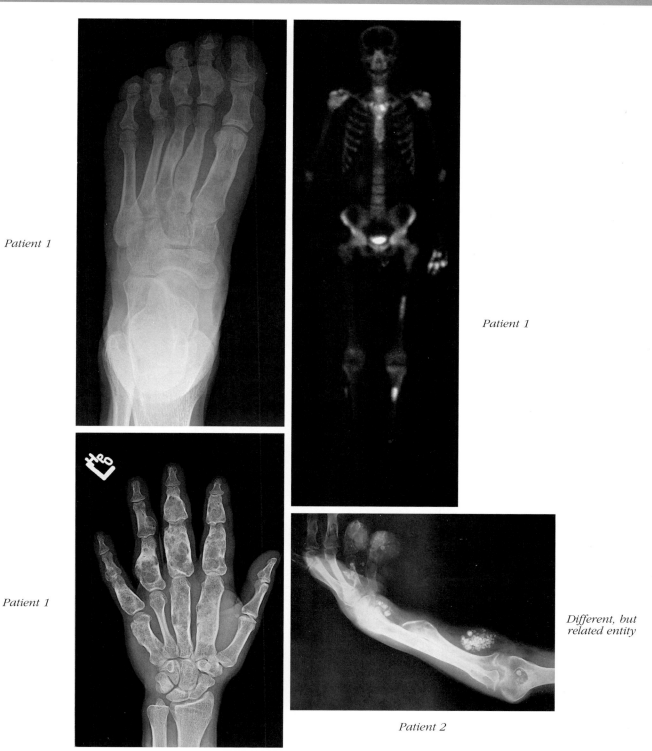

Patient 1

Patient 1

Patient 1

*Different, but
related entity*

Patient 2

1. What is the inheritance of this disorder?

2. Are hand lesions commonly calcified?

3. What is the appearance on MR?

4. Are these lesions hot or cold on bone scan?

Multiple Enchondromatosis (Ollier Disease and Maffucci Syndrome)

1. There is no inheritance, it is nonhereditary.

2. No, they more often do not calcify.

3. Low signal on T1, high signal on T2, Lesions appear characteristically lobular.

4. Hot, as there is enchondral ossification, hyperemia, and active bone formation.

References

Flach HZ, Ginai AZ, Oosterhuis JW: Best cases from the AFIP: Maffucci syndrome: radiologic and pathologic findings. *Radiographics* 21:1311–1316, 2001.

Mainzer F, Minagi H, Steinbach HL: The variable manifestations of multiple enchondromatosis. *Radiology* 99:377–388, 1971.

Cross-Reference

Pediatric Radiology: THE REQUISITES, p 209.

Comment

Enchondromas are benign tumors of cartilage rests that are deposited within the medullary cavity by the growth plate as it marches away from the diaphysis in normal growth and development. Enchondromas are the most common of the intraosseous cartilage tumors and are commonly found in the metaphysis of long bones (bones that undergo enchondral ossification), especially those of the feet and hands. The lesions may either be solitary or multiple. If multiple sites are affected asymmetrically throughout the body the entity is referred to as Ollier disease or multiple enchondromatosis. Alternatively, symmetric involvement of the body with cranial lesions is referred to as generalized enchondromatosis. If soft tissue hemangiomas are present the eponym changes from Ollier to Maffucci syndrome. Malignant degeneration (chondrosarcoma) may occur in a third of patients presenting as a sudden onset of pain or increase in lesion size.

Radiographically, multiple lucent metaphyseal lesions often contain either dense punctate, floccular calcifications, or rings and arcs. Lucency, most often in the hands and feet, is secondary to replacement of bone by nonossified cartilage. The lesions are slowly expansile, yielding a thinned cortex without cortical penetration. Eventually these lesions may result in angular limb deformities.

Notes

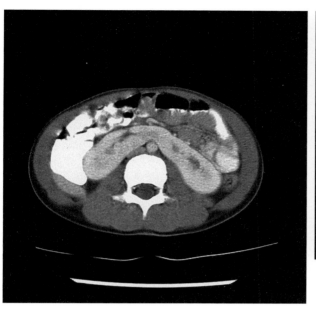 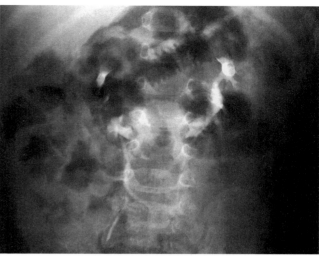

1. What is the most common congenital anomaly of the GU tract?

2. What is the incidence of bladder exstrophy?

3. Is bladder exstrophy associated with epispadia or hypospadias?

4. Which of the following is not associated with bladder exstrophy: rectal prolapse, bifid or unicornuate uterus, ectopic ureterocele, spinal anomalies?

C A S E 132

Renal Ectopia

1. Ureteropelvic junction obstruction.

2. 1:50,000 is the incidence of bladder exstrophy (rare).

3. Bladder exstrophy is always associated with epispadia.

4. Ectopic ureteroceles are not associated with bladder exstrophy.

Cross-Reference

Pediatric Radiology: THE REQUISITES, p 157.

Comment

Ectopia denotes an abnormal organ/tissue address. In this instance the kidneys, which normally migrate superiorly to the renal fossa, may rest anywhere along their path. Ectopic kidneys are malpositioned, usually in the pelvis, and demonstrate abnormal architecture with loss of renal sinus fat readily recognizable by ultrasound. Crossed fused ectopia involves the affected kidney residing on the contralateral side fused to the orthotopic or normally positioned kidney. Crossed fused ectopia is often associated with anorectal malformation, renal dysplasia, or VUR. In horseshoe kidney, fusion of the lower poles prevents complete ascent of the kidneys as they are "hooked" on the inferior mesenteric vein. The collecting system is complex and often prone to urine stasis leading to infection, stone formation, and scarring. Plain films (or formerly EU) will show a "W" (lower poles closer than upper poles) axis to the kidneys instead of a normal "M" (upper poles closer than lower poles) position. The horseshoe kidney carries with it an increased risk of adenocarcinoma, Wilms tumor, and renovascular hypertension. Horseshoe patients are also at risk for serious bleeding secondary to trauma as the isthmus is sandwiched between the abdominal wall and the vertebral column. Patients are counseled to cut down on the roller derby and rugby.

Notes

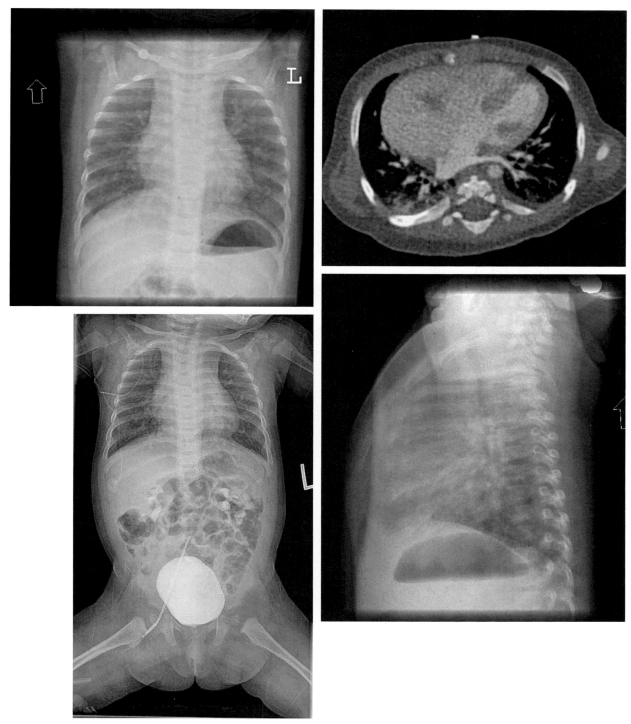

Noncyanotic patient

1. Is there increased or decreased pulmonary vascularity?

2. If the vascularity was normal what is your differential?

3. If the vascularity was increased what is your differential?

4. What is the classic angiogram finding?

Endocardial Cushion Defects

1. It is increased.

2. Acyanotic with normal vascularity: aortic stenosis, pulmonic stenosis, coarctation, and interrupted aortic arch.

3. Endocardial cushion defect, atrial septal defect (ASD), patent ductus arteriosus (enlarged LA and enlarged aorta), and ventricular septal defect (VSD) (enlarged LA and normal aorta).

4. The "gooseneck deformity" representing the LV outflow track.

Reference

Rauzzino M, Oakes WJ: Chiari II malformation and syringomyelia. *Neurosurg Clin N Am* 6(2):293–309, 1995.

Cross-Reference

Pediatric Radiology: THE REQUISITES, 2nd edn, p 58.

Comment

Endocardial cushion defects or atrioventricular (AV) defects are anomalies of development at the interface of the atria and ventricles that lead to a wide variety of cardiac abnormalities. They are strongly associated with Down syndrome (40%). Sixty-five per cent of Down patients have congenital heart disease with one-third of those having an AV canal.

The endocardial cushions contribute to the formation of the lower atrial septum as well as the upper portion of the ventricular septum, the AV septa, tricuspid, and mitral valves. Abnormalities include absence or malformation of the AV septum, mitral and tricuspid valve anomalies, ostium primum ASD, high VSD, cleft mitral valve, cleft tricuspid valve, common AV valve, and insertion of the chordae tendineae on the intraventricular septum. The endocardial cushion cells are derivatives of the neural crest cells and are often associated with facial anomalies. An ostium primum defect in the low atrial septum will lead to a left-to-right shunt. A complete AV canal is the most severe anomaly with malformation of all septa that lead to significant clinical symptomatology. Shunting of blood can occur at multiple levels with a wide variety of hemodynamic abnormalities.

Clinically, these patients present according to their defect. Isolated ostium primum defects are detected on physical exam by auscultation of a murmur. Complete AV canal with left-to-right shunting across both the ASD and VSD present with congestive heart failure, dyspnea, recurrent pneumonia, and failure to thrive.

Radiographically, the ostium primum defect may demonstrate a normal or slightly enlarged heart. Complete AV canal will appear as right-sided enlargement and shunt vascularity with prominence of the pulmonary arteries. The left atrium is usually of normal size unless there is mitral regurgitation. The aorta is frequently not seen. On angiogram a 30° right anterior oblique demonstrates the classic "gooseneck" deformity of the LV outflow tract, a finding most often appreciated in Kentucky motels.

The prognosis is variable as early surgical repair is vital in preventing development of pulmonary hypertension.

Notes

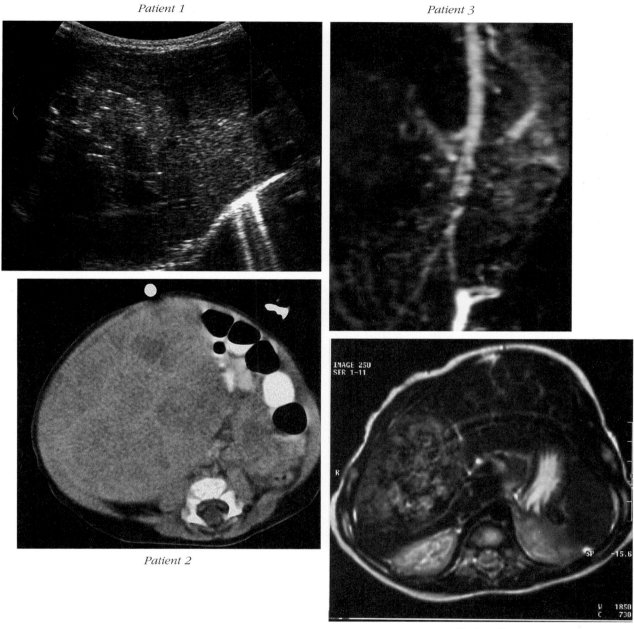

Patient 1

Patient 3

Patient 2

Patient 3

1. What is the most common primary hepatic tumor in pediatrics?
2. Is this lesion most commonly single, multiple, or diffuse?
3. What is the most common presentation of this entity?
4. Would this lesion enhance early or late on a dynamic scan?

Hepatocellular Carcinoma (HCC)

1. Hepatoblastoma.

2. Multiple, approximately 50%.

3. Abdominal mass.

4. Early, blood supply is arterial.

Reference

Siegel MJ. Pediatric liver imaging. *Semin Liver Dis* 21(2): 251–269, 2001.

Cross-Reference

Pediatric Radiology: THE REQUISITES, 2nd edn, p 134.

Comment

Hepatoma is the second most common primary hepatic tumor in children. It occurs between 10 and 15 years of age with a rare early peak at 1–4 years. Males are affected more often than females. There is an association with chronic liver disease (cirrhosis, glycogen storage, tyrosinemia, biliary atresia, and hepatitis). In Japan, Asia, and Africa there is a high association with hepatitis B and aflatoxin exposure.

On CT, hepatoma can either appear as a focal mass or a diffusely infiltrative process. There may be a single large lesion (40%), multiple lesions affecting both lobes of the liver (50%), or diffuse infiltration (10%). The lesion is heterogeneous with necrosis, cyst, and hemorrhage. Vascular invasion is common, whereas biliary is not. On MR, common findings include a capsule, central scar, and septae. The tumor may appear hyper, hypo, or isointense on T1 and hyperintense on T2. The ultrasound appearance is variable with some hepatomas appearing hyper, hypo, or isoechoic. HCC cannot be differentiated from hepatoblastoma by imaging alone. Alpha-fetoprotein levels are elevated.

Three percent of hepatoma is of the fibrolamellar type. It occurs in young adults approximately 20 years of age. There is no association with chronic liver disease. Fifty to sixty per cent are resectable at presentation with therefore a better prognosis than other HCC sybtypes. Only complete resection is curative. Pathologically, these lesions have a central scar with dystrophic calcification. Necrosis and hemorrhage are rare. The lesions are solitary homogeneous and well demarcated. A calcified central scar is pathognomonic. The main differential is focal nodular hyperplasia. Alpha-fetoprotein is not elevated.

Treatment for HCC consists of surgical resection. By contrast the prognosis is worse than hepatoblastoma with only 15–30% resectable at presentation.

Notes

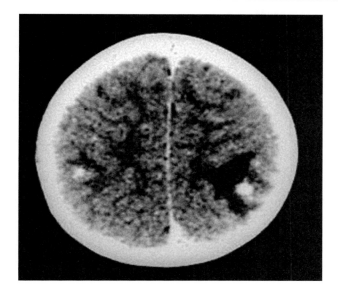

1. How might one increase the sensitivity to calcification on MR?

2. A 180° refocusing pulse is employed in gradient or spin echo imaging?

3. Adjusting the flip angle is a parameter of gradient or spin echo imaging?

4. Patients with cochlear implants may not be scanned by MR, true or false?

Cysticercosis

1. Gradient echo imaging is relatively sensitive to susceptibility artifact. So-called "blooming" will indicate the presence of calcification.

2. Spin echo.

3. Gradient echo.

4. True. Cochlear implants are an absolute contraindication.

Reference

Zee CS, Go JL, Kim PE, et al.: Imaging of neurocysticercosis. *Neuroimaging Clin N Am* 10(2):391–407, 2000.

Cross-Reference

Pediatric Radiology: THE REQUISITES, p 278.

Comment

Neurocysticercosis is the most common parasitic infection of the central nervous system. Eggs are ingested via contaminated water or food and penetrate through the intestine to spread hematogenously to the CNS, muscle, or eye. The larva lodges itself in the brain parenchyma and forms a cyst. Viable cysts tend to be asymptomatic and form little local reaction. Only when the cyst dies is there significant inflammatory edema and mass effect. The infection may involve the subarachnoid space, ventricles, and spinal cord as well as the brain parenchyma.

As stated, the initial infection is silent, as only dying cysts will induce an inflammatory reaction. Clinically, patients present with seizures, neurologic deficits, and headache. Hydrocephalus develops due to either direct obstruction by the cysts or to meningitis, which impairs resorption.

On imaging, CT is most sensitive to detection of calcification. Calcification represents a marker for longstanding infection as calcification requires at least 3 years to develop. Cysts are located most commonly in the cortex followed by the brainstem, cerebellum, and spinal cord. Intraparenchymal cysts may appear either cystic or solid. Solid lesions often contain calcification, while cystic lesions demonstrate rim enhancement. The symptomatic dying cystercircus induces an inflammatory reaction and vasogenic edema easily detectable as a high T2 signal. Infection of the subarachnoid space will demonstrate marked enhancement. Hydrocephalus may gradually develop as a result of inflamed arachnoid granulations, while acute sudden hydrocephalus may result from a cyst obstructing at the level of the fourth or less commonly at Monro and the aqueduct. A soft tissue density representing the head (scolex) may be best visualized on a T1 MR sequence.

Patients are treated with albendazole and steroids to reduce edema. Obstructing intraventricular lesions may require surgical shunting.

Notes

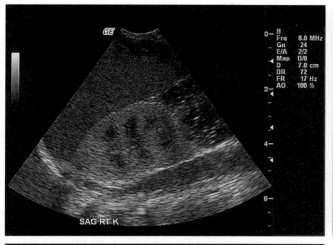

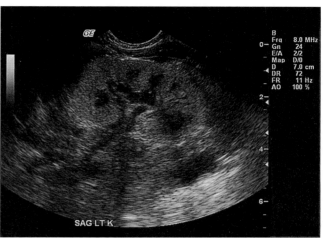

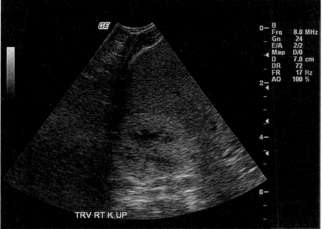

1. Are stones formed in this process?

2. What is the differential for a dilated collecting system?

3. Patients may present with pneumothorax. True or false?

4. What is the resolution of abdominal ultrasound?

Autosomal Recessive Polycystic Kidney Disease

1. Stone formation is a feature of the juvenile type.

2. Obstruction, papillary necrosis, congenital megacalyces, calyceal diverticulum, reflux.

3. True. Pneumothorax is secondary to abnormal lung development due to oligohydramnios and the extrinsic compression of the enlarged kidneys on the thorax.

4. 1.2 mm, hence 1 mm cysts will not be visualized.

Reference

Lonergan GJ, Rice RR, Suarez ES: Autosomal recessive polycystic kidney disease: radiographic-pathologic correlation. *Radiographics* 20:837–855, 2000.

Cross-Reference

Pediatric Radiology: THE REQUISITES, pp 168–169.

Comment

Autosomal recessive polycystic kidney disease (ARPKD) is a rare entity that produces small epithelial-lined cysts derived from renal tubules, the so-called medullary ductal ectasia. These changes lead to loss of concentrating ability, tubular atrophy, and eventual systemic hypertension. For reasons that are not entirely understood, hepatic involvement is seen as well. Congenital hepatic fibrosis is invariably encountered in all forms of ARPKD. Arrested biliary development leads to abnormally enlarged ducts with consequent periportal fibrosis and later, portal hypertension. Congenital hepatic fibrosis has been seen in the absence of ARPKD.

ARPKD is divided into four classes: perinatal, neonatal, infantile, juvenile. The perinatal form demonstrates prominent tubular involvement with minimal hepatic involvement, while the juvenile form demonstrates just the opposite: minimal renal tubular involvement with extensive hepatic involvement. As a rule, the less severe the renal involvement the more severe the hepatic involvement.

Presentation varies from still birth secondary to pulmonary hypoplasia (remember, the lungs require renally produced amnion to develop) to renal insufficiency and eventually systemic hypertension.

On imaging, ultrasound demonstrates enlarged and hyperechoic kidneys. You won't see large cysts on ultrasound as the tubular ectasia is on the order of 1 mm. IVU/IVP/EU is characterized by a prolonged pyelogram and may show brush-like tubules and linear contrast streaks radiating from the papillae into the cortex (not unlike medullary sponge kidney).

Notes

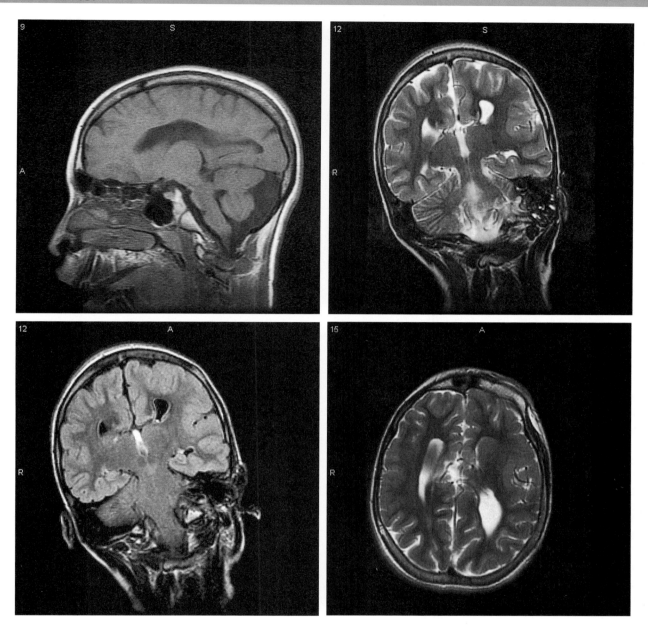

1. Name some common entities associated with this disorder.

2. What is colpocephaly?

3. Is there an association with interhemispheric cysts?

4. Is the cingulate gyrus present?

Agenesis of Corpus Callosum

1. Dandy–Walker malformation, encephalocele, Aicardi syndrome, fetal alcohol syndrome, gray matter heterotopias, polymicrogyria, choroids, plexus papillomas.

2. Colpocephaly is bilateral expansion of the trigones and occipital horns and is seen in agenesis of the corpus collusum.

3. Yes.

4. No, the cingulate gyrus remains everted due to agenesis of the corpus callosum.

Reference

Wright LB, James CA, Glasier CM: Congenital cerebral and cerebrovascular anomalies: magnetic resonance imaging. *Top Magn Reson Imaging* 12(6):361–374, 2001.

Cross-Reference

Pediatric Radiology: THE REQUISITES, p 274.

Comment

Neuroradiology attendings seem to pay quite a bit of attention to the corpus callosum (CC) during case conferences, and for good reason. Due to the CC's characteristic programmed staged development it is possible to infer diagnoses by noting the size, presence, or absence of the four parts that make up the CC. The CC is divided into four sections: the rostrum, genu, body, and splenium. Formation begins at the genu followed by the body, splenium, and finally the rostrum.

Agenesis or absence of the CC is thought to result from gene mutation involved in neuron migration. Agenesis is rarely isolated and most often associated with Dandy–Walker malformation, encephaloceles, and midline facial abnormalities. Seizure microcephaly, and retardation are typical presentations.

On ultrasound, radiation of the medial hemispheric sulci into the third ventricle (Probst bundles) is a useful sign to detect agenesis in newborns who normally have a thin CC. On axial MR the lateral horns appear to run parallel rather than their expected "bow-tie"-like configuration. The third ventricle will ride high into the interhemispheric fissure. There is dilatation of the trigones and occipital horns (colpocephaly). On coronal MR one can see the characteristic "longhorn" appearance of the ventricles.

In cases in which segments of the CC are absent, look for the rostrum, the last developing portion. If the rostrum is intact then most likely some event has destroyed an already formed corpus, so think ischemia or infection instead of developmental abnormality. An interesting exception is holoprosencephaly, which will demonstrate a malformed anterior (genu and body) CC but normal posterior CC (body and splenium).

Notes

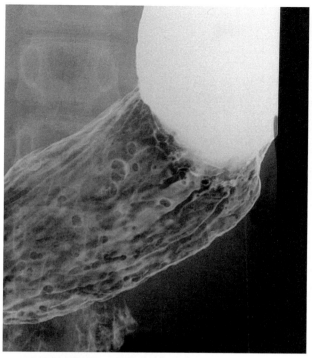

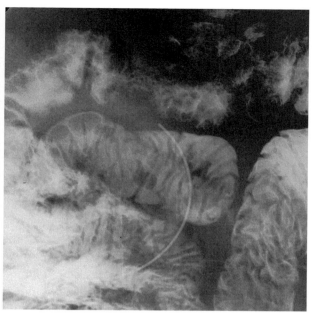

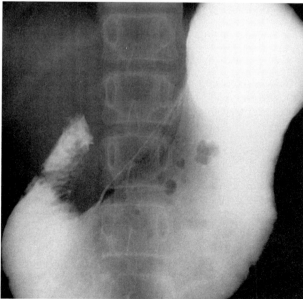

1. What is the most common cause for rectal bleeding in a teenager?

2. Is perioral pigmentation an indication for a barium study?

3. Are there associated bony abnormalities?

4. Can inflammatory bowel disease present with bleeding?

Polyps

1. Juvenile polyp.

2. Yes, Peutz–Jeghers.

3. Osteoma/Gardner syndrome, Juvenile polyposis/ hypertrophic pulmonary osteoarthropathy.

4. Yes, but be aware that unlucky IBD patients may also have polyps.

Reference

Buck JL, Harned RK, Lichtenstein JE, Sobin LH: Peutz-Jeghers syndrome. *Radiographics* 12:365–378; 1992.

Cross-Reference

Pediatric Radiology: THE REQUISITES, 2nd edn, pp 123–124.

Comment

Polyps are classified into four groups: isolated juvenile polyps, inherited polyposis syndromes, inherited adenomatous polyposis syndromes, and noninherited polyposes. The three big hitters for kids include isolated juvenile polyps, juvenile polyposis, and Peutz–Jeghers syndrome.

Isolated juvenile polyps are inflammatory in nature and often appear either solitary or in clusters of four or five within the colon. They are prone to bleeding; hence the most common presentation is painless rectal bleeding. Their malignant potential is exceedingly low. They are easily spotted by first-year residents as large filling defects with stalks on double contrast study.

Six polyps in your colon or other parts of your GI tract earns you the diagnosis of polyposis. These autosomal dominant inherited adenomatous polyps usually make themselves known by the teen years. Patients need to be scoped regularly as there is a high risk for colon carcinoma. A second-year resident can easily spot these small sheets of polyps blanketing the colon.

Peutz–Jeghers syndrome is the most common small-bowel polyposis syndrome. Any third-year resident would be able to tell you that the syndrome consists of mucocutaneous lesions, benign hamartomatous polyps, GI hamartomas, and increased risk of stomach, duodenal, and ovarian cancer.

In short, polyps need your attention.

Notes

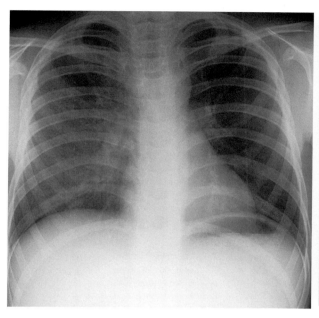 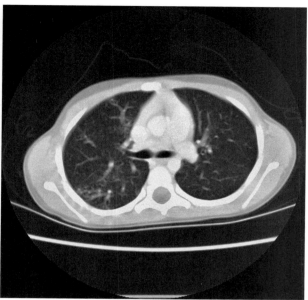

1. What is Westermark's sign?

2. What is the differential diagnosis?

3. What is Hampton's hump?

4. Is a right-sided sequestration more common than left?

Swyer–James Syndrome

1. Pleural-based wedge-shaped area of oligemia secondary to pulmonary embolism.

2. Foreign body aspiration, hypoplastic lung, mucus plugging, pulmonary sling.

3. Radiographic appearance of increased density secondary to pulmonary infarction.

4. Left is more common, a right-sided sequestration is almost always intralobar.

References

Macpherson RI, Cumming GR, Chernick V: Unilateral hyperlucent lung: a complication of viral pneumonia. *J Can Assoc Radiol* 20:225–231, 1969.

Image interpretation session: 1998. Swyer-James (Macleod) syndrome. *Radiographics* 19(1):231–233, 1999.

Cross-Reference

Pediatric Radiology: THE REQUISITES, 2nd edn, p 24.

Comment

Swyer–James is an acquired entity leading to unilateral hyperlucency thought to be a sequela of viral pneumonia, most commonly adenovirus. The infection causes a necrotizing bronchiolitis leading to fibrotic deposition and scarring of the bronchi and bronchioles. The alveoli are spared and remain inflated due to collateral ventilation.

The chest film demonstrates a small, hyperlucent lung. Hyperlucency occurs due to decreased pulmonary blood volume secondary to bronchiolar obliteration. Classically, there is air tapping during expiration. Bronchography would demonstrate abrupt cutoffs consistent with bronchial obstruction, the so-called "pruned tree appearance." The differential diagnosis for hyperlucent lung consists of foreign body, pneumothorax, congenital lobar emphysema, pulmonary artery hypoplasia or occlusion. Other causes of acquired pulmonary hypoplasia are rare yet may include thromboembolism with infarction of the lung, postirradiation therapy, severe dehydration, and nephrotic syndrome.

A small minority of children die within weeks of symptom onset, although most survive with chronic disability.

Notes

Patient 1

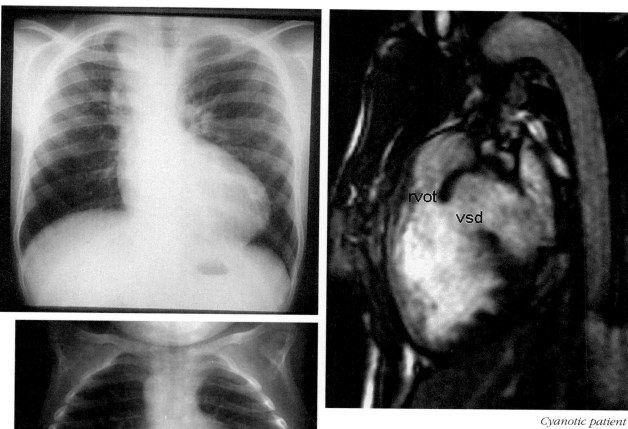

Cyanotic patient

Patient 2

1. Is there increased or decreased pulmonary vascularity?
2. If the vascularity was decreased what is your differential?
3. If the vascularity was increased what is your differential?
4. What percentage of these patients have a right-sided arch?

Tetralogy of Fallot

1. Decreased pulmonary vascularity.

2. Cyanotic with decreased vascularity: tetralogy of Fallot (normal heart size), Ebstein anomaly, pulmonic atresia, and tricuspid atresia (the latter three with enlarged heart).

3. Cyanotic with increased vascularity: five Ts, transposition of the great arteries, truncus, total anomalous pulmonary venous return, and single ventricle.

4. 25% of tetralogy patients have a right-sided arch.

Reference

Rauzzino M, Oakes WJ: Chiari II malformation and syringomyelia. *Neurosurg Clin N Am* 6(2):293–309, 1995.

Cross-Reference

Pediatric Radiology: THE REQUISITES, 2nd edn, pp 64–65.

Comment

Tetralogy of Fallot is defined by four findings: (1) right ventricular outflow obstruction, (2) right ventricular hypertrophy with resultant (3) overriding aorta as well as (4) a ventricular septal defect (VSD). Tet is the most common cyanotic disease in childhood and the only cyanosis without increased pulmonary flow. Right ventricular outflow obstruction and VSD are the big players in tet with the RV obstruction most commonly due to infundibular stenosis. The VSD allows the blood that would normally flow out of the PA to divert to the aorta, which in many cases is enlarged and overriding—a right-to-left shunt. To summarize, a small RV outflow tract increases RV pressure to where it overcomes the LV pressure and a right-to-left shunt develops with non-oxygenated blood exiting the aorta. The degree of obstruction determines the degree of right-to-left shunting.

Clinically, cyanotic and dyspneic symptoms arise earlier with more severe obstruction and shunting. Classically, cyanosis would improve with the child in the fetal (squatting) position as systemic resistance increases, thereby reversing the shunt and forcing blood through the pulmonary artery. Less severe obstruction will initially yield a left-to-right shunt—a pink tet. Pink tets eventually reverse to right-to-left shunting and frank cyanosis.

Radiographically, the heart is normal in size and has a typical "boot" or "clog" shape with uplifting of the ventricular apex due to right ventricular hypertrophy. The pulmonary trunk is not visualized, leaving a suspicious concavity where the LA meets the mediastinum.

Pulmonary vascularity is decreased as the blood is shunted through the VSD to the aorta. Right-sided aortic arches are present in 25% of cases. Currently, MR is utilized to define the anatomy in preparation for surgery.

The classic initial treatment for tetralogy was the Blalock–Taussig shunt in which the left subclavian artery is connected to the pulmonary artery feeding the blood starved lungs. Today surgery of the RV outlet obstruction and VSD repair shows greatly improved prognoses.

Notes

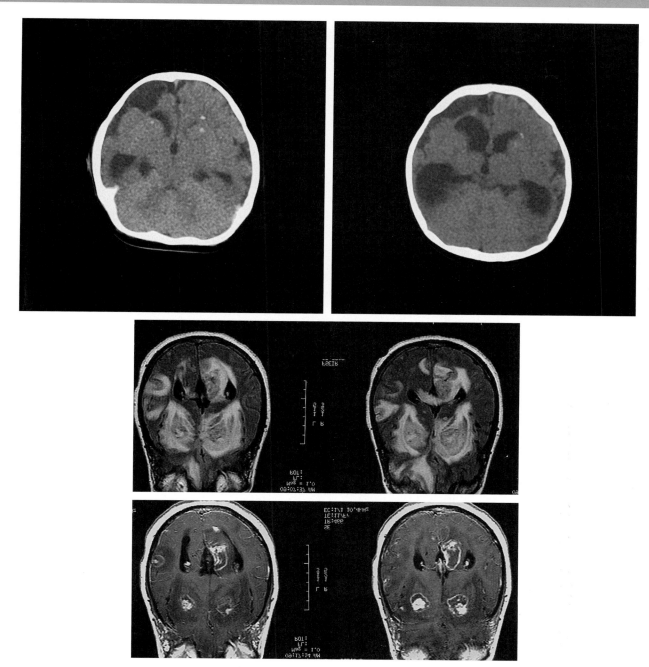

1. Could this represent cytomegalovirus infection?

2. Basal ganglia calcification in this age group is suggestive of what diagnosis?

3. Periventricular calcification in neonates is suggestive of what diagnosis?

4. Will these calcifications resolve following therapy?

Toxoplasmosis

1. No, CMV demonstrates only periventricular calcification, and is associated with lissencephaly and polymicrogyra. There are no cortical developmental abnormalities in toxo, just brain destruction.

2. Toxoplasmosis.

3. CMV.

4. Yes.

References

Chang KH, Han MH: MRI of CNS parasitic diseases. *J Magn Reson Imaging* 8(2):297–307, 1998.

Ramsey RG, Gean AD: Neuroimaging of AIDS. I. Central nervous system toxoplasmosis. *Neuroimaging Clin N Am* 7(2):171–186, 1997.

Cross-Reference

Pediatric Radiology: THE REQUISITES, p 278.

Comment

Toxoplasmosis is caused by an intracellular protozoan parasite that is ingested with tainted fruit or inadequately cooked meat that contain oocytes. Normally, maternal antibodies convey immunity preventing transplacental infection. Fetal infection occurs when either the mother is newly infected and an antibody response has yet to be mounted, or the mother is chronically infected but immunocompromised with resultant low antibody titers. Timing is important as the earlier in gestation the infection the more severe the sequelae. Infection may either be limited to the CNS or generalized. Ependymitis will obstruct CSF flow through the aqueduct, leading to hydrocephalus. Clinically these patients present several days after birth with seizures, chorioretinitis, and hydrocephalus.

On imaging the main findings are multifocal calcifications involving the basal ganglia, periventricular white matter, and cerebral cortex. Areas of ventricular dilatation secondary to hydrocephalus and encephalomalacia are common. Large areas of parenchymal destruction are present as well. CMV is a classic differential and can be distinguished by the predominance of periventricular calcification and presence of polymicrogyra and lissencephaly absent in toxoplasmosis.

Prognosis depends on promptness of treatment with antibiotics and ranges from mild to severe neurologic symptoms characterized by mental retardation, seizures, and spasticity.

Notes

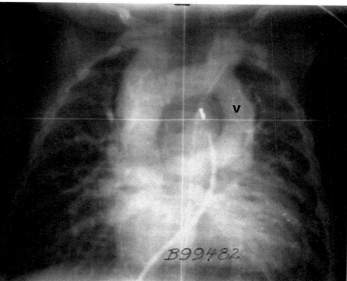

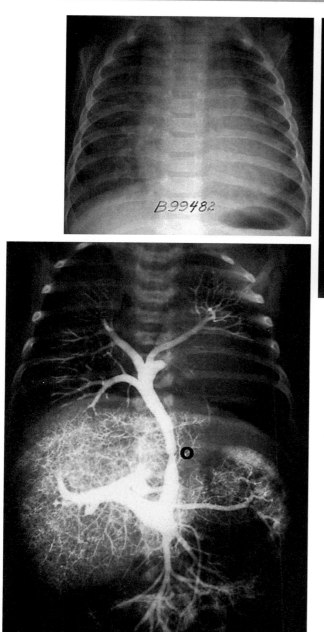

Cyanotic patient

1. Is there increased or decreased pulmonary vascularity?

2. If the vascularity was decreased what is your differential?

3. If the vascularity was increased what is your differential?

4. What is the classic sign that describes the mediastinal and cardiac silouhette for this entity?

Total Anomalous Pulmonary Venous Return (TAPVR)

1. Increased pulmonary vascularity.

2. Cyanotic with decreased vascularity: tetralogy of Fallot (normal heart size), Ebstein anomaly, pulmonic atresia, and tricuspid atresia (the latter three with enlarged heart).

3. Cyanotic with increased vascularity: five Ts, transposition of the great arteries, truncus, TAPVR, and single ventricle.

4. The "snowman" sign.

Reference

Rauzzino M, Oakes WJ: Chiari II malformation and syringomyelia. *Neurosurg Clin N Am* 6(2):293–309, 1995.

Cross-Reference

Pediatric Radiology: THE REQUISITES, 2nd edn, p 63.

Comment

Total anomalous pulmonary venous return is a developmental failure of the common pulmonary vein at the left atrium. During development, the branch pulmonary veins find one of three alternative locations to link up with the circulation—supracardiac, cardiac, and infracardiac. Supracardiac connections are the most common (50%) and involve drainage into the left innominate vein via a left vertical vein. This configuration yields the "snowman" appearance. The cardiac connection is either to the coronary sinus or RA. The infracardiac dives below the diaphragm and joins with either the portal system, hepatic veins, or IVC.

Both the systemic venous and pulmonary circulations drain to the right atrium. The elevated pressure within the right atrium keeps the foramen ovale patent with resultant right to left shunting and cyanosis. Enlargement of the RA and RV follow. Pulmonary venous obstruction is encountered with the infracardiac type as its long course passes through the diaphragm and other potentially obstructing normal anatomic structures. The increased pressure is transmitted back to the capillaries and although the right heart no longer has to contend with increased volume, increased pressure causes pulmonary edema with eventual pulmonary arterial hypertension and developing RV failure.

Clinically, patient presentation depends on the presence of obstruction. Obstructed patients present early with cyanosis and metabolic acidosis. Nonobstructed patients develop mild cyanosis with predominantly a left-to-right physiology.

Radiographically, each of the three forms appears distinct. The supracardiac, type I, and most common form appears as a snowman. The upper half of the snowman is the dilated superior vena cava on the right and the left vertical vein on the left. The body of the snowman represents the enlarged RA. Increased pulmonary flow yields shunt vascularity. Type II, or the cardiac form, demonstrates an enlarged RA as the veins hook directly into either the coronary sinus or the RA itself. Shunt vascularity is present due to the increased flow. Obstructed patients with infracardiac type III demonstrate a normal-sized heart and severe pulmonary edema due to increased hydrostatic pressure.

Surgery is mandatory and most difficult in the infracardiac type. Prognosis has markedly improved over the last two decades.

Notes

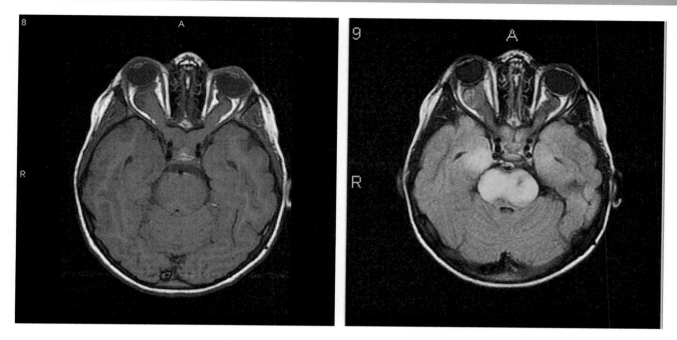

1. Does this entity more commonly affect the optic nerve or optic chiasm?

2. Is there heritability?

3. Does this entity involve the brain surfaces or cranial nerves?

4. Are the thalami and basal ganglia spared?

Neurofibromatosis Type 1

1. Gliomas more commonly affect the optic nerves than optic chiasm.

2. A fair number are spontaneous mutations but there is also autosomal dominant inheritance (50%).

3. Trick question. CN II is involved, although technically CN II is a white matter extension of the brain. NF-2 involves the meninges and peripheral nerves. NF-1 is primarily an intra-axial process.

4. No, they are commonly involved.

Reference

Smirniotopoulos JG, Murphy FM: The phakomatoses. *Am J Neuroradiol* 13(2):725–746, 1992.

Cross-Reference

Pediatric Radiology: THE REQUISITES, pp 271–272.

Comment

Neurofibromatosis type I is a neurocutaneous disorder caused by a mutation of a gene on chromosome 17 that codes for the protein neurofibromin that appears to act as a growth suppressor. Common features include cutaneous café au lait spots, neurofibromas, hamartomas of the iris, white matter and deep gray matter signal abnormalities, optic gliomas, and astrocytomas. Bone involvement includes macrocephaly, dysplasia of the greater and lesser sphenoid, pseudarthrosis, anterior bowing of long bones, scoliosis, and dural ectasia. Associations with NF-1 include Wilms tumor, rhabdomyosarcoma, leukemia, melanoma, pheochromocytoma, and medullary thyroid carcinoma.

Clinically there are a wide range of presentations as expression of the disease is highly variable. The first signs of NF-1 are café au lait spots that may appear between the first and the teen years. Cutaneous neurofibromas will form in childhood and continue to develop. A neurofibroma is a tumor consisting of intermixed neurons, Schwann cells, fibroblasts, mast cells, and vascular elements. Fifteen per cent of patients will demonstrate CNS abnormalities such as blindness due to optic glioma, seizures, and mental retardation. Optic glioma is in fact an astrocytoma, which might make you wonder as you've probably never heard of an astrocytoma in a peripheral nerve. Optic nerves are not peripheral nerves but white matter extensions of the brain.

On imaging the most common MR abnormality is increased T2 signal in the white and deep gray matter. No one is quite sure what is responsible for these changes but myelin vacuolization has been suggested in recent studies. Signal changes may range from punctate to 2 cm and may be located in the basal ganglia, cerebellar peduncles, brain stem or white matter. Enlargement of the optic nerves with increased signal on T2 and mild enhancement are consistent with optic nerve glioma. Astrocytomas in the thalami and basal ganglia as well as brainstem gliomas are commonly present.

Brain tumors are treated with surgery or radiotherapy. Prognosis is variable with expression and ranges from early death to normal life span.

Notes

Patient 1

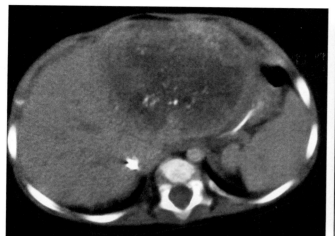

Patient 2

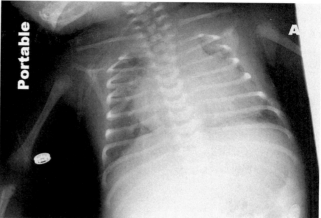

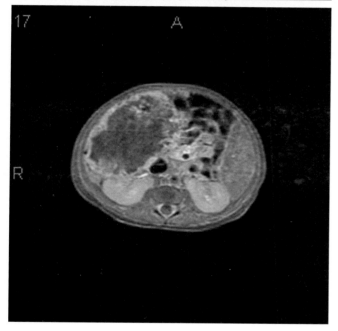

Patient 2

1. What is the differential diagnosis?
2. What is the differential for hepatic central scar?
3. What presentation might suggest this lesion?
4. How might ultrasound be useful in follow-up?

Hemangioendothelioma

1. Metastatic neuroblastoma, multiple arteriovenous malformation, hepatoblastoma (large solitary mass).

2. Focal nodular hyperplasia, giant cavernous hemangioma, fibrolamellar hepatocellular carcinoma (HCC), well-differentiated HCC, hypervascular mets, intrahepatic cholangiocarcinoma.

3. Right upper quadrant mass with cutaneous hemangiomas. Pulmonary edema secondary to high-output congestive heart failure (CHF).

4. Following embolization or ligation, documenting reduced flow via Doppler ultrasound will document therapy success.

Reference

Keslar PJ, Buck JL, Selby DM: From the archives of the AFIP. Infantile hemangioendothelioma of the liver revisited. *Radiographics* 13:657–670, 1993.

Cross-Reference

Pediatric Radiology: THE REQUISITES, 2nd edn, pp 133–134.

Comment

Hemangioendotheliomas or infantile cavernous hemangiomas result from an abnormal proliferation of endothelial cells leading to vascular steal and AV shunting. These lesions typically present under 6 months of age (most common tumor in this age group) with the classic triad of hepatomegaly, CHF (10–50%), and cutaneous hemangiomas (50%). Platelet sequestration (Kasabach–Merritt) is also present in 50% of cases in conjunction with anemia and jaundice. CHF is high-output secondary to AV shunting.

Ultrasound will typically show a large complex hepatic mass with enlarged celiac and hepatic arteries. The aorta will appear reduced in caliber distal to the take off of the hepatic artery. Hemangioendothelioma is highly vascular. Contrast-enhanced CT will demonstrate early peripheral enhancement with delayed centripetal fill-in. The lesion is isointense on delayed imaging. A tagged RBC scan may also be used to detect concurrent lesions within the liver.

These lesions all regress spontaneously as do the cutaneous hemangiomas. However, treatment may be necessary in the symptomatic patient. Inotropes, diuretics, high-dose steroids, alpha-2a interferon, and embolization are all treatment options if symptomatic. In the event of failed medical therapy, surgical resection, radiation therapy, hepatic artery ligation, and embolization have demonstrated effectiveness.

Notes

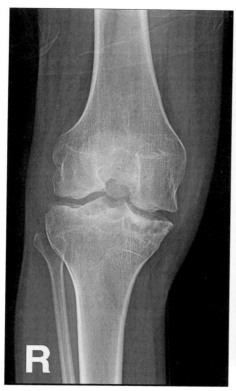
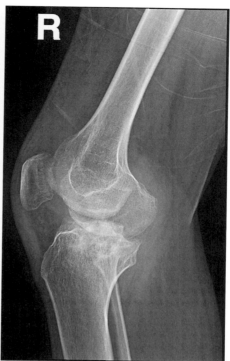

1. What are the most commonly affected joints?
2. What is the differential diagnosis?
3. Is this process more often bilateral or unilateral?
4. What differentiates this entity from degenerative arthritis?

Hemophilia

1. Knee, elbow, and ankle in order of frequency.

2. Septic arthritis, juvenile chronic arthritis, and sickle cell.

3. Unilateral.

4. No bony ankylosis, no growth inhibition, and the frequent presence of pseudotumors in hemophilia.

Reference

Lan HH, Eustace SJ, Dorfman D: Hemophilic arthropathy. *Radiol Clin N Am* 34(2):446–450, 1996.

Cross-Reference

Pediatric Radiology: THE REQUISITES, pp 217–218.

Comment

Bleeding into joints leads to proliferation of synovium, the cells that line the joint space and produce oxygen-rich fluid that bathes the avascular cartilage. Synovium reacts to repetitive bleeding by proliferating and subsequently dissolving articular cartilage. Following cartilage destruction, joint space narrowing and sclerosis follow, appearing indistinguishable from juvenile rheumatoid arthritis.

Radiographically, the initial monoarticular hemorrhage will appear as fullness or distention of the joint capsule. The knee will demonstrate periarticular osteoporosis, effusion, widening of the intercondylar notch secondary to overgrowth of the condyles and squaring of the patella due to bony overgrowth. Findings of chronic hemophilic arthropathy occur after repeated bleeds and include joint space narrowing, subchondral or subarticular cyst, and osteophyte formation. Increased flow to the epiphysis and physis may produce epiphyseal overgrowth or early closure of the growth plate.

MR will demonstrate a low to intermediate signal on both T1 and T2 of the hemosiderin-stained synovium, similar to pigmented villonodular synovitis. The articular surfaces will appear denuded of cartilage.

Notes

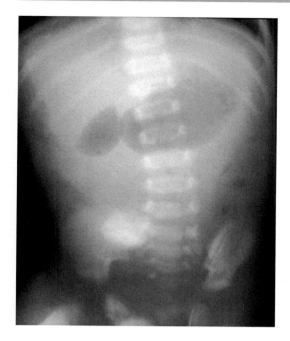

1. What is the differential diagnosis of double bubble?

2. What is the most common cause of high obstruction in the newborn?

3. What is the etiology?

4. Are alpha-fetoprotein levels elevated in omphalocele?

Double Bubble Pattern/Duodenal Atresia

1. Malrotation, duodenal-jejunal atresia, annular pancreas, duodenal web, preduodenal portal vein.

2. Duodenal atresia.

3. A fetal vascular accident precipitated by embolus, volvulus, or intussusception.

4. No, only in gastroschisis, as the covering of omphalocele does not allow communication with the amnion. Note that all bets are off if the omphalocele ruptures.

Reference

Berrocal T, Torres I, Gutiérrez J, et al.: Congenital anomalies of the upper gastrointestinal tract. *Radiographics* 19:855–872, 1999.

Cross-Reference

Pediatric Radiology: THE REQUISITES, 2nd edn, pp 108–110.

Comment

At 5 weeks the primitive gut undergoes epithelial proliferation, producing a solid lumenless tube that normally recanalizes at 10 weeks. Failed recanalization is considered the etiology for duodenal atresia. Complete failure causes complete obstruction, while incomplete recanalization causes duodenal stenosis due to a web or duplication. Other causes of stenosis include annular pancreas, choledochocele, or very rarely a preduodenal portal vein. Twenty-five per cent of patients with duodenal atresia have associated congenital heart disease, a tracheo-esophageal fistula, or an imperforate anus. A third of patients have Down syndrome.

Clinically, atresia presents with bile-stained vomitus in the first 24 hours. Preampullary stenosis (20%) will obviously be bile free. Severity of the presentation is directly proportional to the degree of stenosis.

Lack of distal bowel gas with a large air-distended stomach and duodenal bulb (the "double-bubble" sign), ought to raise your suspicion of atresia. A stenotic duodenum will allow some air to pass to the distal bowel. An upper GI will illustrate the obvious cutoff.

Prenatal ultrasound demonstrates polyhydramnios in 25% of cases as duodenal atresia prevents normal absorption of amniotic fluid by the gastrointestinal tract.

Notes

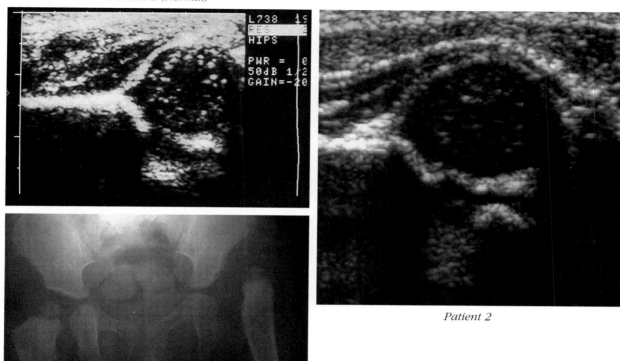

Patient 1 (Normal)

Patient 2

Patient 2

1. What is the male to female ratio?
2. What entities have increased acetabular angles?
3. What entities have decreased acetabular angles?
4. The acetabular angle decreases over time. True or false?

Developmental Dysplasia of the Hip

1. Males:females 1:9. Presumably, endogenous estrogens are responsible for ligamentous laxity. A defect in estrogen metabolism has been suggested.

2. Developmental dysplasia of the hip, neuromuscular disorder.

3. Down syndrome, achondroplasia, osteogenesis imperfecta hypophosphatasia, and sacral agenesis.

4. True. The alpha angle decreases with age.

Reference

Eich GF, Babyn P, Giedion A: Pediatric pelvis: radiographic appearance in various congenital disorders. *Radiographics* 12:467–484, 1992.

Cross-Reference

Pediatric Radiology: THE REQUISITES, pp 251–253.

Comment

For the normal hip to form, the femoral head and acetabulum must be in proper alignment and contact. Developmental dysplasia of the hip is thought to occur due to ligamentous laxity that permits the femoral head to drop out of the acetabulum. Several etiologies have been proposed, including oligohydramnios and breech presentation. Maternal estrogen responsible for ligamentous laxity necessary for childbirth has a similar effect on the fetal joint capsules as well.

As stated, proper positioning of the hip and acetabulum are necessary for proper articular formation in subluxation of the femoral head. A false acetabulum forms while the native acetabulum develops as a shallow dish. Pressure of the subluxed head on the labrum may cause the labrum to invert into the acetabulum, a condition referred to as limbus deformity. Therapy is guided at repositioning the head into the acetabulum thus reestablishing the normal physiologic position, which often induces normal development. The shorter the period of subluxation the more successful the treatment.

Diagnosis is made with ultrasound of the hip as there is very little calcified cartilage or osteoid at birth in the femoral heads and acetabula. The abnormal "clunk" of the neonatal hip examination, or asymmetric buttock folds, provide the indication for ultrasound. Two methods are currently in use, the Graf and dynamic techniques.

The Graf technique uses a single coronal view of the hip with the infant in the lateral decubitus position. The normal femoral head in the coronal plane should resemble a "lollipop" or "golf ball on a tee." A more quantitative approach employs the use of three lines. The A line is drawn from the superior joint capsule insert to the most superior aspect of the ossified acetabulum, the "osseus convexity." The B line connects the aforementioned osseus convexity to the lateral labrum. The C line parallels the ossified acetabulum. Intersection of the A and C lines yields the alpha angle. An abnormal alpha angle is greater than 60°. The beta angle is determined by the intersecting angle of the A and B lines and should not be less than 55°. Greater than 55° indicates lateral displacement. The configuration on the transverse view in the flexed hip should resemble a seagull or rising sun. The alpha angle measures acetabular depth, that ought to normally measure 55–65°.

The dynamic method employs multiple views in stress, flexion, and neutral positions to evaluate anatomy and stability. Ligamentous laxity under stress, subluxation, dislocation, and reducibility may be evaluated with the dynamic method.

Hip dysplasia and subluxation is treated with a cast that places the infant in flexion and abduction. A follow-up ultrasound at 6 weeks is obtained. If no subluxation is detected the cast will be removed after a total of 10 weeks and a radiograph is used to evaluate the therapy.

On the radiograph there are two lines to remember. A horizontal line (Hilgenreiner) is drawn through the triradial cartilage, while a vertical line (Perkins) is drawn perpendicular at the lateral margin of the acetabular roof. The humeral head ought to lie in the lower inner quadrant. The acetabular angle measures the relative socket depth. Draw a line along the roof of the acetabulum to the horizontal Hilgenreiner line and you've defined the acetabular angle, normally 15–30° depending on age. The normal angle decreases with age.

Hip dislocation is treated with a harness as well. Ultrasound is obtained weekly until there is sustained femoral head reduction. Patients then have two additional scans 3 weeks apart to confirm proper alignment, followed by 10 weeks in the harness.

Notes

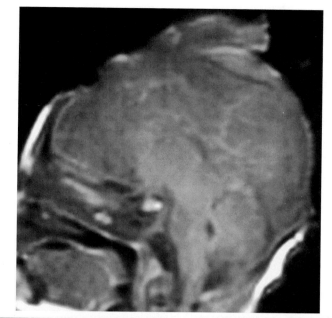

Patient 1

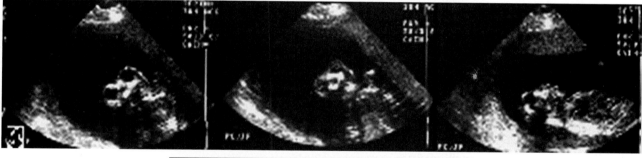

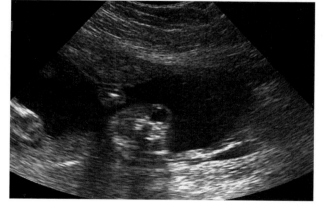

Patient 2

1. What is hypertelorism?

2. What are some causes of hypertelorism?

3. What is hypotelorism?

4. What are some causes of hypotelorism?

Cranioschisis (Anencephaly)

1. Hypertelorism is defined by an increase in the interorbital distance.

2. Hypertelorism is caused by cleidocranial dysostosis, Crouzon disease, Hunter or Hurler syndrome, cephalocele, and thalassemia.

3. Hypotelorism is decreased interorbital distance.

4. Hypotelorism is caused by arhinencephaly, holoprosencephaly, microcephaly, trigonocephaly, and sagittal craniosynostosis.

Reference

Goldstein RB, Filly RA: Prenatal diagnosis of anencephaly: spectrum of sonographic appearances and distinction from the amniotic band syndrome. *Am J Roentgenol* 151(3):547–550, 1988.

Cross-Reference

Pediatric Radiology: THE REQUISITES, pp 261, 268.

Comment

Proper neural tube development is essential for normal organization and function of the nervous system. During organogenesis (3–8 weeks) a portion of the primitive neural ectoderm invaginates, fusing at the cervical region. Fusion proceeds in both opposite cranial and caudal directions. The last portion to close at the cephalic end is the anterior neural pore at 25 days—complete failure will produce anencephaly.

Anencephaly is the most common CNS neural tube abnormality, 1 to 5 in 1000 live births with a 4:1 female predominance. As with any neural tube defect, increased alpha-fetoprotein, a product of the fetal liver, will demonstrate increased maternal blood serum and amniotic fluid levels. Forebrain development is stunted with the absence of the prosencephalon or future cortex as well as the cranial vault. The mesencephalon (midbrain) and rhombencephalon (brainstem) are present. The appearance of anencephaly on ultrasound is similar to that of a frog (frog sign), with pronounced eyes and an absent calvaria. *Tip:* do not call anencephaly before 14 weeks as the skull has yet to ossify. Anencephaly is incompatible with life.

Notes

Patient 1

Patient 2

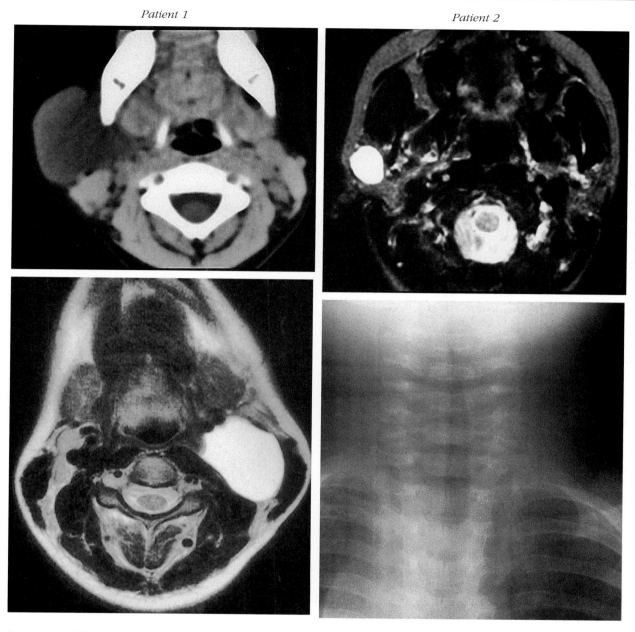

1. What is the differential diagnosis?

2. Where is the lesion?

3. Name the suprahyoid neck compartments.

4. What is the most common parotid tumor?

Branchial Cleft Cyst

1. Second branchial cleft cyst, thyroglossal duct cyst, external laryngocele, cystic hygroma, and adenopathy.

2. Parapharyngeal space, anterior triangle.

3. Parapharyngeal, pharyngeal, masticator, parotid, retropharyngeal, perivertebral, posterior cervical.

4. Mixed type.

Reference

Benson MT, Dalen K, Mancuso AA, et al.: Congenital abnormalities of the branchial apparatus: embryology and pathologic anatomy. *Radiographics* 12:739–748, 1992.

Cross-Reference

Pediatric Radiology: THE REQUISITES, 2nd edn, pp 12–13.

Comment

What are the branchial clefts? Mesenchymal tissue, a derivative of mesoderm, appears in the embryo at the fourth to fifth week, creating pillars separated by spaces or clefts. These nubbins of mesenchyme separated by clefts represent the proto-architecture of the neck and face. During development, migration of embryonic tissues may pinch off and isolate clefts along the anterior margin of the sternocleidomastoid, the normal axis for arch migration. This process may produce a spectrum of defects ranging from sinuses or fistulae to cysts. Clinically, fistulas and sinuses present soon after birth due to drainage. Cysts present in older patients.

CT reveals an ovoid thin-walled cystic-appearing structure. Infected cysts demonstrate wall thickening, septations, and high attenuation. MR appearance is variable depending upon the presence of infection. The most common anomaly is the second branchial cyst that arises at the angle of the mandible and may extend from the level of the clavicles to the tonsillar fossa along the anterior belly of the sternocleidomastoid. Communication with the skin may also be seen.

Notes

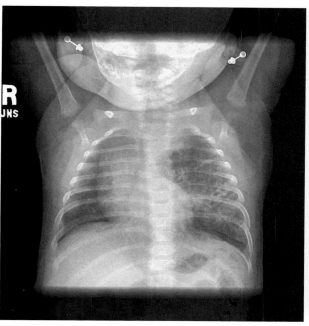
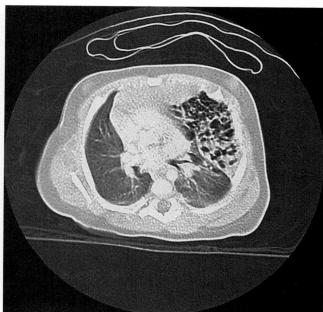

1. How is this disease categorized?
2. Which category holds the poorest prognosis?
3. Which lobes are most commonly affected?
4. What is the prenatal radiographic appearance?

Congenital Cystic Adenomatoid Malformation

1. Categorized by cyst size.

2. Type III, the diffuse cysts.

3. The upper lobes.

4. Solid as opposed to cystic.

Reference

Siegel BA, Proto AV, eds.: *Pediatric Disease (Fourth Series) Test and Syllabus*. Reston, VA: American College of Radiology, 1993, pp 102–106.

Cross-Reference

Pediatric Radiology: THE REQUISITES, 2nd edn, pp 26, 28.

Comment

Congenital cystic adenomatoid malformation is characterized by anomalous fetal development of terminal respiratory structures—either too many bronchioles or not enough alveoli. Cysts develop in utero that later interfere with normal alveolar development. Respiratory distress in the first month of life is the usual presentation—90% are less than 1 year of age.

	Features	Prognosis	Related abnormalities
Type I 50%	>2 cm One dominant cyst	Excellent	Rare
Type II 40%	1–2 cm Smaller cysts, air filled with variable solid tissue	Intermediate	Renal, intestinal, cardiac, skeletal
Type III 10%	<1 cm Microcysts, solid mass	Poor	Fetal hydrops, maternal polyhydramnios

The disease is classified into three types. On plain film type I lesions appear as one or more dominant cysts, type II as diffuse smaller cysts, and type III as a solid mass. The disease has an upper lobe predominance. The differential includes staphylococcal pneumonia, complicated bronchogenic cyst, and diaphragmatic hernia. Surgery is curative.

Notes

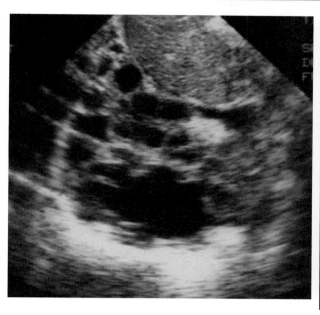

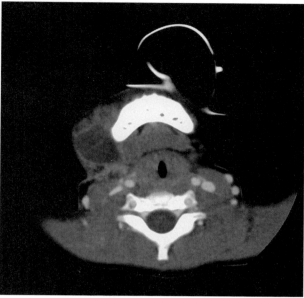

1. What are the histologic types of this entity?

2. Are there any congenital lesions associated with this entity?

3. Name the infrahyoid neck compartments.

4. What is the differential diagnosis?

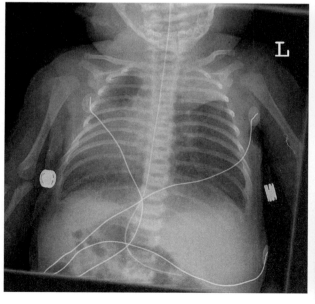

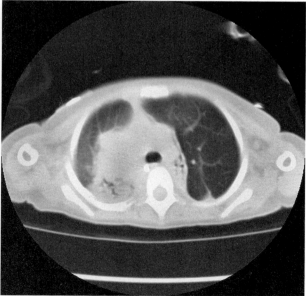

1. What are the associated findings?

2. What are the genetics?

3. What chromosome is cystic fibrosis carried on?

4. Is there an association with infertility?

Cystic Hygroma

1. Capillary, cavernous, and cystic.

2. Turner syndrome, fetal alcohol syndrome, and Noonan syndrome.

3. Visceral, carotid, posterior cervical, retropharyngeal, perivertebral.

4. Branchial cleft, thyroglossal duct, cavitating abscess.

Reference

Koeller KK, Alamo L, Adair CF, et al.: Congenital cystic masses of the neck: radiologic-pathologic correlation. *Radiographics* 19(1):121–146, 1999.

Cross-Reference

Pediatric Radiology: THE REQUISITES, 2nd edn, p 12.

Comment

Cystic hygromas are lymphatic malformations consisting of dilated lymph channels referred to as lymphangiomas. Lymph channels develop from the embryonic venous system. If communication is lost between the two systems, a lymphatic malformation develops as there is no route for drainage. Small lymphatic sequestrations lead to hydrops as in this case. Large lymphatic sequestrations are incompatible with life. Clinically they often appear as painless, compressible neck masses.

On CT cystic hygromas appear as thin-walled multiloculated cystic masses with septations. Previous infections may demonstrate thickened septae. The vast majority develop within the posterior triangle (sternocleidomastoid, trapezius, and clavicle). These lesions are prone to hemorrhage and may show a dramatic increase in size or fluid–fluid levels on MR. A noninfected cystic hygroma will be dark on T1 and bright on T2.

Reaccumulation of cystic hygromas is common following needle aspiration. Complete surgical excision is indicated but difficult. An alternative to surgery, bleomycin injections have demonstrated promising results.

Notes

Kartagener Syndrome

1. Situs inversus, sinusitis, and bronchiectasis.

2. Autosomal recessive.

3. Chromosome 7, autosomal recessive.

4. Yes, microtubule dysfunction leads to immotile spermatozoa.

Reference

Fonte JM, Varma JD, Kuligowska E: Thoracic case of the day. Kartagener syndrome. *Am J Roentgenol* 173(3): 822, 826–827, 1999.

Cross-Reference

Pediatric Radiology: THE REQUISITES, 2nd edn, p 42.

Comment

Kartagener syndrome is caused by a deficiency in the dynein arms of cilia yielding abnormal cilia motion. All organs containing cilia are affected. Respiratory immotility causes bronchiectasis and sinusitis, auditory dysmotility causes deafness and spermatocyte cilia dysfunction causes infertility. Studies have suggested that normal ciliary motility of differentiating epithelial cells plays a critical role in the determination of visceral situs. It has been theorized that disarrayed ciliary motion leads to an equal chance of levorotation or dextrorotation (situs inversus). Impaired mucociliary clearance in the respiratory tract leads to chronic pulmonary infections, bronchiectasis, chronic sinusitis, and otitis media.

Patients in early childhood typically present with recurrent pneumonias, chronic otitis media, nasal polyps, productive cough, hemoptysis, and eventual respiratory and cardiac failure. Bacterial agents include *Hemophilus*, *Neisseria*, and *Streptococcus*. Bronchiectasis is the hallmark of Kartagener syndrome and is characterized by persistent bronchial dilatation secondary to bronchial muscle and elastic tissue destruction. The frequency of bronchiectasis in patients with immotile cilia is approximately 30%.

CT findings of bronchiectasis include thick-walled cystic spaces (bronchi) grouped together in parallel clusters. The vessels in the involved areas of lung are poorly defined and crowded reflecting volume loss of the affected lung segments. Conventional radiographs demonstrating situs inversus and pneumonia ought to raise the possibility of cilia dysmotility syndrome. If, in addition, you are shown a positive sinus film, pull out your Louisville slugger and crush it to the Executive Inn across the street.

Notes

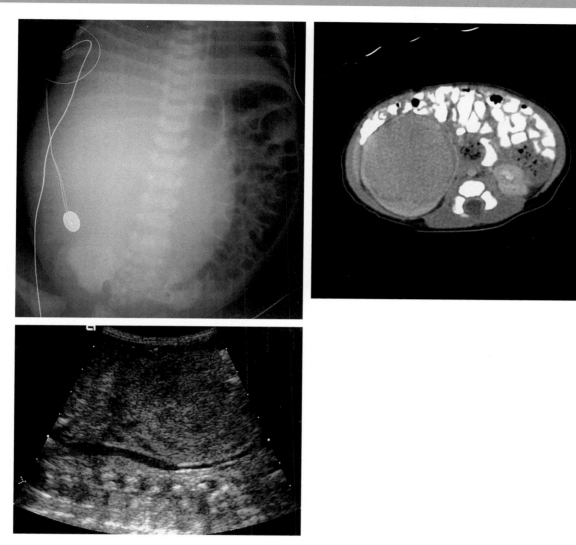

1. Is this disorder commonly diagnosed before or after age 2?

2. Are these lesions commonly exophytic?

3. Are these lesions distinguishable from Wilms tumor?

4. Does this lesion have malignant potential?

Mesoblastic Nephroma

1. It is commonly diagnosed in the neonatal period.

2. Yes, they are commonly exophytic.

3. No, mesoblastic nephroma commonly mimics a Wilms tumor.

4. No, mesoblastic nephroma does not have malignant potential.

Reference

Lowe LH, Isuani BH, Heller RM, et al.: Pediatric renal masses: Wilms tumor and beyond. *Radiographics* 20:1585–1603, 2000.

Cross-Reference

Pediatric Radiology: THE REQUISITES, pp 171–173.

Comment

Mesoblastic nephroma is the most common neonatal mesenchymal neoplasm. This benign tumor arises from the metanephric blastema giving the histologic appearance of a hamartoma—normal tissues in abnormal arrangements. The tumor does not invade the renal pedicle. Presentation is typically a large nontender abdominal mass in neonates less than 3 months. Patients may also have hematuria, hypertension, and anemia.

A mass may be present on conventional radiograph. Enhanced CT will show nonfunctional intrarenal masses. Ultrasound will demonstrate a large, solid, hypoechoic, homogeneous mass replacing most of the renal parenchyma. A heterogenous appearance on ultrasound may be observed in the infrequent event of hemorrhage or necrosis. Cystic change is rare but may resemble multilocular cystic nephroma. Unfortunately, imaging cannot differentiate this lesion from the rare neonatal Wilms tumor necessitating surgical excision.

Notes

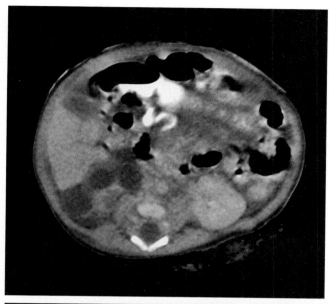

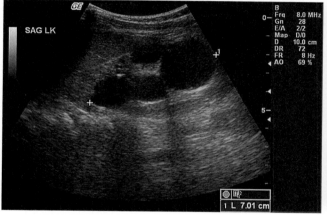
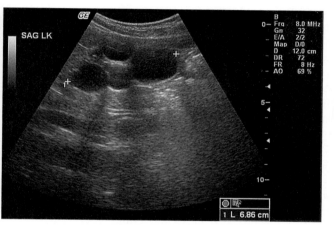

1. Is this disorder inherited?

2. How may this entity appear in adulthood?

3. Is there function in the affected kidney?

4. Renal arteries demonstrate compensatory hypertrophy of both the adventitia and media but not the intima. True or false?

Multicystic Dysplastic Kidney

1. No inheritability.

2. A nubbin of renal tissue or complete dissapearance.

3. There is no function in the multicystic dysplastic kidney.

4. Ridiculously false. The renal vessels are atretic as there is no flow to a congenitally obstructed kidney.

Reference

Strife JL, Souza AS, Kirks DR, et al.: Multicystic dysplastic kidney in children: US follow-up. *Radiology* 186(3): 785–788, 1993.

Cross-Reference

Pediatric Radiology: THE REQUISITES, p 160.

Comment

Multicystic dysplastic kidney (MCDK) is the result of in utero urinary obstruction secondary to a developmentally atretic or stenosed collecting system. MCDK is the severe form of congenital ureteropelvic junction (UPJ) obstruction. The noncommunicating cysts are usually dilated calyces accompanied by nonfunctioning renal atrophic tissue. The entity is divided into two types: the more common pelvoinfundibular-atretic ureter and pelvis with resultant multiple cysts, and the hydronephrotic-atretic ureter only, with one large renal pelvic cyst. The use-it-or-lose-it maxim prevails as obstruction prevents normal function, yielding atrophic parenchyma as well as a hypoplastic renal artery. In 15% of cases there is contralateral UPJ obstruction. Half of the cases demonstrate congenital heart disease and facial anomalies.

Patients present with an abdominal mass at birth. Ultrasound will demonstrate multiple noncommunicating cysts (pelvoinfundibular type) with thick septae, absence of normal parenchyma and renal sinus fat, and multiple small echogenic foci of primitive mesenchyme. Patients are followed up every 6 months for 3 years to ensure the diagnosis and monitor the decrease in size of the cysts. Surgical removal is necessary if growth occurs. A cystic form of Wilms tumor will grow larger rather than involute in the case of MCDK.

Notes

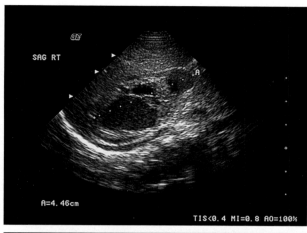

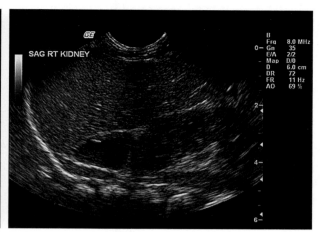

1 Month Follow Up Exam

4 Month Follow Up

1. What is the differential diagnosis?

2. What is the most common etiology for adrenal calcification?

3. Describe the normal venous drainage of the adrenal glands?

4. Does this lesion grow hyperechoic or hypoechoic with time?

C A S E 155

Neonatal Adrenal Hemorrhage

1. Neuroblastoma or exophytic Wilms.

2. Previous bleed.

3. The left adrenal vein drains into the left renal vein. The right adrenal vein drains directly into the aorta.

4. Hypoechoic.

Reference

Westra, SJ, Zaninovic AC, Hall TR, et al.: Imaging of the adrenal gland in children. *Radiographics* 14:1323–1340, 1994.

Cross-Reference

Pediatric Radiology: THE REQUISITES, p 177.

Comment

Neonatal adrenal hemorrhage presents with anemia or jaundice and has been linked to birth trauma, stress, anoxia, and dehydration. The adrenal glands are large and hypervascular as they carry the androgenesis load during the final trimester of pregnancy. Increases in arterial flow or increased venous pressure may cause hemorrhage. The right gland (70%) is more susceptible than the left due to its direct drainage into the IVC. Hemorrhage occurs bilaterally in 10% of cases.

Ultrasound demonstrates a suprarenal echogenic heterogenous mass. To differentiate from neuroblastoma, a scan 3–5 days later will show a shrinking hypoechoic hemorrhage, while the neuroblastoma may show no change or even enlargement. Doppler may show relative hypovascularity compared with neuroblastoma.

Notes

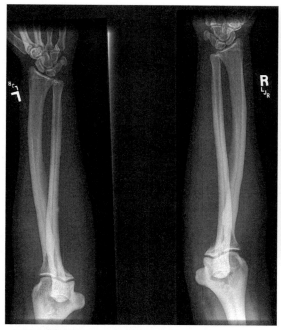
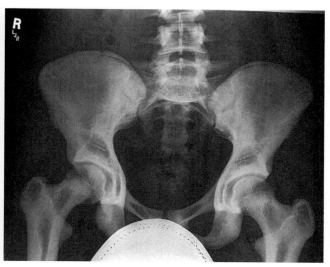
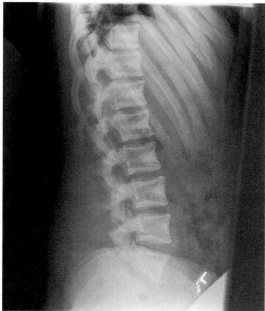

1. How many forms of this disease are there?

2. Which types demonstrate anemia and organomegaly?

3. What is the genetic defect?

4. Are the patient's bones under or overtubulated?

Osteopetrosis

1. Four: a congenital or precocious form, a delayed or tarda form, an intermediate form, and a tubular acidotic form.

2. The congenital or precocious type but not the delayed type.

3. An enzymatic defect that causes failure of primary spongiosa resorption.

4. Undertublated (Erlenmeyer flask deformity).

Reference

Greenspan A: Sclerosing bone dysplasia–a target-site approach. *Skeletal Radiol* 20:561–583, 1991.

Cross-Reference

Pediatric Radiology: THE REQUISITES, p 211.

Comment

Osteopetrosis refers to a group of disorders that all demonstrate diffuse osteosclerosis secondary to dysfunctional osteoclasts. Osteoclast dysfunction is thought to occur from a number of different genetic defects that prevent bone resorption. Currently, there have been four types that have been identified: precocious, delayed, intermediate recessive, and tubular acidotic.

The precocious type, a.k.a. the lethal type, is an AR inherited disorder presenting with failure to thrive, hepatosplenomegaly, and cranial nerve dysfunction. The marrow space fills, destroying bone, platelet, and blood precursors, leading to anemia, immunocompromise, infection, and death. Radiographically, the bones are chalky, osteosclerotic, and poorly modeled. The bone within bone appearance has been reported. A thickened skull with obliteration of the marrow space is seen. Patients improve with bone marrow transplant.

The delayed type, AD, a.k.a. Albers–Schönberg disease, is for the most part asymptomatic. The findings are similar but less severe than the precocious or lethal type.

The intermediate recessive type is between the precocious AR and the delayed AD type with respect to clinical severity and radiographic findings.

Osteopetrosis with tubular acidosis is secondary to a carbonic anhydrase deficiency, leading to failure to thrive, renal tubular acidosis, muscle weakness, and hypotonia. Pathologic fractures and obliterated medullary cavities in the setting of diffuse osteosclerosis is characteristic. Calcification is also present within the basal ganglia. This entity is AR with long-term survival and mental retardation.

Notes

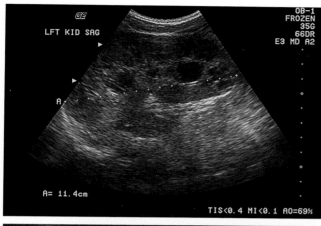
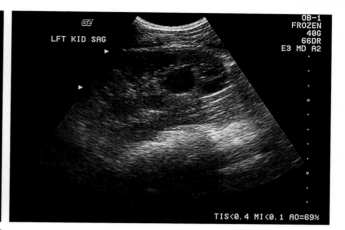
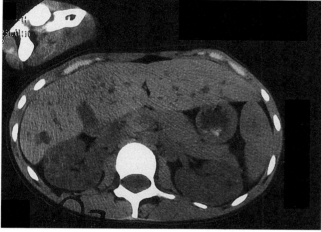

1. What disease entities are associated with congenital hepatic fibrosis?

2. What is the incidence of this entity?

3. Is there a genetic basis for this disorder?

4. Is this disease potentially fatal?

Autosomal Dominant Polycystic Kidney Disease

1. Autosomal dominant polycystic kidney disease (most common), autosomal recessive polycystic kidney disease (ARPKD, uncommon), multicystic dysplastic kidney, Caroli, choledochocele.

2. 1:1000, common compared with ARPKD (1:10,000).

3. Yes, it is caused by a mutation of the gene that encodes polycystin, a membrane protein.

4. Yes, in adulthood a burst of an associated Berry aneurysm of the cerebral circulation may lead to death.

Reference

Choyke PL: Inherited cystic diseases of the kidney. *Radiol Clin N Am* 34(5):925–946, 1996.

Cross-Reference

Pediatric Radiology: THE REQUISITES, p 169.

Comment

Autosomal dominant polycystic disease is caused by a mutation to the gene that encodes polycystin, an integral membrane protein important in basement membrane production and modulating cellular differentiation. Cyst formation is poorly understood yet it is thought that the epithelium is arrested during development producing epithelial hyperplasia, cellular proliferation, and blocked tubules. Subsequent cyst formation with active secretion causes enlargement over time. Cysts are also seen within the liver, although rarely associated with hepatic fibrosis in contradistinction to ARPKD. The spleen, testes, pancreas, ovaries, and lungs may also demonstrate cysts. Berry aneurysms are noted in 35% of patients and require screening with MRA for those with the disease or family history.

Clinically, the majority of these patients present with renal insufficiency, pain, and hematuria during adulthood. The hematuria is produced by bleeding cysts that may form clots leading to renal colic. Death following ruptured cerebral aneurysm occurs in 10% of cases.

On ultrasound, bilaterally enlarged hyperechoic kidneys are present as in ARPKD, yet macroscopic cysts varying in size on the order of 3 cm may be noted. Cysts within other organs are not detected by ultrasound in the child. Normal function with gross distortion ("Swiss cheese nephrogram") due to mass effect characterizes the calyceal system on IVU.

Notes

Challenge Cases

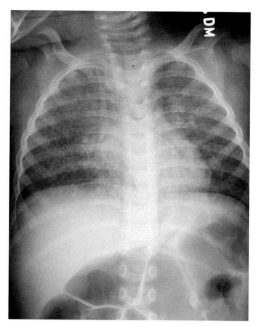

Hypoxemic and HIV⁺

1. What is the therapy for this entity?
2. Are you likely to see a drop in the A-a gradient?
3. What is the differential of thymomegaly?
4. What is the differential diagnosis?

Lymphocytic Interstial Pneumonitis

1. Steroids.

2. Yes!

3. Hyperthyroidism, Addison disease, lymphoma, leukemia, and Langerhans cell histiocytosis.

4. Miliary TB, varicella, thyroid cancer mets, neuroblastoma mets.

Reference

Lynch JL, Blickman JG, ter Meulen DC, et al.: Radiographic resolution of lymphocytic interstitial pneumonitis (LIP) in children with human immunodeficiency virus (HIV): not a sign of clinical deterioration. *Pediatr Radiol* 31(4):299–303, 2001.

Cross-Reference

Thoracic Radiology: THE REQUISITES, pp 284–285.

Comment

Lymphocytic interstitial pneumonitis (LIP) is a disease of unknown etiology present in perinatally infected HIV babies. Thirty to forty per cent of those infected newborns will develop LIP, a diffuse lymphocytic infiltration of the alveolar septa, interlobular septa, and subpleural and peribronchial lymph channels. Clinically, the infant presents with mild hypoxemia. The hypoxemia develops due to the deposition of cells on the interstitium, thereby obstructing oxygen diffusion from the alveoli to the capillaries. Nonproductive cough with associated findings of salivary gland enlargement, generalized lymphadenopathy, and digital clubbing are present in the 2–3-year age group.

Radiographically, LIP appears as a diffuse, symmetric, reticulonodular, or nodular infiltrate with or without the presence of hilar and mediastinal adenopathy. Nodules may appear 2–3 mm in size and are usually at the bases and lung periphery. Eventually, air space consolidation, bronchiectasis, cystic lung disease, and bacterial superinfection may develop. Patients have shown improvement on steroid therapy.

Notes

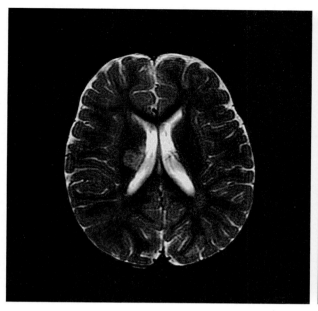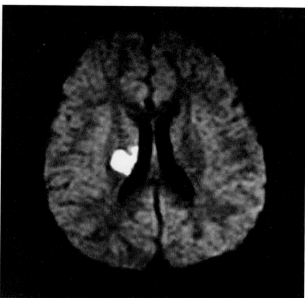

1. Is multiple sclerosis monophasic?

2. How might imaging suggest a monophasic entity?

3. Is thalamic involvement rare or common in MS?

4. What is the mortality associated with this entity?

Acute Disseminated Encephalomyelitis (ADEM)

1. No, it occurs over time, unlike ADEM, which is monophasic.

2. You would expect to see enhancement of all the lesions.

3. Thalamic involvement is rare in MS but not uncommon in ADEM.

4. 10–30% mortality in ADEM.

Reference

Hynson JL, Kornberg AJ, Coleman LT, et al.: Clinical and neuroradiologic features of acute disseminated encephalomyelitis in children. *Neurology* 22;56(10): 1308–1312, 2001.

Cross-Reference

Pediatric Radiology: THE REQUISITES, p 211.

Comment

Acute disseminated encephalomyelitis is a demyelinating disease caused by an autoimmune mechanism. It has been hypothesized that a viral antigen from either infection or vaccination cross-reacts with myelin, inducing the immune system to target the body's own nerve sheaths. Confluent areas of demyelination occur within the white matter. Clinically, patients may present with a fulminant case characterized by seizures and focal neurologic signs, or less dramatically with headache, fever, drowsiness, vomiting, and irritability. Resolution of neurologic signs and symptoms occurs within a few weeks with 90% of patients showing no sequelae. The remaining unlucky 10% show permanent damage.

On imaging, areas of low density in the white matter tracts may be present on CT. On MR, patchy areas of high signal intensity on T2 are present in the subcortical and deep white matter. There is variable enhancement of these lesions. Lesions may have a hemorrhagic or cavitary appearance. There are three big differentials to consider: multiple sclerosis, Lyme disease, and subacute sclerosing panencephalitis (SSPE). MS is characterized by a more insidious onset and will rarely involve the thalamus as is common in ADEM. Lyme most often involves a tic bit history, rash, and cranial nerve enhancement. SSPE has greater cortical involvement and does not demonstrate abnormal enhancement.

Steroids are the mainstay of therapy.

Notes

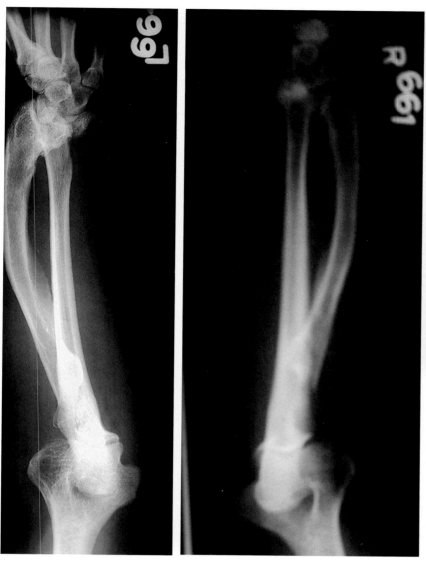

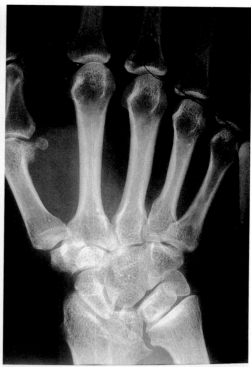

1. What is the differential diagnosis?

2. What are the long-term sequelae of this skeletal deformity?

3. What is the eponym for this disorder?

4. What is the typical age of presentation of dyschondrosteosis?

C A S E 160

Dyschondrosteosis (Mesomelic Dwarfism)

1. Post-traumatic Madelung deformity, multiple exostoses with Madelung deformity, Turner syndrome, and acromesomelic dysplasia.

2. Spontaneous rupture of extensor tendons.

3. Leri–Weill disease.

4. Between 8 and 9 years.

Reference

Beals RK, Lovrien EW: Dyschondrosteosis and Madelung's deformity. Report of three kindreds and review of the literature. *Clin Orthop* (116):24–28, 1976.

Cross-Reference

Pediatric Radiology: THE REQUISITES, p 205.

Comment

Short stature can be symmetric or asymmetric. Asymmetric forms include short-limb, short-trunk, and proportional dwarfism. Short-limbed dwarfs are subdivided on the basis of distribution: rhizomelic, mesomelic, and acromelic. Rhizomelic involves the proximal appendicular skeleton (humeri and femura), mesomelic the middle skeleton (radius–ulna and tibia–fibula) and acromelic the distal skeleton (metacarpals, metatarsals, and phalanges).

Dyschondrosteosis is the most common form of mesomelic dwarfism and demonstrates autosomal dominant inheritance. Clinically, patients have shortness of both forearms and lower legs. There is dorsal and external bowing forearms and limited range of motion at the elbows and wrists. Associations include ligamentous laxity, retardation, Turner syndrome, and systemic lupus erethematous.

Radiographically, there is bowing and shortening of both radii with triangulaton of the distal radial ephiphysis—bilateral Madelung deformity. Madelung deformity describes a variety of disorders that lead to premature closure of the radial growth plate and subsequent shortening and bowing of the diaphysis. The abnormality is thought to arise from premature closure of the medial aspect of the distal radial physis secondary to trauma or an anomalous ligament associated with dysplasia. The bowing of the radius leads to shortening, while the ulna develops normally, leading to distal dorsal subluxation. The radial epiphysis assumes a triangular configuration. The carpal bone relationships are abnormal and lead to early degenerative changes. Clinically, patients present with pain, fatigue, and limited range of motion at adolescence. Progression eventually ceases and pain may decrease. Surgery is required in some cases.

Notes

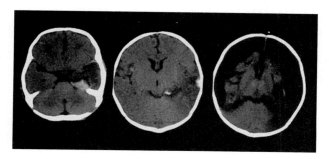

1. What is the differential diagnosis?
2. What is the treatment?
3. Is imaging of low or high priority?
4. Would you expect a temporal lobe predominance in this entity?

Neonatal Herpes Encephalitis

1. Bacterial meningitis, congenital toxoplasmosis, congenital cytomegalovirus, congenital rubella.

2. Antiviral drugs.

3. High, as timely diagnosis and efficacy of treatment depend greatly on prompt therapy.

4. No, unlike adult infection neonatal herpes causes diffuse brain involvement.

Reference

Noorbehesht B, Enzmann DR, Sullender W, et al.: Neonatal herpes simplex encephalitis: correlation of clinical and CT findings. *Radiology* 162:813–819, 1987.

Cross-Reference

Pediatric Radiology: THE REQUISITES, p 278.

Comment

Neonatal herpes infection is transmitted via two routes; transplacental and delivery. The majority of infections occur at delivery as the newborn comes into contact with an active lesion in the vagina. The brain is involved in approximately 30% of infections. The etiologic agent is herpes simplex virus type 2. The distribution of brain involvement differs from reactivated latent HSV1 or HSV2 in adults. While adults and older children demonstrate involvement of the temporal lobes and insular cortex, neonatal herpes causes diffuse brain destruction with multiple areas of focal hemorrhagic necrosis.

Clinically, patients present with symptoms within the first 2–4 weeks of life. Focal or generalized seizures, lethargy, cyanosis, fever, jaundice, and respiratory distress are presenting signs. The CSF will show a negative Gram stain with mononuclear pleocytosis.

As changes are dramatic and rapid in congenital HSV1 infection, the imaging findings vary with timing of the study. Early disease will demonstrate patchy areas of hypodensity within the periventricular white matter and cortex on CT. MR will demonstrate T2 hyperintensity, gyral swelling, and loss of gray-white contrast, indicating cerebral edema. Meningeal enhancement is highly suggestive of the diagnosis. Several days later petechial hemorrhage in the cortex, progressive atrophy, profound cortical thinning, and multicystic encephalomalacia of white matter are apparent on CT. MR changes include focal hemorrhagic necrosis and extensive T2 hyperintense cystic changes with parenchymal loss yielding a "Swiss cheese" appearance.

Antiviral drugs are the treatment of neonatal HSV1 infection, which holds a 15% mortality rate and 75% neurologic sequelae rate.

Notes

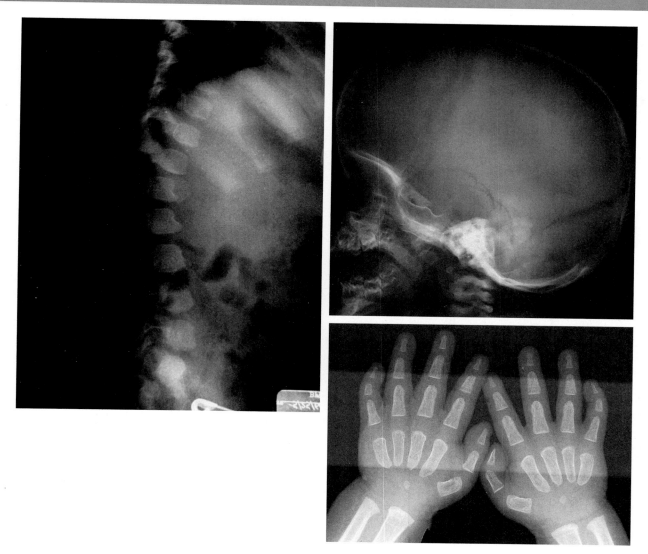

1. What is the inheritance pattern of this disorder?
2. Are ovoid vertebral bodies noted early or late in this process?
3. In Sanfilippo syndrome what type of anterior vertebral beaking is present?
4. Mucolipidosis radiographic skeletal changes are present at birth, true or false?

Hurler Syndrome

1. Hurler inheritance is autosomal recessive.

2. Ovoid vertebral bodies are noted early, while vertebra plana is noted late.

3. Sanfilippo sydrome is suggested by central and inferior anterior vertebral beaking.

4. True. Mucolipidosis, unlike mucopolysaccharidoses, demonstrate skeletal changes on radiographs at birth.

Reference

Schmidt H, Ullrich K, von Lengerke HJ, et al.: Radiological findings in patients with mucopolysaccharidosis I H/S (Hurler-Scheie syndrome). *Pediatr Radiol* 17(5):409–414, 1987.

Cross-Reference

Pediatric Radiology: THE REQUISITES, pp 208–209.

Comment

Hurler syndrome or mucopolysaccharidosis type I-H is the result of an enzyme deficiency that leads to the deposition of large amounts of mucopolysaccharides within multiple tissues of the body. Clinically, patients present within the first 2 years of life and may progress to mental retardation, deafness, corneal opacities, hepatosplenomegaly, cardiomegaly, and murmurs. Heparin sulfate and dermatin sulfate are detected in the urine.

Radiographically, most of the mucopolysaccharidoses are indistinguishable. Osteoporosis, macrocephaly, thick calvaria, wide ribs with narrowing at the costovertebral junction (canoe paddle), beaked oval vertebral bodies, thickened trabeculae, femoral head dysplasia, coax valga, narrow iliac wings, shortened tubal bones, and tapering of the second to fifth metacarpal bones represent many of the features common to the dysotosis multiplex syndromes encompassing both the mucopolysaccharidoses and mucoliposises. Distinctive in Hurler syndrome is the thickened metacarpals with proximal tapering described as a "bullet" appearance. In addition, inferior beaking of the vertebral bodies suggests Hurler or Hunter, while central beaking is noted in Morquio syndrome.

MR findings include delayed myelin formation (dysmyelination) yielding indistinct gray-white differentiation and atrophy with hydrocepahus. Cystic changes are noted within the peri and supraventicular white matter, corpus callosum, and basal ganglia. These cysts are likely to represent accumulations of mucopolysaccharides within the perivascular spaces. Infarcts and demyelination follow with progression of the disease.

Hurler syndrome is the most severe of the mucopolysaccharidoses. Therapy is primarily supportive. Bone marrow transplant has demonstrated some promise in recent studies. Life expectancy is 10 years.

Notes

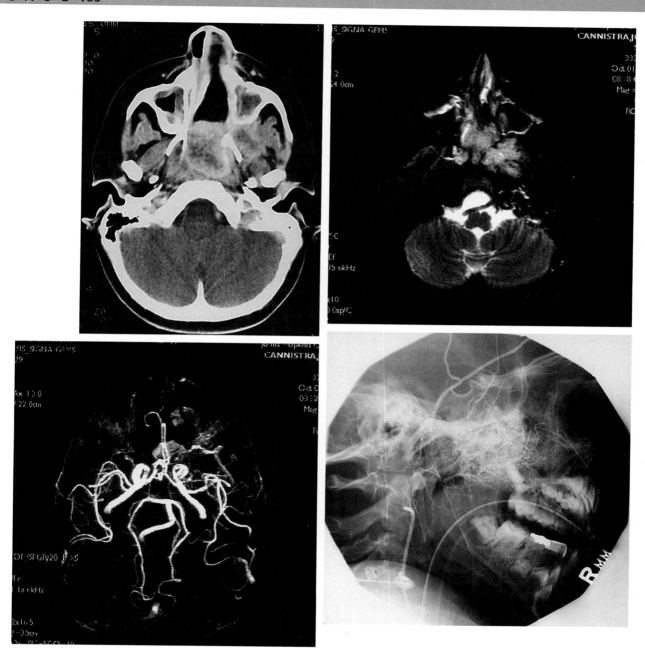

1. What is the differential diagnosis?
2. What percentage of cases involve intracranial spread?
3. How does this mass gain access to the cranium?
4. The majority of cases involve adolescent girls, true or false?

Juvenile Nasopharyngeal Angiofibroma

1. Chordoma, rhabdomyosarcoma, schwannoma of the fifth cranial nerve, nasopharyngeal carcinoma, angiomatous polyp.

2. 20%.

3. Through the pterygopalatine fossa (vidian canal and foramen rotundum).

4. False. It is almost exclusively seen in adolescent boys.

Reference

Chong VF, Fan YF: Radiology of the nasopharynx: pictorial essay. *Australas Radiol* 44(1):5–13, 2000.

Cross-Reference

Neuroradiology: THE REQUISITES, p 560.

Comment

Juvenile nasopharyngeal angiofibroma is a benign vascular tumor of the nasopharynx thought to arise from malformation of vasculature in or near the sphenopalatine foramen. The tumor grows along the vasculature expanding foramina and fissures while recruiting vessels from the external carotid artery and then later the internal carotid. Intracranial extension is most commonly seen within the infratemporal fossa via the pterygomaxillary fissure, the orbital apex through the inferior orbital fissure, or the middle cranial fossa via foramen rotundum. Clinically, adolescent boys present with epistaxis or nasal obstruction. This finding is rare in females.

CT will demonstrate a heterogeneous mass in the nasopharynx adjacent to the pterygopalatine fossa. Anterior bowing, thinning, and erosion of the posterior wall of the maxillary antrum without destruction may be present. MR will demonstrate enhancement, signal voids, and areas of T1 iso to hypointensity.

Patients are treated with preoperative embolization followed by surgery.

Notes

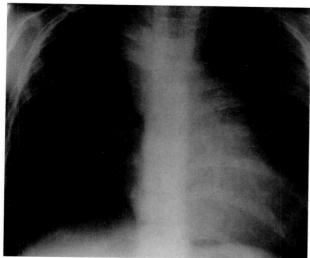

Cyanotic patient

1. Is there increased or decreased pulmonary vascularity?

2. If the vascularity was decreased what is your differential?

3. If the vascularity was increased what is your differential?

4. A right arch and cyanosis ought to make you think of what two diagnoses?

Truncus Arteriosus

1. Increased pulmonary vascularity.

2. Cyanotic with decreased vascularity: tetralogy of Fallot (normal heart size), Ebstein anomaly, pulmonic atresia, and tricuspid atresia (the latter three with enlarged heart).

3. Cyanotic with increased vascularity: transposition of the great arteries, truncus, total anomalous pulmonary venous return, and single ventricle.

4. Tetralogy of Fallot and the less common truncus arteriosus.

Reference

Allen HD, Gutgesell HP, Clark EB, et al.: *Moss and Adams Heart Disease in Infants, Children and Adolescents: Including the Fetus and Young Adult*, 6th edn. Baltimore: Lippincott Williams & Wilkins, 2000, pp 910–923.

Cross-Reference

Pediatric Radiology: THE REQUISITES, 2nd edn, pp 61–63.

Comment

Truncus arteriosus is an uncommon anomaly in which there is failure of the primary truncus to divide into the pulmonary artery and aorta. One large vessel supplies the coronary, systemic, and pulmonary circulations. A ventricular septal defect (VSD) is always present. There are four types: Type I, the aorta and PA share the truncus; Type II, no pulmonary trunk as the PA arises from the aorta; Type III, complete absence of the PA with lung circulation arising from the patent ductus arteriosus; Type IV, PA dominance with a hypoplastic proximal aorta and a PDA that perfuses the systemic circulation. There is a mild increase in flow to the pulmonary circulation as the systemic circulation presents greater resistance.

Clinically, cyanosis and heart failure occur early in life. Bounding peripheral pulses and a widened pulse pressure are due to the heart's attempt at increasing systemic circulation as the blood diverts to the lungs.

Radiographically, cardiomegaly and increased pulmonary circulation are present. The increased flow is transmitted to the left atrium as the left ventricle decompresses through the VSD. A prominent aorta is present and right sided in three-quarters of cases. In summary, cyanosis with shunt vascularity, cardiomegaly, and a prominent aortic arch are highly suggestive of truncus arteriosus. Surgical correction is recommended in the first few days of life.

Notes

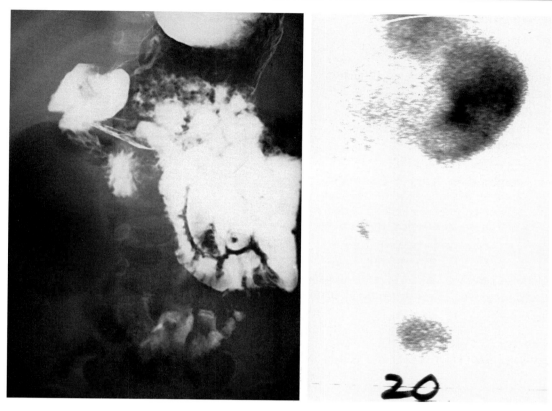

1. How large can this entity get?
2. What is the differential diagnosis for GI bleeding?
3. Who was JLA Peutz?
4. Who was Jeghers?

Meckel Diverticulum

1. 5 to 6 cm long.

2. Anal fissure, gastric mucosa containing Meckel diverticulum, juvenile polyp, inflammatory bowel disease, peptic ulcer disease

3. A Dutch pediatrician who in 1921 described a family with intestinal polyps as well as oral cutaneous pigmentation.

4. An American internist born in Jersey City, NJ. Jeghers completed residency at Boston City Hospital and in 1939 described the second case of intestinal polyps with oral cutaneous pigmented lesions and published a paper citing Peutz's case.

Reference

Khati NJ, Enquist EG, Javitt MC: Imaging of the umbilicus and periumbilical region. *Radiographics* 18:413–431, 1998.

Cross-Reference

Pediatric Radiology: THE REQUISITES, 2nd edn, p 111.

Comment

The vitelline duct is a tubular structure that runs within the umbilical cord connecting the midgut (at the site of the future terminal ileum) to the extraembryonic sac. The duct involutes at the sixth week. Persistence of the duct can manifest as a sinus, fistula, cyst, or diverticulum of the small bowel (Meckel diverticulum). Twenty per cent of these diverticula contain gastric mucosa or pancreatic rests that may cause ulceration. The most common presentation is GI bleeding ranging from hemoccult positive stools to hematochezia. Meckel diverticulum may also be a lead point for intussusception.

On imaging, conventional radiographs may show obstruction, intussusception, volvulus, or pneumoperitoneum from perforation. Definitive diagnosis is obtained through injection with 99mTc pertechnetate. The nuclear imaging study takes advantage of the normal uptake of pertechnetate by gastric mucosa, but will only be positive if gastric mucosa is present (20% of cases).

Notes

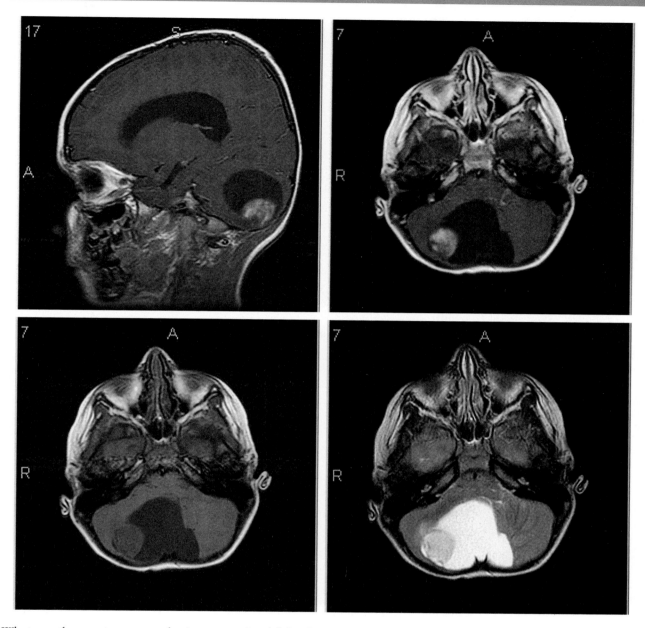

1. What are the most common brain tumors in children?

2. In what regions of the brain are these lesions found?

3. Is there a genetic etiology?

4. Is surgery curative?

Cerebellar Astrocytoma

1. Astrocytomas (40–50% of intracranial neoplasms).

2. 60% in the posterior fossa (40% in the cerebellum, 20% in the brainstem).

3. Juvenile pilocytic astrocytoma has been associated with long-arm deletions of chromosome 17.

4. Yes, in those cases that are surgically accessible.

Reference

Fulham MJ, Melisi JW, Nishimiya J, et al.: Neuroimaging of juvenile pilocytic astrocytomas: an enigma. *Radiology* 189:221–225, 1993.

Cross-Reference

Pediatric Radiology: THE REQUISITES, p 286.

Comment

Juvenile pilocytic astrocytoma (JPA) is a low-grade glial tumor that occurs in the under-10 age group. More than half of cases arise in the posterior fossa with the cerebellum and brainstem being the most common locations. Clinically, these patients present with early morning headache, vomiting, irritability, and ataxia as a result of mass effect causing obstructive non communicating hydrocephalus.

On CT, JPA appears as a well-circumscribed midline mass with a large cyst and focal mural nodule. Alternatively, the mass may be a rim of solid tumor surrounding necrotic debris. In either form there is little surrounding edema or calcification. There is intense enhancement of the solid portion or mural nodule. The intense enhancement is thought to be due to a special property of pilocytic astrocytomas that distinguishes them histologically from low-grade astrocytomas. JPAs, unlike astrocytomas, contain endothelial cells with open tight junctions and fenestrations allowing contrast to escape. Naturally, there is no enhancement of the cystic structure.

On MR the solid component of the tumor is isohypointense as opposed to medulloblastoma, which is hyperintense on T1 due to its high nucleus-to-cytoplasm ratio. On T2 JPA is hyperintense. The cystic components are bright on T2 but variable on T1 due to protein content.

If complete surgical resection is not possible, chemo and radiation are used. Prognosis is good relative to other forms of astrocytoma.

Notes

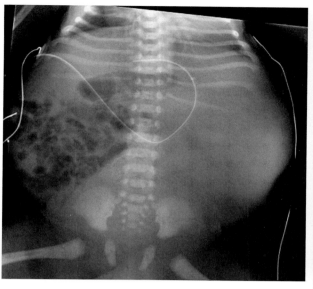 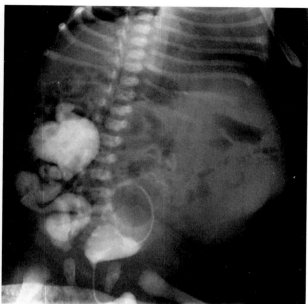

1. What is the frequency of this entity?

2. Is this entity inherited?

3. Is there a gender predominance?

4. Why is cryptorchidism coexistant with this entity?

Prune Belly (Eagle–Barrett) Syndrome

1. 1:40,000.

2. There is no inheritability.

3. Exclusively male.

4. The large bladder interferes with the normal descent of the testes.

Reference

Das Narla L, Doherty RD, Hingsbergen EA, et al.: Pediatric case of the day. Prune-belly syndrome (Eagle–Barrett syndrome, triad syndrome). *Radiographics* 18:1318–1322, 1998.

Cross-Reference

Pediatric Radiology: THE REQUISITES, p 164.

Comment

A classic triad of hypoplasia of the abdominal musculature, cryptorchidism, and marked dilatation of the urinary tract compose the Eagle–Barrett or prune belly syndrome. The etiology is related to abnormal musculature of the ureters as well as the abdominal wall. The entity is present exclusively in boys. Associated anomalies include: hypoplasia of the lungs, polydactyly or syndactyly, malrotation, scoliosis, congenital heart disease, pneumothorax, microcephaly, and imperforate anus. Twenty per cent of patients die in infancy.

Voiding cystourethrogram may demonstrate a hypertrophied bladder. Severe VUR often occurs, leading to tortuous dilated ureters and renal dysplasia. A large patent urachus is commonly present as it functions to decompress the pressure from reflux as well as urethral atresia. Excretory urography or a renogram is used to assess renal size, shape, and position. Scintigraphy may be employed to measure residual function prior to surgery as well.

Notes

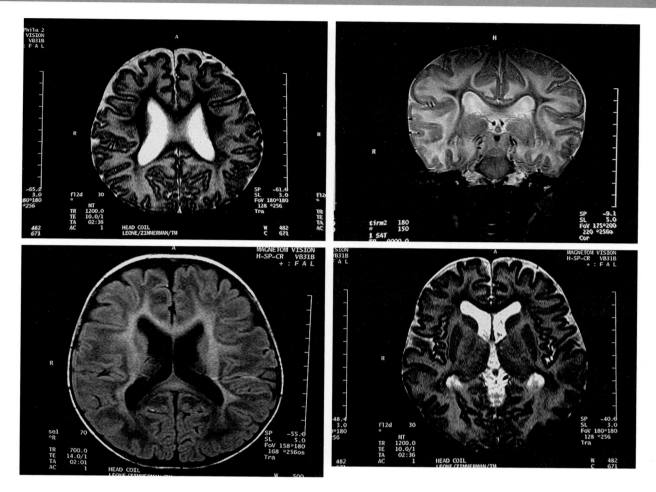

1. Which ethnic group is generally linked to carrying this disease?

2. Is MR spectroscopy useful in this disorder?

3. Are the internal capsules commonly spared or involved?

4. What similar disease presenting with macrocephaly demonstrates internal capsule involvement?

Canavan Disease

1. Askenazi Jews (eastern European descent) are carriers for Canavan. Sfardic Jews are of western European (mainly Spanish) descent.

2. Yes, MR spectroscopy can detect high levels of *N*-acetylaspartate.

3. The internal capsules are commonly spared.

4. Alexander disease typically demonstrates internal capsule involvement.

Reference

Brismar J, Brismar G, Gascon G, et al.: Canavan disease: CT and MR imaging of the brain. *Am J Neuroradiol* 11(4):805–810, 1990.

Cross-Reference

Pediatric Radiology: THE REQUISITES, p 361.

Comment

Canavan disease is an autosomal recessive inherited white-matter disease caused by the deficiency of the enzyme *N*-acetylaspartase. The disease presents in early infancy with hypotonia followed by spasticity, cortical blindness, and macrocephaly. There is an accumulation of *N*-acetylaspartic acid in the urine, brain, and blood. Three types have been identified: neonatal, infantile, and juvenile. Canavan disease is rapidly progressive.

On imaging, subcortical white matter demonstrates hypodensity on CT and hyperintensity on T2-weighted imaging. Canavan is unique among the leukodystrophies as it initially involves the subcortical white matter and then spreads to the deep white matter. Gyral expansion and cortical thinning are present. Involvement tends to be symmetric with areas of ventriculomegaly late in the disease. Low-intensity T1 signal is demonstrated as a result of demyelination. MR spectroscopy demonstrates high levels of *N*-acetylaspartate. Diffusion-weighted imaging demonstrates restricted diffusion in affected regions.

Prognosis is poor with death by 5 years.

Notes

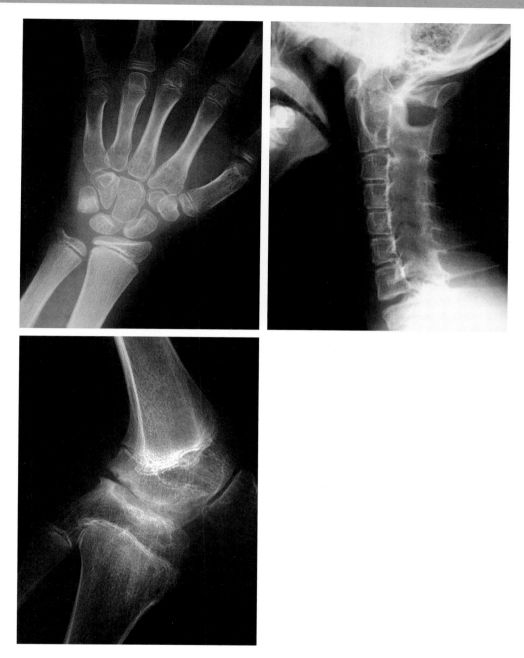

1. Are there extra-articular manifestations of this process?

2. Assuming you answered yes to the previous question, what are they?

3. If you had answered no to question 1, do not delay and proceed directly to Louisville.

4. What is the differential diagnosis?

Juvenile Chronic Arthritis (JCA)

1. Yes, JCA affects many systems as its central pathophysiology is vasculitis.

2. Pulmonary fibrosis, pericarditis, myocarditis, glomerulonephritis, and uveitis.

3. The three-letter airport code is SDF.

4. Juvenile chronic arthritis (Still disease), hemophilia, trauma, infection.

Reference

Johnson K, Gardner-Medwin J: Childhood arthritis: classification and radiology. *Clin Radiol* 57(1):47–58, 2002.

Cross-Reference

Pediatric Radiology: THE REQUISITES, pp 225–226.

Comment

Rheumatoid arthritis is a chronic systemic inflammatory disorder thought to be triggered by exposure to an arthrogenic antigen in patients that are immunologically susceptible. Genetic susceptibility has been linked to various haplotypes that have a specific antigen binding cleft adjacent to the T-cell receptor on macrophages that induces the autoimmune response. It is thought that Epstein–Barr virus cross-reactivity with type 2 collagen or specific cell surface glycoproteins may play a role as the initiating etiology. There is subsequent infiltration of inflammatory cells, notably T-cells, in the synovial lining of the joint. The cytokine and immunologic mediators induce angiogenesis with resultant increased blood flow to the joint. Eventually, a mass of synovium mixed with fibroblasts and inflammatory cells, the pannus, erodes the underlying cartilage and produces a fibrous and eventual bony bridge with the opposing bone. Adult rheumatoid is defined clinically as containing four of the following criteria: (1) arthritis in three or more areas, (2) arthritis of hand joints, (3) rheumatoid nodules, (4) morning stiffness, (5) symmetric arthritis, (6) serum rheumatoid factor, (7) radiographic inflammatory synovitis changes. Other areas affected by rheumatoid include the skin and vascular system with nodules and vasculitis the central manifestations.

Juvenile chronic arthritis is a blanket term covering juvenile-onset ankylosing spondylitis, psoriatic arthritis, arthritis of inflammatory bowel disease, juvenile-onset adult type seropositive rheumatoid arthritis, and seronegative chronic arthritis (Still disease—70% of cases).

Juvenile chronic arthritis begins before 16 with a 2:1 female predominance. JCA differs from adult rheumatoid as oligoarthritis is more common, and there is large joint predominance, systemic onset predominance, absent rheumatoid nodules, absent rheumatoid factor, and antineutrophillic cytoplasmic antibody (ANCA) positivity. The knees, wrists, elbows, and ankles are commonly affected.

Still disease is divided into three categories, (1) systemic disease, (2) polyarticular disease with moderate systemic involvement, and (3) mono or oligoarticular disease with little systemic involvement. The monoarticular variant is most common and often presents in the knee. Still disease presents earlier than the other forms of JCA. Radiographically, soft tissue swelling, osteoporosis, periostitis, erosions, ankylosis, and growth disturbances are present. Growth disturbances such as epiphyseal overgrowth secondary to hyperemia or distal ulna undergrowth due to erosions depend on the nature of the process.

Many patients fully recover by adulthood, while a fair number have permanent sequelae characterized by degenerative arthritis, growth deformity, muscle wasting, and loss of function.

Notes

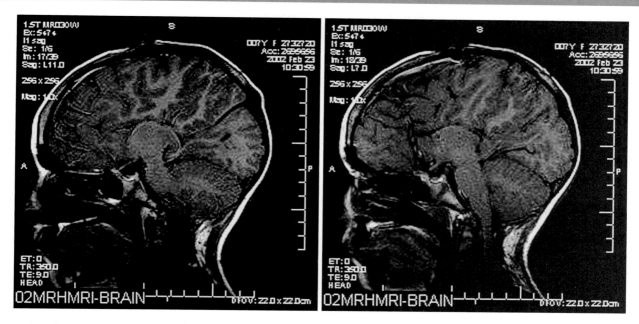

1. Which infectious agent is linked with this disorder?

2. What is the distinction between pachygyria and this entity?

3. What part of the brain is most often affected?

4. What percentage of cases demonstrate calcification?

Polymicrogyria

1. Cytomegalovirus.

2. Pachygyria is a migrational abnormality. In polymicrogyria the neurons are in the proper cortical layer but are disordered and miswired.

3. Posterior aspect of the sylvian fissure.

4. Less than 5%.

Reference

Barkovich AJ, Kuzniecky RI: Neuroimaging of focal malformations of cortical development. *J Clin Neurophysiol* 13(6):481–494, 1996.

Cross-Reference

Pediatric Radiology: THE REQUISITES, p 274.

Comment

Polymicrogyria (PMG) translates as too many small gyri and is thought to occur due to either an ischemic or infectious insult during the second trimester. There are varying degrees of cortical disorganization depending on the timing of the event. Clinically, patients present with seizures, hemiplegia, and developmental delay with age of onset directly related to the degree of malformation.

On CT, PMG appears very close in appearance to pachygyria (a smooth brain devoid of cortical sulci). Calcification may be noted secondary to TORCH infection. On MR the cortical surface will appear bumpy and irregular. Signal characteristics of the affected areas follow normal cortical signal on all sequences. A high T2 signal in white matter may be seen in 20% of cases, presumably from gliosis secondary to the ischemic event. Large draining veins may be noted as the underlying cortical disorganization leads to abnormal outflow pathways.

Treatment is medical for seizures, with variable prognosis depending on severity of involvement.

Notes

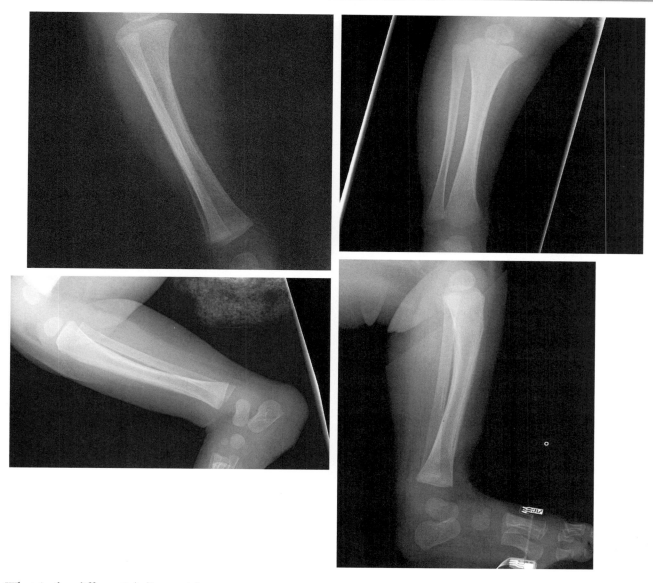

1. What is the differential diagnosis?

2. Would you be surprised to find that the patient had a patent ductus arteriosus (PDA)?

3. Soft tissue swelling is commonly seen overlying which bone?

4. Is this entity more commonly monostotic or polyostotic?

Infantile Cortical Hyperostosis
(Caffey Disease)

1. Infection, trauma, hypervitaminosis A, malignancy, and prostagladin therapy.

2. No, long-term prostaglandin therapy for PDA has been implicated as a cause.

3. Mandible.

4. Polyostotic.

Reference

Kocher MS, Kasser JR: Radiologic case study. Infantile cortical hyperostosis (Caffey's disease). *Orthopedics* 22(7):712, 707–708, 1999.

Cross-Reference

Pediatric Radiology: THE REQUISITES, pp 213–214.

Comment

Caffey disease or infantile cortical hyperostosis is a rare disorder of unknown etiology occurring during the first 9 weeks of life. Irritability, fever, anemia, increased SED rate, and soft tissue swelling around such areas as the mandible, clavicle, and tubular bones, are common at presentation. The clinical course is variable.

Radiographically, periosteal new bone formation effects the mandible, ribs, clavicle, and ulna in decreasing order of frequency. A lamellated appearance of the cortex is commonly present and may affect multiple or single bones. Resolution occurs over 6–12 months with normalization of the bony appearance. Differential considerations include hypervitaminosis A, long-term prostaglandin E administration, physiologic periostitis, infection, scurvy, and trauma X.

Notes

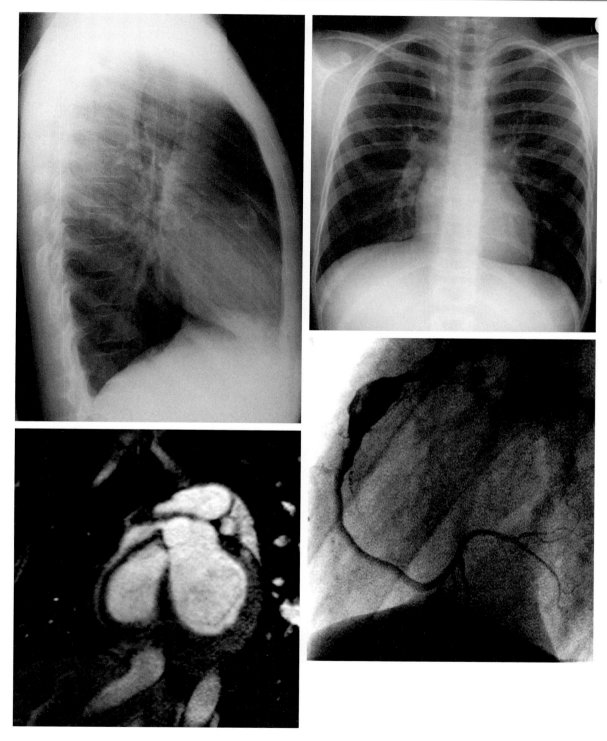

1. What are the clinical manifestations of this disease?
2. What are the complications?
3. What is the suspected etiology of this disease?
4. Infants are more prone to serious disease. True or false?

Kawasaki Disease

1. Conjunctivitis, fever, strawberry tongue, lymphadenopathy, desquamating hands and feet, angular stomatitis.

2. Arthritis, myocarditis, pericarditis, mitral insufficiency, congestive heart failure, uveitis, meningitis, and gallbladder hydrops.

3. The suspected etiology is viral, although the agent has yet to be isolated.

4. True. Infants are at great risk for coronary aneurysms and infarction.

Reference

Rauzzino M, Oakes WJ: Chiari II malformation and syringomyelia. *Neurosurg Clin N Am* 6(2):293–309, 1995.

Cross-Reference

Pediatric Radiology: THE REQUISITES, 2nd edn, pp 70–71.

Comment

Kawasaki disease or mucocutaneous lymph node syndrome is an infectious inflammatory entity that affects mainly infants and children. Kawasaki disease is defined by the presence of five or six signs, including: enanthema, exanthema, extremity changes, conjunctivitis, unremitting fever, and lymphadenopathy. A third of patients develop coronary artery aneurysms in the proximal segments of both left and right coronary arteries. The aneurysms place the infant at great risk for myocardial infarction.

Radiographically the chest film is normal, although the coronary arteries may calcify and severe myocarditis may cause cardiac enlargement. Echocardiogram is the test of choice and will easily delineate the large aneurysm seen at the proximal coronary arteries. The aneurysms may appear saccular, cylindric, fusiform, or segmental. If coronary artery bypass is considered, coronary angiogram will define the precise anatomy.

Treatment in the acute period includes intravenous gamma globulin and salicylates to prevent aneurysm development. Coronary bypass has been performed with patients demonstrating ischemia.

Notes

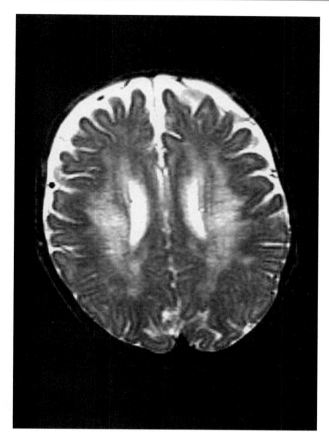

1. What are bulbar signs?

2. What muscles are innervated by the motor nuclei of the lower brainstem?

3. How is the diagnosis of this entity made?

4. What is the enzyme deficiency in this disorder?

Krabbe Disease

1. Bulbar is an old term referring to the obdula oblongata. Bulbar signs refer to weakness and wasting of muscles innervated by the motor nuclei of the lower brainstem.

2. Muscles of the jaw, face, tongue, larynx, and pharynx are innervated by the motor nuclei of the lower brainstem.

3. Diagnosis is based on an assay for beta-galactosidase activity from skin fibroblasts.

4. Beta-galactosidase deficiency.

Reference

Sasaki M, Sakuragawa N, Takashima S, et al.: MRI and CT findings in Krabbe disease. *Pediatr Neurol* 7(4):283–288, 1991.

Cross-Reference

Neuroradiology: THE REQUISITES, p 362.

Comment

Globoid cell leukodystrophy, or Krabbe disease, is an entity caused by the deficiency of beta-galactosidase, with resultant accumulation of galactoceramide and psychosine, substances highly toxic to developing myelin-producing oligodendrocytes. Clinically, patients present with irritability, fever, feeding problems, hyperreflexia, and delayed development. Optic atrophy leading to blindness may develop. There are four types: infantile, late infantile, juvenile, and adult.

On CT, diffuse areas of high attenuation are present in the thalami, corona radiata, and caudate and dentate nuclei. Diffuse white-matter disease follows with low density seen thoughout the white-matter tracts and ever increasing atrophy. MR demonstrates low signal on T1 and high signal on T2 throughout the white matter with a predominance in the parietal lobes. The splenium of the corpus callosum and the posterior limb of the internal capsule are characteristic for involvement. Thalamic involvement is present late in the course of the disease.

Treatment is supportive; however, some progress has been shown in bone marrow transplant in patients at the early onset of symptoms. Prognosis varies with type: infantile average 13 months, late infantile 2 years, juvenile and adult are highly variable.

Notes

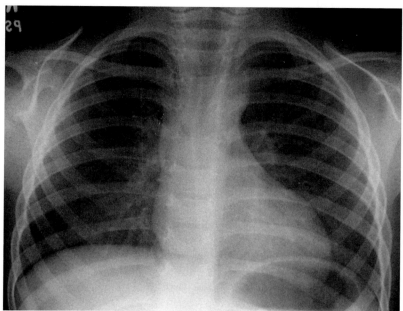

Noncyanotic patient

1. Is there increased or normal pulmonary vascularity?
2. If the vascularity was normal what is your differential?
3. If the vascularity was increased what is your differential?
4. What is the most common congenital cardiac abnormality?

Congenital Aortic Stenosis

1. Normal, ascending aorta is prominent at an early age (<10 years).

2. Acyanotic with normal vascularity: aortic stenosis, pulmonic stenosis, coarctation, and interrupted aortic arch.

3. Endocardial cushion defect, atrial septal defect, patent ductus arteriosus (PDA) (enlarged LA and enlarged aorta), and ventricular septal defect (VSD) (enlarged LA and normal aorta).

4. Bicuspid aortic valve.

Reference

Rauzzino M, Oakes WJ: Chiari II malformation and syringomyelia. *Neurosurg Clin N Am* 6(2):293–309, 1995.

Cross-Reference

Pediatric Radiology: THE REQUISITES, 2nd edn, pp 66–67.

Comment

The most common congenital anomaly is not VSD but a bicuspid aortic valve. Although initially asymptomatic, bicuspid valves become stenotic with time during adolescence or adulthood. Aortic stenosis (AS) is associated with other cardiac anomalies in a quarter of cases. Anomalies include PDA and coarctation. There is male predominance.

AS is divided into four anatomic types: valvular (75%), supravalvular, subvalvular membranous, and subvalvular muscular. Most valvular stenoses develop from turbulent blood flow through bicuspid valves that grow thickened, rigid, and deformed over time. The ventricle compensates by hypertrophying, although progressive valvular disease leads to eventual failure. Flow to the coronaries is compromised and patients are at risk for sudden death at times of increased activity. Patients are at risk for endocarditis as well.

Radiographically, the chest film may be normal or may show left ventricular hypertrophy on the lateral. The LV comprises the lower half of the posterior cardiac border on the later view. The posterior heart border ought to cross the IVC 2 cm above the diaphragm. An intersection below this point suggests LV enlargement. Post-stenotic dilatation may be present in the enlarged ascending aorta. Treatment involves either balloon dilatation or valve replacement. The ascending aorta should not be border-forming before 10 years.

In supravalvular stenosis there is congenital narrowing of the ascending aorta. The entity is usually associated with Williams syndrome. Williams syndrome is idiopathic infantile hypercalcemia: mental retardation, elfin facies (friendly demeanor), supravalvular aortic stenosis, and pulmonic stenosis. Chest radiographs are normal. Patients may have a diffuse coarctation manifested as a segment of narrowing from the subclavian to the ductus. An hourglass appearance to the proximal aorta is seen on angio in some cases.

Subvalvular stenosis is divided into membranous or muscular types. The membranous type is caused by the formation of an abnormal membrane that develops just below the valve, obstructing the outflow tract. The muscular variety obstructs the outflow tract due to left ventricular hypertrophy.

Notes

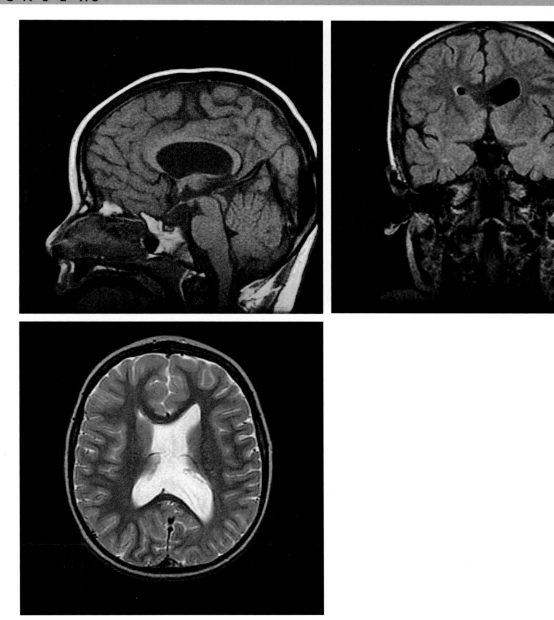

1. Is this entity more common in males or females?
2. What vascular territory is thought to be involved?
3. What is Kallman syndrome?
4. What cranial nerves are involved in this disorder?

Septo-optic Dysplasia

1. Septo-optic dysplasia is more common in females.

2. Anterior cerebral.

3. Holoprosencephaly and septo-optic dysplasia.

4. CN I and II.

Reference

Lau KY, Tam W, Lam PK, et al.: Radiological cases of the month. Septo-optic dysplasia (de Morsier syndrome). *Am J Dis Child* 147(1):71–72, 1993.

Cross-Reference

Pediatric Radiology: THE REQUISITES, p 269.

Comment

Septo-optic dysplasia or de Morsier syndrome consists of hypoplasia or aplasia of the septum pellucidum and hypoplasia of the optic nerves. The syndrome is thought to be a result of in utero ischemia with a genetic component. Heritability has been suggested as there are familial cases described. One variant has been associated with schizencephaly and hypothalamic—pituitary dysfunction. Patients are of short stature as a result of growth hormone deficiency. Other variants include ectopic pituitary and holoprosencephaly type hypoplasias of the falx and corpus callosum.

Clinically, patients present with nystagmus and blindness. Patients with hypothalamic involvement are short. Seizure disorder is seen in up to 50% of patients.

On CT there is an absent septum pellucidum; small optic canals and thin optic nerves. MR will demonstrate hypoplasia or complete absence of the septum pellucidum. On coronal sections, the frontal horns may have a box-like configuration. The optic nerves will appear thin, most pronounced in the area of the optic chiasm, a good place to look. Schizencephaly, polymicrogyra, and gray-matter heterotopias are findings that ought to provoke closer examination of the optic nerves.

Patients are treated with seizure meds and for growth hormone deficiency.

Notes

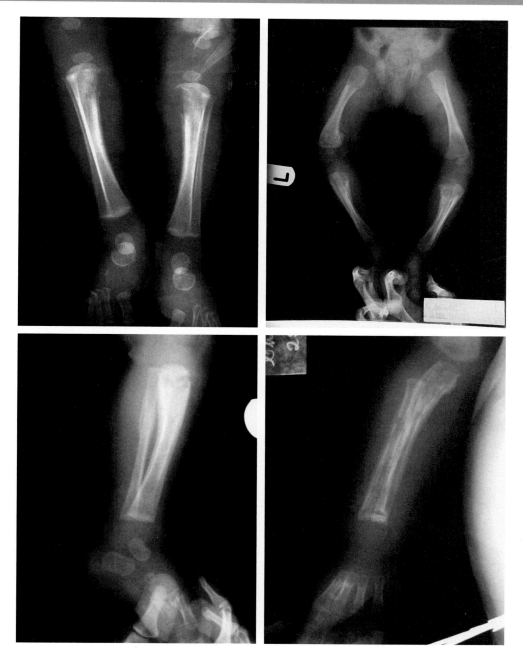

1. Is this entity an increasing public health worry?

2. How is a frog-leg lateral positioned and what does it demonstrate?

3. Is Wimberger's ring characteristic in this entity?

4. What is the differential diagnosis?

Congenital Syphilis

1. Congenital syphilis incidence is decreasing.

2. It is an A-P film with the hips flexed and abducted. The view allows for physeal evaluation and the relative position of the epiphyses and metaphyses as in slipped capital femoral epiphysis.

3. No, Wimberger's ring is seen in scurvy. Wimberger's sign is seen in syphilis.

4. TORCH infections, hypervitaminosis A, or Caffey disease.

References

Dalinka MK, Lally JF, Koniver G, et al.: The radiology of osseous and articular infection. *CRC Crit Rev Clin Radiol Nucl Med* 7(1):1–64, 1975.
Parish JL: Treponemal infections in the pediatric population. *Clin Dermatol* 18(6):687–700, 2000.

Cross-Reference
Pediatric Radiology: THE REQUISITES, p 225.

Comment

Congenital syphilis is usually acquired from an infected mother during the second or third trimester. Clinically, rhinorrhea, rash, anemia, hepatosplenomegaly, ascites, and nephrotic syndrome are manifested. Skeletal changes, present in 90% of cases, become apparent at 6–8 weeks. The spirochetes directly infiltrate the bone, periosteum, and cartilage via the blood thereby favoring the region with greatest vascularity, the metaphysis. The spirochetes inhibit and eventually destroy osteoblasts, arresting enchondral bone formation and leading to widened irregular growth plates.

Radiographically, symmetric involvement of enchondral ossification sites is the rule. Widened metaphyses with fraying and fragmentation reflect the physeal growth disturbance. Erosive changes appearing as notches on the medial proximal metaphysis of the tibia are classic and referred to as Wimberger's sign. Diffuse periostitis is present and thought to occur as either a result of direct infection of the periosteum or as a reparative response.

Notes

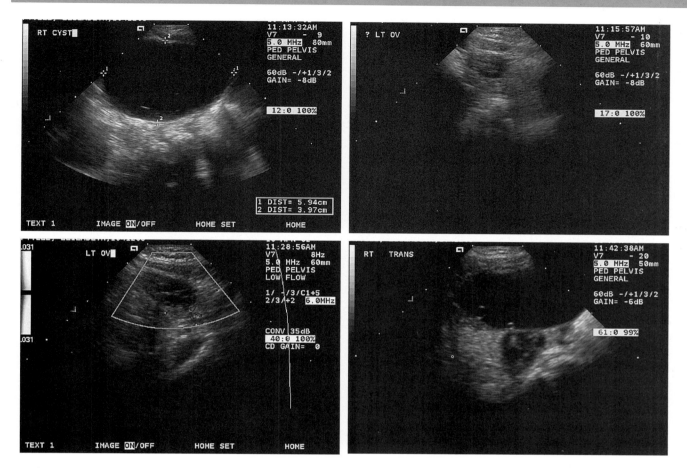

1. What is the most common ovarian mass in adolescence?

2. Which diseases are associated with this entity?

3. Can this entity pose a danger at delivery?

4. Pre-eclampsia, diabetes, and RH isoimmunization have all been implicated as etiologies; why?

Neonatal Ovarian Cyst

1. Simple ovarian cyst.

2. Cystic fibrosis, congenital juvenile hypothyroidism, McCune–Albright syndrome, and sexual precocity.

3. Yes, mechanical complications during delivery have been reported.

4. They are associated with higher levels of gonadotropin.

Reference

Schmahmann S, Haller JO: Neonatal ovarian cysts: pathogenesis, diagnosis and management. *Pediatr Radiol* 27(2):101–105, 1997.

Cross-Reference

Pediatric Radiology: THE REQUISITES, p 188.

Comment

Ovarian cysts during the neonatal period may present as large abdominal masses and are thought to be Graafian follicles that enlarge secondary to stimulation by maternal chorionic gonadotropin. Ultrasound will show large, simple cysts that are para midline. Differential considerations include hydronephrosis (be sure to positively identify normal kidneys), urachal cyst (midline), and an enteric duplication cyst (a hyperechoic rim representing the muscular layer). Most simple ovarian cysts resolve spontaneously, while those greater than 6 cm predispose to ovarian torsion and require surgery or percutaneous drainage.

Notes

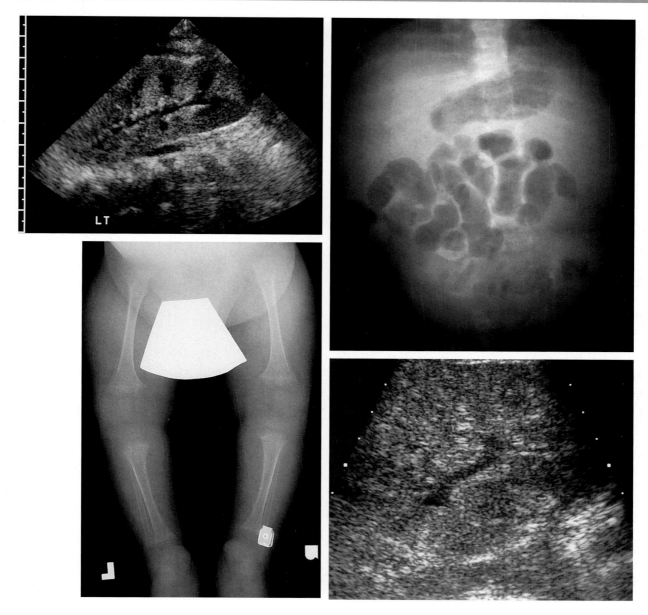

1. What is the distinction between gallbladder hydrops and acalculous cholecystitis?

2. What is the differential for fatty liver?

3. Name causes of cirrhosis.

4. Are these patients at increased risk for hepatocellular carcinoma?

Tyrosinemia

1. Both show dilated gallbladders, but there is no wall thickening in hydrops, as there is no inflammatory component.

2. Cystic fibrosis, malnutrition, hyperalimentation, glycogen storage disease, steroid therapy.

3. Biliary atresia, cholestasis secondary to total parenteral nutrition, tyrosinemia, galactosemia and alpha-1-antitrypsin deficiency, hepatitis.

4. Yes, they are at increased risk for hepatocellular carcinoma

Reference

Dubois J, Garel L, Patriquin H, et al.: Imaging features of type 1 hereditary tyrosinemia: a review of 30 patients. *Pediatr Radiol* 6(12):845–851, 1996.

Cross-Reference

Pediatric Radiology: THE REQUISITES, 2nd edn, p 133.

Comment

Tyrosinemia is an inborn error of metabolism with autosomal recessive inheritance. The defect involves the final step in catabolism of tyrosine leading to abnormal accumulation of tyrosine within the liver and kidneys. An infant with hepatic dysfunction, rickets, and renal disease should be suspected of having tyrosinemia. Ultrasound and CT will show an enlarged liver with a heterogeneous echotexture. Nodule formation has been reported. Renal findings on ultrasound include enlargement, hyperechogenecity, and nephrocalcinosis.

Tyrosinemia may lead to cirrhosis. Cirrhosis is defined as a diffuse process characterized by fibrosis and the conversion of normal liver architecture into structurally abnormal nodules. The pathophysiology centers around three processes: cell death, fibrosis, and regeneration. The imaging findings demonstrate enlargement of the left and caudate lobes, and nodularity and compression of intrahepatic vessels. Ultrasound will show increased echogenicity. Regenerating nodules will follow normal liver parenchyma on MR sequences.

Notes

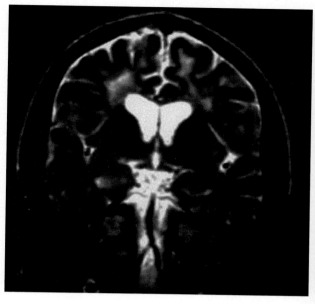 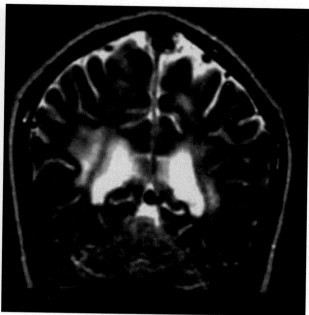

1. What is the differential diagnosis?
2. What are the CT findings?
3. When do MRI findings begin to develop relative to clinical findings?
4. Findings are bilateral and symmetric, true or false?

Subacute Sclerosing Panencephalitis

1. MS, Lyme, acute disseminated encephalomyelitis (ADEM).

2. Diffuse atrophy with multifocal areas of low attenuation in the white matter.

3. 3–4 months after clinical findings.

4. False, bilateral and asymmetric.

Reference

Bohlega S, al-Kawi MZ: Subacute sclerosing panencephalitis. Imaging and clinical correlation. *J Neuroimaging* 4(2):71–76, 1994.

Cross-Reference

Pediatric Radiology: THE REQUISITES, p 278.

Comment

Subacute sclerosing panencephalitis (SSPE) is a disorder of neurologic deterioration caused by reactivation of latent measles virus. Onset of SSPE is usually seen between ages 5 and 15 years. Clinically, patients present with behavioral changes, mental decline, myoclonus ataxia, and seizures.

On imaging, MR may be normal within the first 3–4 months. Eventually an abnormally high T2 signal is seen within the cortex and subcortical white matter of the temporal and parietal lobes. Over time the high T2 signal extends to the ventricle with involvement of the periventricular white matter and corpus callosum. In later stages the abnormal T2 signal extends to the brainstem and diffuse atrophy occurs. Enhancement is present early on. Differentials include MS (very little cortical involvement), Lyme (history and cranial nerve involvement), and ADEM (white matter involvement and history).

Prognosis is poor with the development of dementia, quadriparesis, and autonomic instability. Patients die within 2–6 years.

Notes

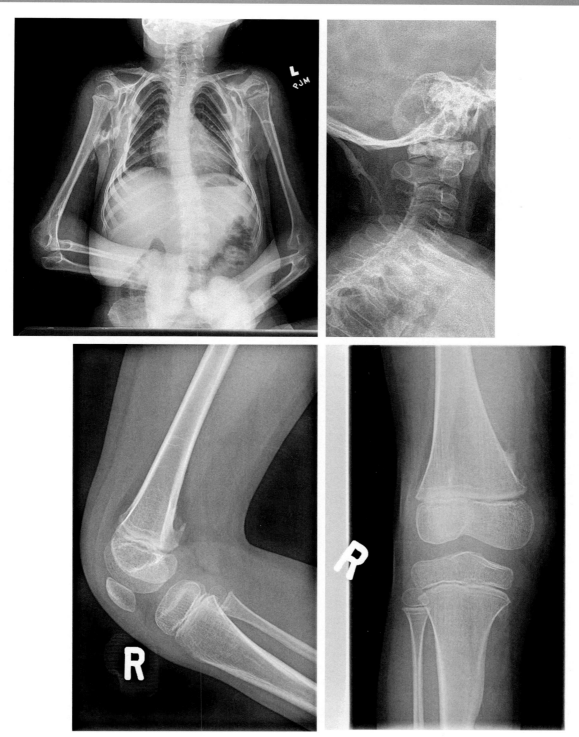

1. Is this disorder heritable?

2. Are the teeth involved?

3. What are the differential diagnostic considerations?

4. Is there commonly an initiating event?

Fibrodysplasia Ossificans Progressiva

1. Yes, it is transmitted via autosomal dominance.

2. Yes, patients may be missing incisors.

3. Klippel–Feil (c-spine), myositis (extremity), rheumatoid (c-spine), multiple exostosis (extremity), and extraskeletal osteosarcoma (extremity).

4. There is usually a history of traumatic injury.

Reference

Kocyigit H, Hizli N, Memis A, et al.: A severely disabling disorder: fibrodysplasia ossificans progressiva. *Clin Rheumatol* 20(4):273–275, 2001.

Comment

Fibrodysplasia ossificans progressiva (FOP) is a rare hereditary disorder in which muscle, tendons, ligaments, and fascia progressively ossify. This entity ought not be confused with myositis ossificans, a disorder characterized by soft tissue calcification usually following a traumatic injury. FOP is not calcification but rather ossification of the soft tissues. The etiology is not well understood but appears to be mapped to chromosome 4, which codes for a bone morphogenic growth protein. It appears that trauma to the soft tissues initiates the proliferation of fibroblasts and replacement of muscle tissue by bone.

Clinically, congenital malformations of the hands and feet (hallux valgus deformity) are present. In early infancy patients have episodes of soft tissue swelling followed 3–4 weeks later by ectopic bone formation in the musculature. Over time, the ligaments, fascia, tendons, and joint capsules become involved. Patients report of painful, tender soft tissue indurations following trauma. Eventually involvement of the limbs and chest wall leads to restrictive lung disease, pneumonia, and death before 40.

Radiographically, multifocal heterotopic ossification is present within muscle and subcutaneous tissue. Ankylosis is a common feature with involvment of the interphalangeal, carpometacarpal, and metatarsophalangeal joints. Hallux valgus, webbed toes, polydactyly, and phalangeal synostosis are present as well. Vertebral anomalies include early small vertebral bodies with vertebral fusion in later childhood. Fusion occurs from posterior to anterior with involvement of the neural arches followed by vertebral body fusion. Acetabular dysplasia and subluxation are present in the femur in addition to short, broad femoral necks.

Notes

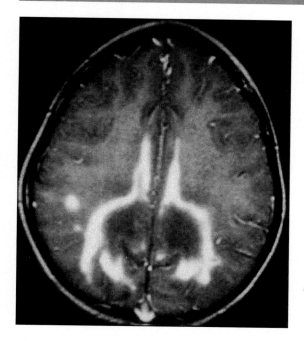

1. Is magnetic transfer imaging sensitive to myelination vs. demyelination?
2. Is diffusion-weighted imaging sensitive to myelination vs. demyelination?
3. What is the etiology of this disorder?
4. Is the corpus callosum spared?

Adrenoleukodystrophy

1. Yes. Increased myelination leads to increased magnetic transfer.

2. Yes. Demyelinated nerves demonstrate unrestricted diffusion in multiple planes rather than just in the longitudinal direction.

3. A deficiency of aryl-coenzyme A synthetase, an enzyme that functions in the beta hydroxylation of fatty acid chains.

4. No, the corpus callosum is usually involved.

Reference

Jensen ME, Sawyer RW, Braun IF, et al.: MR imaging appearance of childhood adrenoleukodystrophy with auditory, visual, and motor pathway involvement. *Radiographics* 10:53–66, 1990.

Cross-Reference

Neuroradiology: THE REQUISITES, p 219.

Comment

Adrenoleukodystrophy is an X-linked disorder due to a perixosomal enzymatic defect in the metabolism of very long-chain fatty acids. It has been proposed that these fatty acids have a direct toxic effect on the brain, triggering an inflammatory response that leads to breakdown of myelin.

Patients usually present between 5 and 10 years initially with learning difficulties, gait disturbance, intellectual impairment, hypotonia, seizures, visual complaints, and swallowing difficulties. Progressive paresis follows until death.

On CT, low attenuation is seen in the occipital white matter and splenium of the corpus callosum. MR is characteristic with confluent T2 hyperintensity present in the occipital white matter surrounding the atria. The hyperintensity extends into the splenium as well. Gadolinium will demonstrate enhancement only in areas of active demyelination. Over time involvement will progress to the frontal white matter. Corticospinal tracts in the pons and medulla as well as the auditory pathways demonstrate high T2 signal.

Patients are treated with steroids, bone marrow transplantation, and dietary fatty acids.

Notes

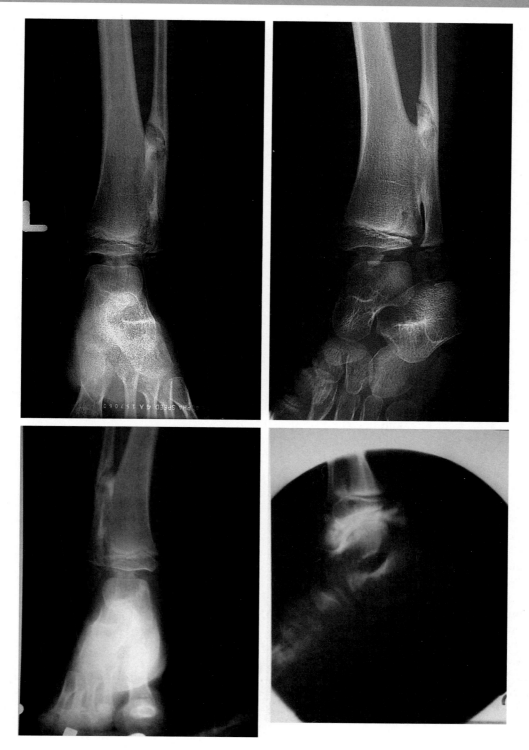

1. How rare is this lesion?

2. Which joints are most commonly affected?

3. What is the differential diagnosis?

4. Is there malignant potential?

Trevor Disease

1. Prevalence is estimated at 1:1,000,000.

2. Knee, talus, and tarsal navicular are most commonly affected.

3. Chondroblastoma, osteochondroma, and enchondroma are differential considerations.

4. No malignant potential has been reported.

Reference

Murphey MD, Choi JJ, Kransdorf MJ, et al.: Imaging of osteochondroma: variants and complications with radiologic-pathologic correlation. *Radiographics* 20(5):1407–1434, 2000.

Cross-Reference

Pediatric Radiology: THE REQUISITES, p 46.

Comment

Trevor disease, or dysplasia epiphysealis hemimelica (DEH), is a rare disorder in which osteochondromas arise at the epiphysis. Osteochondromas are normally found on the metaphyseal side of the physis. The etiology is unknown but thought to involve disturbance of regulation in cartilage-producing cells in the early limb bud. Clinically, patients present with painless swelling, asymmetric mass on one side of the joint, limitation of motion, and recurrent joint locking. The knee, talus, navicular, and cuneiform joints are most often affected, with predilection for the medial aspect of the epiphysis.

Radiographically, the affected epiphysis appears overgrown with a partially calcified projecting mass. The mass may appear extra-articular on projectional radiographs; however, following ossification, a bridge or broad-based attachment is detectable. MR is useful in that it allows direct visualization of the nonossified mass as well as presurgical planning for resection and delineation of the abnormal and normal epiphyseal components. In addition, MR has demonstrated utility in evaluation of the surrounding soft tissue structures. MR findings will demonstrate signal characteristics that follow cartilage on all sequences; intermediate signal intensity on T1-weighted and high signal intensity on T2-weighted images. Areas of low signal intensity on T1- and T2-weighted images correlate with areas of calcification or ossification that progress with skeletal maturity. DEH does not appear to grow beyond skeletal maturity. A full skeletal survey is recommended as multiple sites on one bone or an entire extremity represent one-third of all cases.

Most of these lesions have been treated by surgery with correction of the secondary angular deformity. Complications include early osteoarthritis, loose bodies, and leg length discrepancy.

Notes

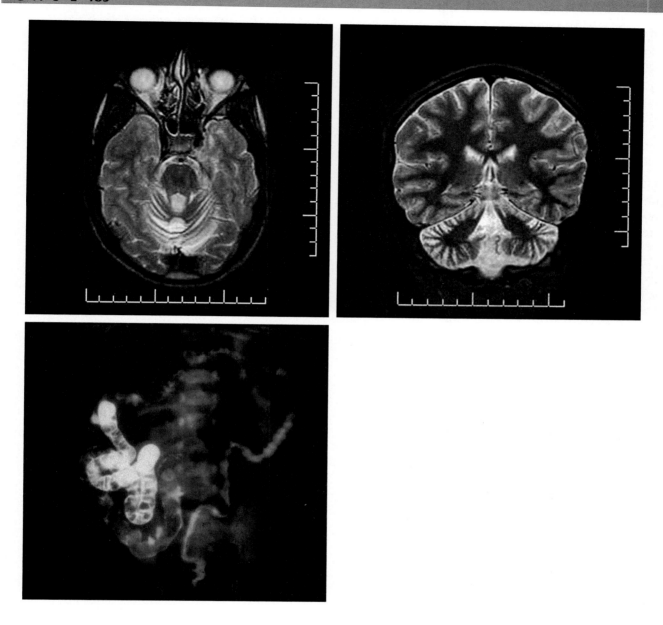

1. Might this patient be referred to a dermatologist?
2. What is the leading cause of death?
3. Might you expect the patient to have splenomegaly?
4. What percentage of these patients develop leukemia or lymphoma?

Ataxia Telangiectasia

1. Yes, multiple capillary telangiectasias of the skin appear between 3 and 6 years.

2. Pulmonary infections secondary to impaired immunity.

3. No, these patients have congenital absence of their spleen.

4. 10% develop lymphoma and leukemia.

Reference

Franquet T, Gimenez A, Caceres J, et al.: Imaging of pulmonary-cutaneous disorders: matching the radiologic and dermatologic findings. *Radiographics* 16:855–869, 1996.

Cross-Reference

Pediatric Radiology: THE REQUISITES, p 273.

Comment

Louis–Barr syndrome or ataxia telangiectasia is a genetically transmitted disorder (AR) that involves mutation of a gene thought to control the cell cycle and DNA repair mechanisms. The syndrome manifests as multiple capillary telangiectasias on the skin and mucous membranes. Progressive cerebellar degeneration and increased risk of lymphoma are the associated CNS entities. Clinically, cerebellar ataxia presents in childhood followed by skin lesions. These patients have cellular immune deficiency as they are congenitally lacking lymphoid tissue: spleen, thymus, and lymph nodes. IgA deficiency contributes to humeral deficiency, making these patients prone to deadly sinus and pulmonary infections that represent the leading cause of death.

On MR, the cerebellum is small with significant atrophy of the anterior vermis. Over time there is progression of cerebellar degeneration. Given the impaired DNA repair mechanism, lymphoma may be seen anywhere in the body.

Notes

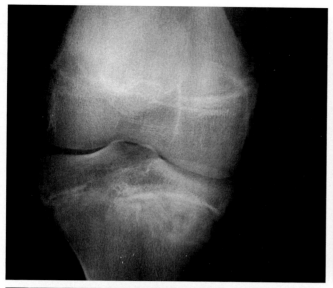

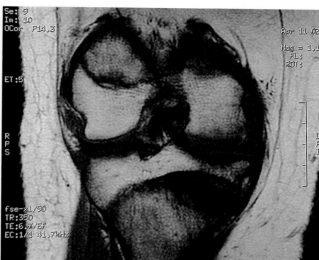

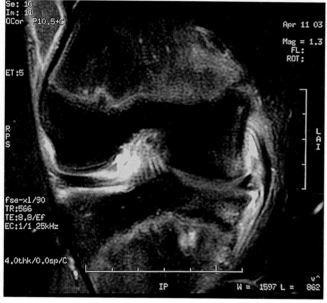

1. What ages are affected?

2. Which of the four types is most common?

3. Is obesity a risk factor?

4. Is this entity more commonly unilateral or bilateral in the infantile form?

Blount Disease (Tibia Vara)

1. The infantile form affects the 2–3 year age group, while the adolescent affects the 8–15 year age group. The third type, late onset, is in slightly older obese black children.

2. The infantile is far more common than the adolescent.

3. Yes, obesity is a risk factor.

4. Tibia vara is more commonly bilateral (60%) in the infantile form and unilateral (90%) in the adolescent form.

Reference

Greene WB. Infantile tibia vara. *J Bone Joint Surg Am* 75(1):130–143, 1993.

Cross-Reference

Pediatric Radiology: THE REQUISITES, p 249.

Comment

Blount disease, or tibia vara, is an osteochondrosis in which there is a local growth disturbance of the medial proximal tibial epiphysis. There are at least three varieties: the infantile, adolescent, and late onset. Normally as toddlers begin to walk their bones will bend medially, a phenomenon known as physiologic bowing. The bowing will normally resolve, in contrast to tibia vara, which progresses to increasing varus deformity. Mechanical factors such as increased growth and weight lead to Blount in patients with a genetic predisposition. As the center of force migrates medially the mechanics of the knee fail, leading to collapse of the medial tibial plateau cartilage. A sharp angle results at the medial side with sparing of the lateral tibial epiphysis. The adolescent and late onset forms are thought to occur due to repeated mechanical stress that leads to cartilage damage.

Radiographically, the infantile form may be distinguished from physiologic bowing by the abrupt angle at the beaked medially tibial metaphysis. In contrast, physiologic bowing will yield a gradual metaphyseal contour. A normal lateral tibial epiphysis, metaphysis, a normal distal femur, in conjuction with genu varus secondary to sharp angulation at the medial epiphysis ought to seal the diagnosis. Physiologic bowing will demonstrate a bent tibia, whereas in tibia vara the tibia shaft is not intrinsically curved. MRI may show articular cartilage hypertrophy, angulation, and an enlarged medial meniscus.

Treatment varies from conservative to surgery and is determined by staging (I–VI). Stages I and II may use a brace with good results. Stage III requires osteotomy with overcorrection, while IV, V, and VI require osteotomy with lateral physeal resection.

Notes

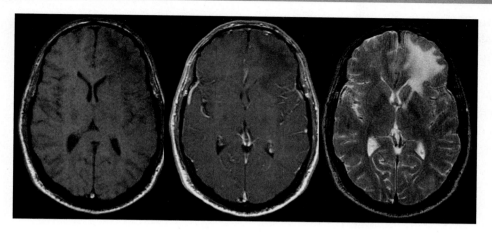

1. What are the etiologies of this entity in the pediatric age group?

2. What is the "heart of the gyrus" pattern?

3. Does this entity involve the spine?

4. The dentate nucleus is a common site of involvement, true or false?

Progressive Multifocal Leukoencephalopathy

1. Immunosuppression, leukemia, transplant, congenital HIV.

2. Sparing of the cortical ribbon with marked subcortical edema.

3. No, the spine is spared, unlike MS and acute disseminated encephalomyelitis.

4. True.

Reference

Vandersteenhoven JJ, Dbaibo G, Boyko OB, et al.: Progressive multifocal leukoencephalopathy in pediatric acquired immunodeficiency syndrome. *Pediatr Infect Dis J* 11(3):232–237, 1992.

Cross-Reference

Pediatric Radiology: THE REQUISITES, p 278.

Comment

Progressive multifocal leukoencephalopathy (PML) is caused by the Jakob–Creutzfeld virus, a papovavirus. Patients with impaired cellular immunity, HIV, congenital immune deficiency, and patients receiving chemo or immune suppressive therapy are affected. Viral infection of oligodendrocytes leads to myelin destruction and lymphocytic infiltration. Clinically, there is insidious onset of sensory deficits, paralysis, ataxia, visual loss, and decreased mentation. The diagnosis is made clinically with a positive polymerase chain reaction of the CSF and supportive imaging findings.

Multiple subcortical areas of increased signal on T2 and decreased signal on T1 within the white matter characterize the MR findings. The lesions do not enhance and show no evidence of mass effect, distinguishing them from metastatic disease. Gyri will appear thickened due to white-matter edema. The lesions are distributed in a multifocal asymmetric pattern with absence of gray-matter involvement. PML is seen most commonly in the frontal and parieto-occipital lobes but may be found in the corpus callosum, thalami, or basal ganglia—anywhere that myelin may live.

Prognosis is exceedingly poor with 6-month survival of 50%. Therapy is supportive.

Notes

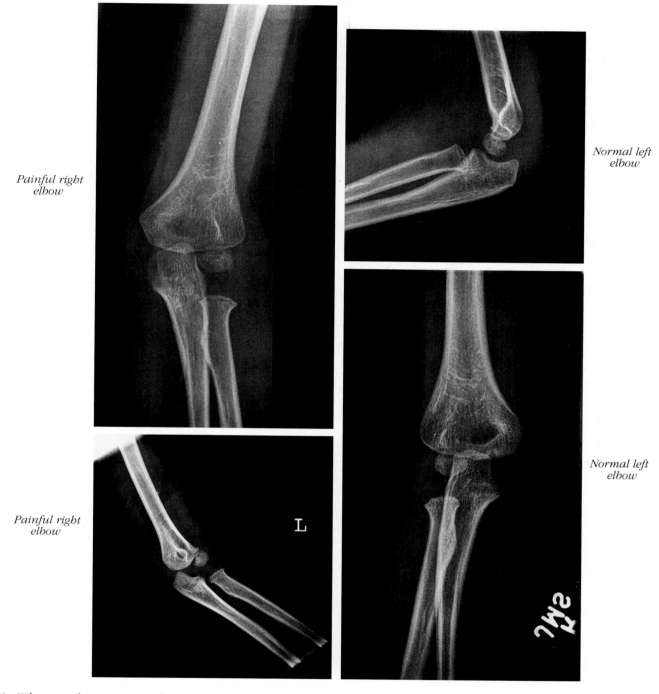

Painful right
elbow

Normal left
elbow

Painful right
elbow

L

Normal left
elbow

1. What are the two main diagnostic possibilities?

2. Is the capitellum completely ossified?

3. What is the age range of this disorder?

4. Is partial involvement of the capitellum seen in this disorder?

Panner Disease

1. Panner disease or osteochondritis dissecans.

2. The capitellum is not completely ossified in Panner disease.

3. Panner = 5–10 years.

4. No, Panner involves the whole capitellum, while osteochondritis dissecans may involve partial to complete involvement.

Reference

Stoane JM, Poplausky MR, Haller JO, et al.: Panner's disease: X-ray, MR imaging findings and review of the literature. *Comput Med Imaging Graph* 19(6): 473–476, 1995.

Cross-Reference

Musculoskeletal Imaging: THE REQUISITES, 2nd edn, p 166.

Comment

Panner disease (PD) is an avascular necrosis of the capitellum occurring primarily in boys from 5 to 10 years commonly associated with baseball and gymnastics. Considered to be largely a product of chronic microtrauma, PD is seen in throwing athletes and has been referred to as "little leaguer's elbow." Clinically, patients complain of restricted range of motion, pain on extension, and joint effusion.

Osteonecrosis of the capitellum occurs between the ages of 5–10 as that is the period in which the capitular nucleus is supplied by only one or two vessels. The vessels enter the nucleus from the posterior aspect of the ephiphysis, a region vulnerable to lateral compression secondary to repetitive valgus stress.

Radiographs demonstrate fragmentation, increased density of the capitellum, resorption of the radial head, and increasing size of the radiohumeral space. Be sure to obtain contralateral elbow films as these findings can be subtle. A radiolucent band may appear at the capitellum similar to the crescent sign seen in hip osteonecrosis. On MR the capitellum will demonstrate a dark signal on T1 and a bright signal on T2 fat sat images involving the entire bone, much like Keinbock disease involves the entirety of the lunate. In addition, the capitellum may demonstrate an irregular contour deformity. Loose body formation is not seen in contradistinction to osteochondritis dissecans, which affects the 12–16 age group.

Osteochondritis dissecans is commonly present in the dominant elbow of throwing athletes. Similar to the talar lesion, the exact etiology is unknown but thought to occur due to osteonecrosis secondary to a compromised blood supply due to repetitive microtrauma. The primary difference between Panner and osteochondritis is not the etiology but rather the substrate. In Panner the incompletely ossified capitellum will reestablish blood supply and heal without long-term deformity. The mature capitellum in osteochondritis dissecans will fragment giving rise to loose bodies and permanent deformity. A suspected loose body case may benefit from a spoiled gradient echo sequence with a three-dimensional acquisition as blooming artifact, and volumetric imaging will maximize conspicuity of a fragment.

Panner disease most often heals without sequelae following reconstitution of the blood supply. A prolonged hyperemia, however, may close the radial growth plate early, leading to radial shortening.

Notes

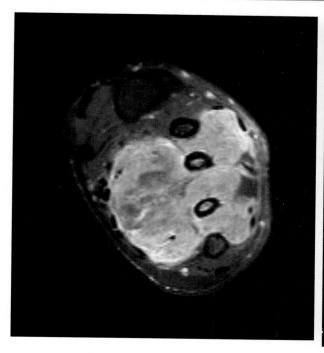
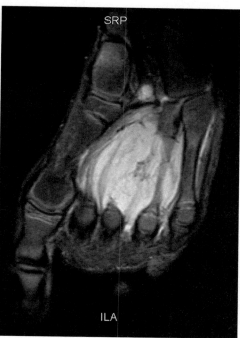

1. Where is the most common anatomic site for involvement of this lesion?

2. What is the most common pediatric soft tissue tumor?

3. What is the treatment?

4. What age group is most commonly affected?

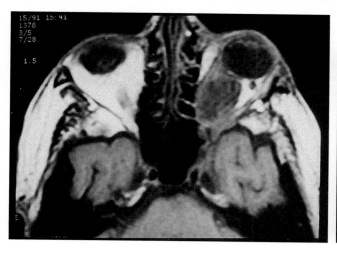
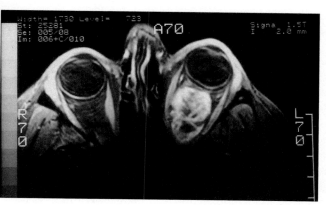

1. What neurocutaneous syndrome with 17 letters is associated with this entity?

2. What percentage of the patients with the syndrome referred to in question 1 are affected by this entity?

3. Are all these lesions genetically inherited?

4. Patients under 5 years with this diagnosis have a better prognosis, true or false?

Rhabdomyosarcoma

1. The neck is the most common anatomic site.

2. Rhabdomyosarcoma.

3. Surgery followed by chemotherapy and radiation.

4. Children between the age of 2 and 6 years.

References

McCarville MB, Spunt SL, Pappo AS: Rhabdomyosarcoma in pediatric patients: the good, the bad, and the unusual. *Am J Roentgenol* 176(6):1563–1569, 2001.

McHugh K, Boothroyd AE: The role of radiology in childhood rhabdomyosarcoma. *Clin Radiol* 54(1): 2–10, 1999.

Cross-Reference

Pediatric Radiology: THE REQUISITES, p 231.

Comment

The approach to soft tissue tumors is similar to that of bone tumors—location, size, margin, and patient age. Location can either be subcutaneous, intermuscular, or intramuscular or intra/periarticular. Rhabdomyosarcoma is an example of an intramuscular soft tissue tumor.

Rhabdomyosarcoma is the most common pediatric soft tissue sarcoma and may arise in any location of the body, excluding the brain. Rhabdo develops from totipotent mesenchymal cells that are presumed to arise from striated muscle progenitors and includes several histologic forms: embryonal, alveolar, pleomorphic and undifferentiated. The most common sites for rhabdomyosarcoma are head and neck, genitourinary tract, and skeletal muscle. The skeletal tumor is of alveolar histology in contrast to the embryonal type linked with the GU type. Presentation is often a painless mass.

Radiographically, noncalcified soft tissue fullness with possible bone erosion and periosteal reaction is typical. MR, with its superb tissue contrast, will clearly delineate the extent of the soft tissue mass—dark on T1 and bright on T2. The masses tend to vary from homogenous to heterogeneous and may undergo central necrosis. Imaging is critical in classifying treatment failure risk. Prognosis is determined by the clinical group, stage, history, and age at presentation. The clinical group is based on tumor respectability, site, size, invasiveness, and lymphadenopathy. Imaging is also used following resection for the detection of tumor recurrence.

Notes

Optic Glioma

1. NF-1, or von Recklinghausen disease.

2. 40%.

3. No, approximately half are. The other half are caused by sporadic mutations.

4. False. Patients under 5 years have a poorer prognosis.

Reference

Kornreich L, Blaser S, Schwarz M, et al.: Optic pathway glioma: correlation of imaging findings with the presence of neurofibromatosis. *Am J Neuroradiol* 22(10): 1963–1969, 2001.

Cross-Reference

Pediatric Radiology: THE REQUISITES, pp 271–272.

Comment

Optic gliomas are low-grade pilocytic astrocytomas involving the optic nerves or, in this case, the optic chiasm, and are better referred to as chiasmal gliomas. The optic nerve isn't really a nerve but rather a white-matter extension of the brain. Glial tumors are strictly confined to the brain and do not involve the peripheral nervous system. In addition to visual symptoms, patients may present with pituitary abnormalities and headaches. Two histologic types predominate, juvenile pilocytic astrocytomas and low-grade fibrillary astrocytomas. Unlike the craniopharyngioma that presents with mass effect, the chiasmal glioma produces visual symptoms early on. Pituitary abnormalities and headache are present as well.

On CT these noncalcified homogenous astrocytomas appear hypodense relative to gray matter. Bone windows may show enlargement of the optic chiasm. MR will demonstrate an enlarged optic chiasm that is isointense on T1, bright on T2, and enhances post contrast. Alternatively, optic gliomas may infiltrate the subarachnoid space encasing a normal-appearing nerve. The lesion may extend to the thalamus, basal ganglia, or frontal lobes.

Treatment involves radiotherapy alone or surgery and radiotherapy. Prognosis is variable.

Notes

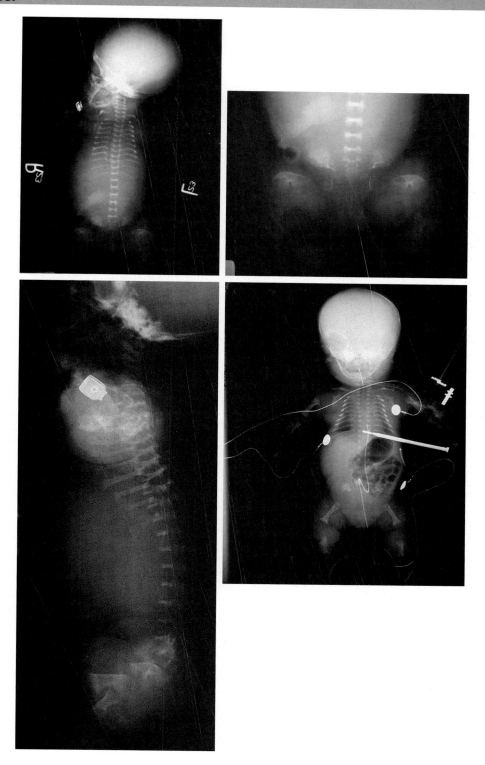

1. What is the differential diagnosis?
2. Which is the most common lethal neonatal skeletal dysplasia?
3. What is the mode of inheritance?
4. What are the findings on head MRI?

Thanatophoric Dysplasia

1. Homozygous achondroplasia, achondrogenesis I and II, short-rib polydactyly, and asphyxiating thoracic dysplasia (Jeune syndrome).

2. Osteogenesis imperfecta type II.

3. Autosomal dominant mutation.

4. Abnormal sulci with polymicrogyia and neuronal heterotopia.

Reference

Taybi H, Lachman L: *Radiology of Syndromes and Metabolic Disorders,* 4th edn. St. Louis: Mosby-Year Book, 1996, pp 939–941.

Cross-Reference

Pediatric Radiology: THE REQUISITES, p 204.

Comment

Thanatophoric dysplasia is the second most common lethal skeletal dysplasia. A mutation in a fibroblast growth factor receptor is thought to interfere with chondrocyte differentiation. Thanatophoric translates as "death-bringing" as it is often lethal in the neonatal period. Patients succumb to respiratory insufficiency from reduced thoracic capacity as well as brainstem compression from a stenotic foramen magnum. Two subtypes exist: the more common, type I, with a normal skull and curved long bones and type II, demonstrating a cloverleaf-shaped skull and straight femora.

Clinically, these patients demonstrate marked short-limb dwarfism, limb curvature, disproportionately large heads, diminutive thoracic cage, and severe developmental and growth delay if they survive the neonatal period.

Most cases are diagnosed in the second trimester via ultrasound. Findings include polyhydramnios, short, curved (I), or straight (II) femora, a large cloverleaf skull (II), small appendages, hypoplastic vertebral bodies, small thorax, and enlarged abdomen. Radiographically, the limbs are symmetrically short. Metaphyseal flaring gives the appearance of "telephone receiver"-shaped femora. The vertebral bodies appear flattened with wide intervertebral spacing. The ribs are shortened and flared. The skull is enlarged and may appear cloverleaf shaped due to early suture closure.

Treatment is supportive with VP shunting and ventilator therapy. Death by respiratory insufficiency usually occurs within the first few days of life.

Notes

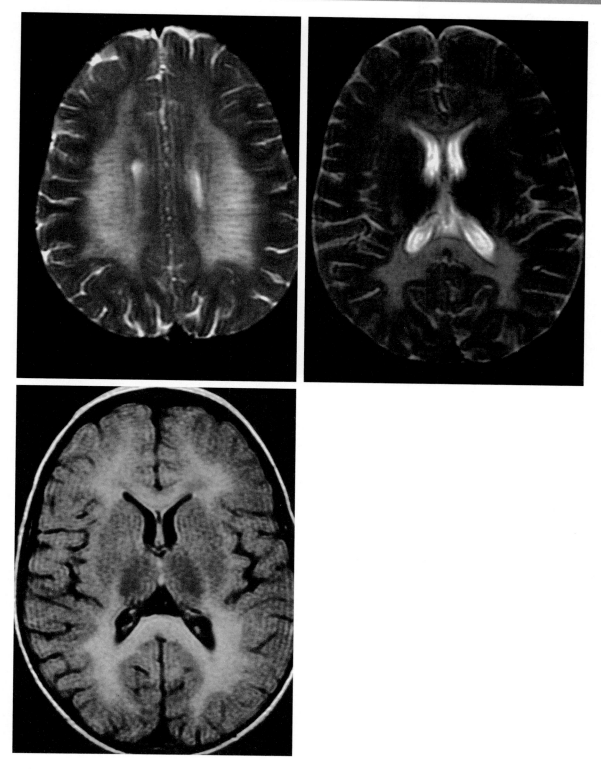

1. What is the genetics of this entity?

2. What is the distinction between demyelination and dysmyelination?

3. Is enhancement common?

4. Myelination begins at the most primitive brain structures, true or false?

Metachromatic Leukodystrophy

1. Autosomal recessive.

2. Demyelination is the breakdown of normally formed myelin. Dysmyelination refers to abnormal or absent myelin formation.

3. No, enhancement is uncommon.

4. True.

Reference
Cheon JE, Kim IO, Hwang YS, et al.: Leukodystrophy in children: a pictorial review of MR imaging features. *Radiographics* 22:461–476, 2002.

Cross-Reference
Neuroradiology: THE REQUISITES, p 219.

Comment
Metachromatic leukodystrophy (MLD) is the most common dysmyelinating disease and is caused by deficiency in the enzyme arylsulfatase A. Arylsulfatase A hydrolyzes sulfates to cerebrosides. Enzyme deficiency produces a toxic overabundance of sulfatides that cause the destruction of forming myelin. The age of onset and severity of the disease vary with the degree of enzymatic deficiency. Clinically, patients may present as infants, adolescents, or adults. Peripheral neuropathies, psychosis, hallucination, delusions, hypotonia, impaired gait, and dementia are the findings.

On imaging, you will see diffuse low density throughout the white matter as well as a high T2 signal on MR. Adults, however, will demonstrate a frontal lobe predominance in contradistinction from adrenoleukodystrophy (ADL), which hugs the periatrial white matter. The lesions tend not to enhance. One other specific finding is the sparring of the subcortical U fibers. MLD is the most common of the dysmyelinating diseases.

Myelination, as everything in pediatrics, has a temporal component. A rise in the quantity of surface membrane glycolipids leads to a corresponding drop in water content and T2 hypointensity. Remember that progression of myelination coincides with neurologic development and follows from the most primitive areas of the brain to the most recently evolved—brainstem, cerebellum, cerebrum. Infants are born with a myelinated thalamus, cerebellar peduncles, and median longitudinal fasciculus. By 3 months, the cerebellar white matter is myelinated, along with the posterior limb of the internal capsule and the paraventricular and paracentral white matter. By 6 months, the optic radiation, and splenium are myelinated, and by 1 year the anterior limbs of the internal capsule and genu or the corpus callosum are myelinated. Finally cerebral lobar myelination achieves the adult appearance by 24 months.

Notes

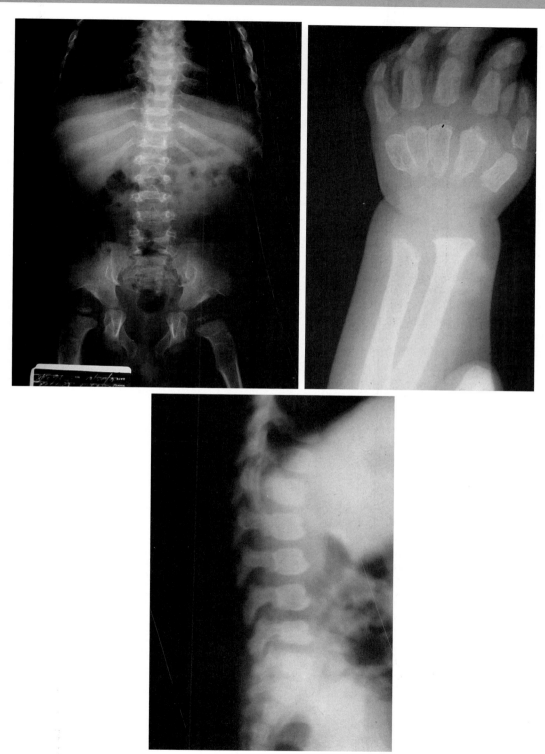

1. What is platyspondyly?

2. What entities demonstrate platyspondyly at birth?

3. What entities demonstrate platyspondyly developing later in childhood?

4. Does platyspondyly imply a congenital condition?

Morquio

1. Platyspondyly is defined as a flattened vertebral body shape with reduced distance between the endplates.

2. Congenital platyspondyly occurs in thanatophoric dysplasia, metatropic dwarfism, and osteogenesis imperfecta type IIA.

3. Platyspondyly developing in later childhood occurs in Morquio disease, spondyloepiphyseal dysplasia tarda, and Kniests dysplasia.

4. Yes, unlike verebra plana (noncongenital Langerhans cell histiocytosis), platyspondyly suggests a congenital etiology.

Reference

Mikles M, Stanton RP: A review of Morquio syndrome. *Am J Orthop* 26(8):533–540, 1997.

Cross-Reference

Pediatric Radiology: THE REQUISITES, p 209.

Comment

Morquio is one of the mucopolysaccharidoses (MPS), a group of closely related diseases resulting from genetic deficiencies of lysosomal enzymatic degradation of mucopolysaccharides. As the mucopolysaccharides build up they are deposited in multiple tissues and organs, most commonly the spleen, liver, bone marrow, lymph nodes, blood vessels, and heart.

Morquio (MPS IVA) is inherited through autosomal recessive transmission as are all the mucopolysaccharidoses with the exception of Hurler syndrome. Clinically, Morquio presents within the first 3 years of life with short-trunk dwarfism secondary to universal platyspondyly. Kyphosis, valgus deformity at the knees, hyperextensible joints, atlantoaxial subluxation, cataracts, pulmonary infections, and valvular disease are some of the clinical findings.

Radiographically, the skull will demonstrate dolichocephaly, with underdevelopment of the mastoids and flat or concave mandibular condyles. The spine demonstrates universal platyspondyly, a finding unique to Morquio within the MPSs. A small or disappearing dens with atlantoaxial subluxation and spinal stenosis are common and often a cause of acute spinal cord compression. "Canoe paddle"-shaped ribs, flared pelvis, and shortened broad bones are present as well.

Morquio leads to death by 2 years of age.

Notes

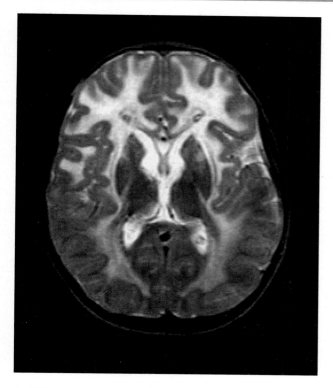

1. What are the three clinical subgroups of this entity?
2. Which is the most common subgroup?
3. Which laboratory test is diagnostic?
4. What is the histologic finding?

Alexander Disease

1. The three clinical subgroups of Alexander disease are infantile, juvenile, and adult.

2. The most common subgroup is infantile.

3. There is no laboratory test. Diagnosis is established by macrocephaly, clinical findings, and imaging.

4. Histologic findings include massive deposition of Rosenthal fibers (dense, eosinophilic, rod-like cytoplasmic inclusions found in astrocytes) in the subependymal, subpial, and perivascular regions.

Reference

Johnson AB: Alexander disease: a review and the gene. *Int J Dev Neurosci* 20(3–5):391–394, 2002.

Cross-Reference

Neuroradiology: THE REQUISITES, p 361.

Comment

Alexander disease or fibrinoid leukodystrophy is an entity of unknown etiology in which patients experience progressive white-matter disease leading to death. The disease has been divided into three clinical subgroups: infantile, juvenile, and adult. The infantile subgroup presents with macrocephaly and developmental delay, spasticity, and seizures within the first few weeks to 1 year of life. The juvenile form (7–14 years) presents with spasticity, while the adult onset is characterized by clinical findings similar to multiple sclerosis.

CT of the head will demonstrate low density in the frontal white matter, often progressing to the parietal lobe and internal capsule. Contrast enhancement at the tips of the temporal lobes may be seen early in the disease. MR will demonstrate T2 hyperintensity at the anterior temporal lobes as well. A similar pattern seen in CT is evidenced on MR with early frontal predominance extending posteriorly with progression of the disease.

The infantile form leads to psychomotor retardation with eventual death in infancy or early childhood.

Notes

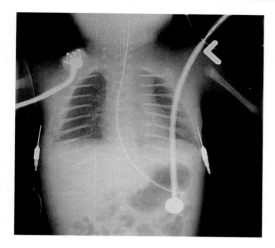

1. Which is the most common defect in this entity?
2. There is often shortening of the second metacarpal, true or false?
3. What is the most common finding in the pelvis?
4. What is the differential diagnosis?

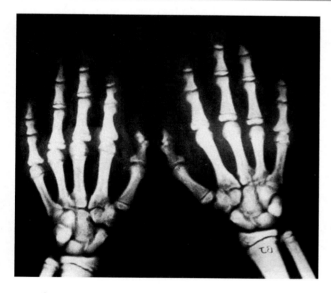

1. What artist is associated with this disease?
2. What is the differential diagnosis for acro-osteolysis?
3. What are the two main imaging features in this entity?
4. These patients are prone to osteomyelitis in what bone?

Cleidocranial Dysostosis

1. Absence of the distal clavicles.

2. False: there may be elongation of the second metacarpal.

3. Widened pubic symphysis.

4. Pyknodysostosis, osteogenesis imperfecta.

Reference
Markowitz RI, Zackai E: A pragmatic approach to the radiologic diagnosis of pediatric syndromes and skeletal dysplasias. *Radiol Clin N Am* 39(4):791–802, xi, 2001.

Cross-Reference
Pediatric Radiology: THE REQUISITES, p 198.

Comment
Enchondral ossification is the developmental mechanism of the long bone growth. Mesenchymal cells differentiate into chondroblasts and lay down a cartilage-containing framework that ossifies (provisional calcification). Osteoblasts invade the framework and replace the zone of provisional calcification with osteoid, the collagen backbone. Alternatively, flatbones develop without the help of the cartilaginous middleman and form directly from mesenchymal precursors. This process is referred to as intramembranous ossification. In cleidocranial dysostosis intramembranous formed bones (skull, clavicles, pubic bone, etc.) fail to ossify sufficiently and instead are replaced by fibrous tissue. The disorder is inherited as an autosomal dominant trait. Clinically, a large head, slender build, shrunken face, long neck, and drooping shoulders are noted. Hearing loss due to ossicular abnormalities is noted.

Radiographically the skull appears poorly calcified with widened sutures and Wormian bones. A large foramen magnum with basilar invagination is often present. In addition, a broad mandible, persistent synchondroses, and poorly formed nasal sinuses are seen. Hypoplasia, or less commonly (10%) aplasia of the clavicles, is noted with the missing segments tending toward the lateral aspects. Findings in the hand include small tapered phalanges, large epiphyses, and poor ossification of the hands.

Notes

Pyknodysostosis (Acromelic Dwarfism)

1. Toulouse-Lautrec, French painter.

2. PINCHFO: **P**soriasis, **I**njury, **N**europathic, **C**ollagen/vascular, **H**yperparathyroidism, **F**amilial, **O**ther (polyvinyl chloride exposure, snake and scorpion bites).

3. Osteosclerosis and abnormal development (hypoplastic facial bones and widened sutures).

4. Mandible.

Reference
Thora S, Nadkarni J, Singh SD, et al.: Pyknodysostosis. *Indian Pediatr* 30(6):796–798, 1993.

Cross-Reference
Pediatric Radiology: THE REQUISITES, pp 205–206.

Comment
Short stature can be symmetric or asymmetric. Asymmetric forms include short-limb, short-trunk, and proportional dwarfism. Short-limbed dwarfs are subdivided on the basis of distribution: rhizomelic, mesomelic, and acromelic. Rhizomelic involves the proximal appendicular skeleton (humeri and femura), mesomeliac the middle skeleton (radius–ulna and tibia–fibula), and acromeliac the distal skeleton (metacarpals, metatarsals, and phalanges).

Pyknodysostosis is an acromelic dwarf variant characterized by generalized osteosclerosis, short stature, short broad hands and bones that fracture frequently. It is inherited as an autosomal recessive trait. Clinically, delayed closure of the anterior fontanel in an enlarged cranium, bulging eyes, a parrot-like nose, and receding chin are reported.

Radiographically there is generalized osteosclerosis with multiple fractures of varying ages. Fractures are often transverse and diaphyseal. Hypoplastic facial bones, hypoplastic sinuses, short distal phalanges, and Wormian bones are present as well. Pyknodysostosis may be differentiated from osteopetrosis by absence of a bone in bone appearance. Patients undergo surgical reconstruction of the mandible and facial bones.

Notes

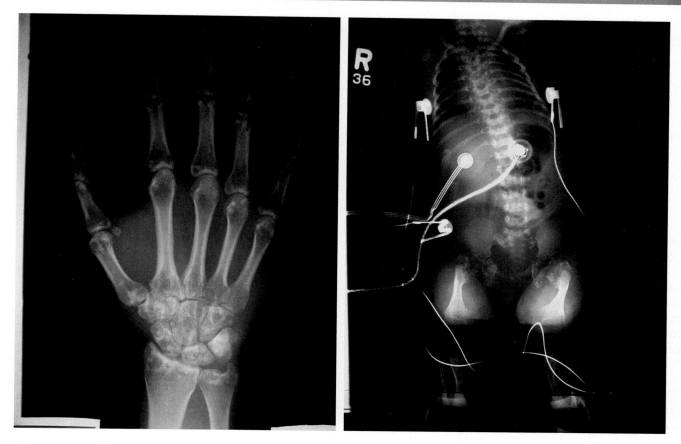

1. How many subtypes of this entity are there?

2. What is the dominant finding?

3. Is limb shortening asymmetric or symmetric?

4. Calcification of the humeral epiphysis normally occurs at what age?

Chondrodysplasia Punctata

1. Five.

2. Ossified epiphyses within the first year of life.

3. Asymmetric.

4. Never. The epiphyses normally undergo ossification!

Reference
Anderson PE: Chondrodysplasia punctata. *Skelet Radiol* 16:223, 1987.

Cross-Reference
Pediatric Radiology: THE REQUISITES, p 206.

Comment
Chondrodysplasia punctata represents a form of multiple epiphyseal dysplasia that demonstrates abnormal calcification of unossified epiphyses during the first year of life. A consensus conference has designated five subtypes. CDP is inherited by varying modes of transmission. Stippled epiphyses appear to form as a result of abnormal matrix with subsequent cyst formation and calcification. The calcification appears to interfere with proper ossification, and leads to developmental sequelae. Clinically, patients have short stature with disproportionate limb shortening. Retardation, cardiac malformations, pulmonary infections, and generalized rashes are seen.

This case represents one of the more common forms, the Conradi–Huermann syndrome subtype, an X-linked inheritance. The C-H subtype is associated with a flat nose and asymmetric limb shortening. Radiographically, punctate calcification is noted within the epiphyses. Calcification may be present within the ends of the short tubular bones, vertebral endplates, cartilage rings of the trachea, and in the cartilage of the pharynx. The more calcification noted the greater the overall severity of skeletal deformities. Calcification decreases with age and is replaced by ossified bone within 2 years. Recovery is variable. Asymmetric epiphyseal dysplasia commonly results leading to long bone shortening, vertebral deformities, and scoliosis.

Alternatively, the rhizomelic form is lethal and characterized by symmetric short-limbed dwarfism, severe pschyomotor retardation, flat face, and vertebral coronal clefting. A milder form, known as the Sheffield type, is characterized radiographically by a stippled calcaneus. The tibial–metacarpal type demonstrates decreased cervical vertebral body ossification, coronal clefts, distal ulna hypoplasia, and a short tibia with a long fibula. Stippling is predominantly found in the tarsal and carpal bones.

Prognosis is highly variable depending upon subtype and ranges from normal to lethality at birth.

Notes

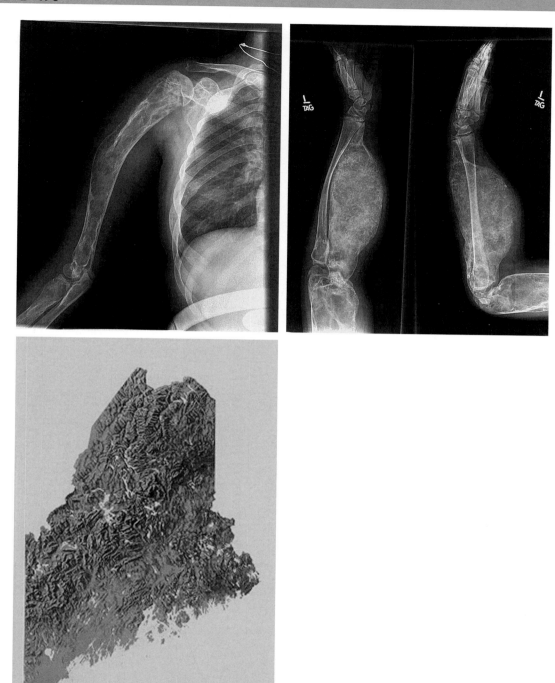

1. Is there a gender predominance?
2. Does fibrous dysplasia have a gender predominance?
3. What bone is described by the "shepherd's crook" deformity?
4. Is there malignant potential in fibrous dysplasia?

McCune–Albright Syndrome

1. Yes, nearly 90% of the cases have involved females.

2. No, fibrous dysplasia is seen equally in males and females.

3. The femur.

4. Yes, but rare; chondrosarcoma has been reported.

Reference
Gurler T, Alper M, Gencosmanoglu R: McCune–Albright syndrome progressing with severe fibrous dysplasia. *J Craniofac Surg* 9(1):79–82, 1998.

Cross-Reference
Pediatric Radiology: THE REQUISITES, p 220.

Comment
Fibrous dysplasia is a nonheritable skeletal developmental anomaly in which fibroblasts proliferate and produce fibrous tissue that combines with immature woven bone trabeculae. The lesion is commonly found in the marrow space but may extend to the cortex. The abnormal trabeculae give the characteristic ground glass appearance on conventional radiograph. A relative dearth of trabeculae will result in a lucent lesion.

Involvement may either be confined to one bone or as in this case to multiple bones. Eighty per cent are monostotic, 20% of cases are polyostotic and 2–3% are associated with endocrine abnormalities—McCune–Albright syndrome. The McCune–Albright syndrome is a triad of fibrous dysplasia, café au lait spots, and endocrine dysfunction. The associated fibrous dysplasia is often unilateral. The endocrine abnormalities commonly include precocious puberty, hyperparathyroidism, and hyperthyroidism. The café au lait spots give the appearance of the coast of Maine. The coast of Maine is thought to interdigitate more than the "smooth" coast of California.

Skin pigmentation may be present with polyostotic fibrous dysplasia in the absence of McCune–Albright. The severity of the bone involvement is much greater in polyostotic versus monostotic disease; severe involvement is unusual for monostotic fibrous dysplasia. Larger segments of bone, a younger patient profile, and more severe clinical symptomatology are seen in polyostotic versus monostotic disease.

Radiographically, unilateral disease or asymmetric large lucent lesions with sclerotic rims are noted. Bowing of weight-bearing bones is common as the structural integrity is compromised. The shepherd's crook deformity and leg length discrepancy are common manifestations of disease. Therapy is aimed at treating the complications of fractures and the endocrine abnormalities in the case of McCune–Albright.

Notes

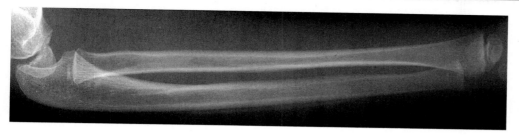

1. Which bones are most commonly affected?
2. Is the growth plate involved?
3. Cartilage is spared with this entity, true or false?
4. What are long-term sequelae in this entity?

Hypervitaminosis A

1. Most commonly the ulna and metatarsals followed by clavicles, tibia, and fibula.

2. Yes, hypervitaminosis may appear similar to rickets with respect to the physis. There may be cupping and splaying of the metaphysis with widening of the growth plate.

3. False, the epiphysis is involved with long-standing disease.

4. Short stature, flexion contractures, and leg length discrepancy.

Reference
Binkley N, Krueger D: Hypervitaminosis A and bone. *Nutr Rev* 58(5):138–144, 2000.

Cross-Reference
Pediatric Radiology: THE REQUISITES, p 217.

Comment
The acute sequelae of a massive dose of vitamin A are clinical: nausea, vomiting, and lethargy. Chronic excessive vitamin A intake results in bony proliferation along the shafts of mainly the ulna and phalanges, causing soft tissue masses and hyperostosis. The hyperostosis is most pronounced at joints and tendinous insertions with the development of entheses that may be associated with pain.

Clinically, these patients present between 1 and 3 years with pruritus, loss of appetite, and painful lumps in the soft tissues. Vitamin A is stopped and the changes reverse themselves. Differentiation from infantile cortical hyperostosis is based on location. Infantile cortical hyperostosis involves the mandible and clavicle while hypervitaminosis more commonly affects the appendicular skeleton. Infantile cortical hyperostosis produces changes by the first 6 months, while hypervitaminosis A begins demonstrating changes no earlier than 12 months.

Notes

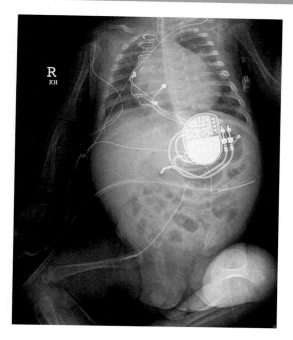

1. What are the cardiac associations in Down syndrome?

2. Which are the embryonic arch origins of the following structures: right subclavian artery, aortic arch, pulmonary arteries, and common carotid?

3. What is the most common congenital heart anomaly?

4. Enlarged heart in an adolescent or young adult + breast shadows = ?

Double Outlet Right Ventricle

1. Endocardial cushion defects, atrial septal defect (ASD), ventricular septal defect (VSD), patent ductus arteriosus, cleft mitral valve.

2. RSA = IV, AA = IV, PA = VI, CC = III.

3. Bicuspid aortic valve.

4. ASD, most common congenital defect presenting in adults.

Reference

Allen HD, Gutgesell HP, Clark EB, et al.: *Moss and Adams Heart Disease in Infants, Children and Adolescents: Including the Fetus and Young Adult,* 6th edn. Baltimore: Lippincott Williams & Wilkins, 2000, pp 1102–1120.

Cross-Reference

Pediatric Radiology: THE REQUISITES, 2nd edn, p 63.

Comment

Double outlet right ventricle is a developmental anomaly in which both the pulmonary artery and aorta arise from the right ventricle. The left ventricle must pump blood through a VSD to supply the systemic circulation with oxygenated blood. Patients may present with varying degrees of cyanosis depending on associated anomalies and the size of septal defects. If pulmonic stenosis is present the vascularity and heart size will appear decreased. If there is no significant pulmonary stenosis, increased vascularity will predominate. Ultimately the radiographic picture will vary on the associated defects.

The Taussig–Bing complex is a second type of double outlet right ventricle in which the aorta lies anterior and to the right of the pulmonary artery. It is considered an incomplete form of transposition in which the pulmonary artery is overriding the ventricular septum. A VSD, subaortic stenosis, and coarctation are present.

Notes

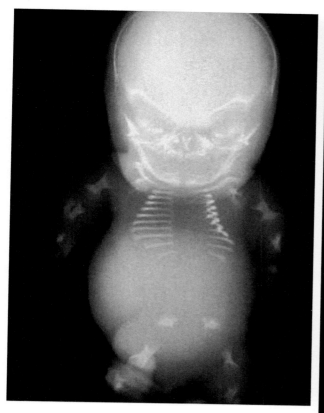
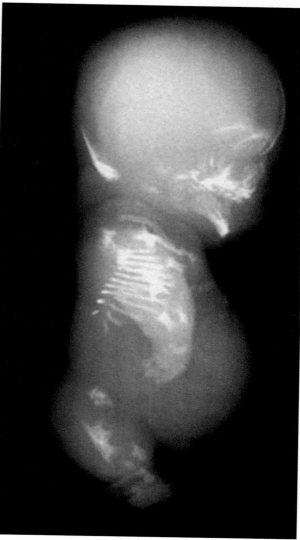

1. How might this entity present prenatally?

2. What is the differential diagnosis?

3. Is this condition lethal?

4. What is micromelic dwarfism?

Achondrogenesis

1. Prenatal presentation includes polyhydramnios, hydrops, and breech presentation.

2. Achondroplasia, hypophosphatasia, osteogenesis imperfecta, thanatophoric dwarf

3. Yes, achondrogenesis is lethal.

4. Micromelic dwarfism is symmetric disproportionately short or small limbs. That is both the proximal and distal aspects of the limbs are shortened.

Reference

Taybi H, Lachman L: *Radiology of Syndromes and Metabolic Disorders,* 4th edn. St. Louis: Mosby-Year Book, 1996, pp 746–748.

Cross-Reference

Pediatric Radiology: THE REQUISITES, p 208.

Comment

Achondrogenesis is a chondrodysplasia caused by a range of mutations that affect the normal formation of cartilage. Four types have been described in the updated system based upon radiologic findings and measurements. Recent progress in genetics has revealed different mutations in the genes that synthesize collagen. Incidence of achondrogenesis is approximately 1 in 40,000.

Type IA (Houston–Harris type) demonstrates lethal neonatal dwarfism. The mode of inheritence is autosomal recessive. Clinically, the head and trunk are disproportionately large, while both the proximal and distal aspects of the limbs are short (micromelia) and flipper-like. Radiographically, the skull is poorly ossified with small of islands of mineralized osteoid. The chest is short, with widened AP diameter, thin ribs with splayed ends, and multiple fractures. The vertebral bodies may appear unossified. An arched ilium and hypoplastic (but ossified) ischium are present. The tibia and fibula are short and flared.

In type IB (Fraccaro) stillbirth is the rule. Mode of inheritance is autosomal recessive. Clinically, the presentation is similar to the type IA: large head and trunk with small extremities. Radiographically, the skull is well ossified unlike IA. The ribs are normal, the vertebral pedicles are ossified, the ischium is unossified, the femora are trapezoidal, the tibia is stellate, and the fibula is unossified.

In type II (Langer–Saldino) the mode of inheritance is autosomal dominant. Clinically, these patients demonstrate micromelic dwarfism, enlarged cranium, and coarctation. Radiographically, the skull is large but ossification is normal. The thorax is bell shaped and intact. The vertebrae are ossified. The limbs are short

and broad with flared, cupped ends. The iliac wings are small.

Types III and IV have recently been considered to be variations of type II.

As there is no treatment for achondrogenesis, gentic counseling is vital in couples who have had a type I affected child. Recurrence risk is 1:4 (AR). Type II has a markedly lower recurrence rate as it is due to a new dominant mutation.

Notes

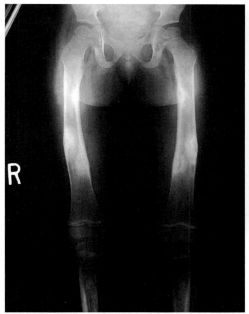
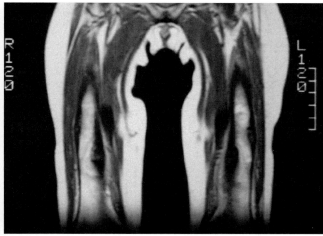
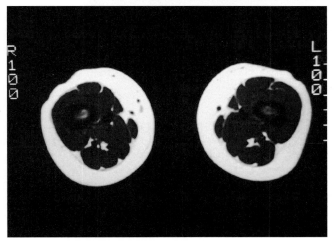

1. Which part of the skull is commonly involved?
2. Is this entity symmetric or asymmetric in most cases?
3. Sclerosis of the anterior vertebral body is a common finding, true or false?
4. What is the differential diagnosis?

Engelmann Disease

1. The skull base, which may lead to cranial nerve impingement.

2. Symmetric involvement is more common.

3. False, the posterior aspect of the vertebral body and neural arches are most often involved. Sclerotic posterior vertebral bodies and neural arches with hepatosplenomegaly on CT should get you thinking about the diagnosis.

4. Paget disease, familial hyperphosphatemia, craniodiaphyseal dysplasia, and melorrheostosis.

Reference

Vanhoenacker FM, De Beuckeleer LH, Van Hul W, et al.: Sclerosing bone dysplasias: genetic and radioclinical features. *Eur Radiol* 10(9):1423–1433, 2000.

Cross-Reference

Pediatric Radiology: THE REQUISITES, p 213.

Comment

Englemann disease or diaphyseal dysplasia is an autosomally dominant transmitted entity of unknown etiology. Defective haversian bone formation or deficient cortical vascular supply have been implicated as a possible cause. Clinical onset usually begins in the first decade with waddling gait, loss of muscle mass, muscular weakness, and extremity pain. Radiographically, diaphyseal dysplasia is characterized by irregular and inhomogenous thickening and sclerosis of the dyaphyseal corticies leading to expansion of the shaft with narrowing of the medullary cavities. Medullary cavities may be compromised to the degree that extramedullary hematopoesis develops. The epiphyses and metaphyses are characteristically spared. Involvement is largely symmetric and demonstrated most commonly in the decreasing order of frequency: tibia, femur, humerus, ulna, radius, fibula clavicle, and ribs. Skull base sclerosis is common and significant as it often leads to cranial nerve encroachment.

The disease course is highly variable and therapy is largely supportive.

Notes

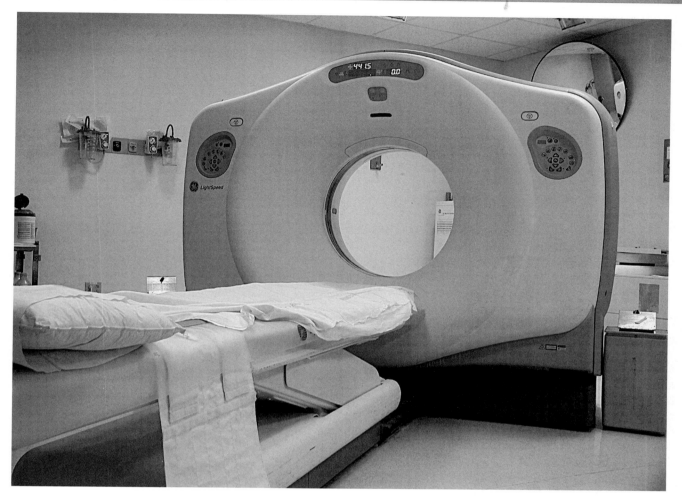

1. What is the adult exposure of a chest X-ray?

2. What is the adult exposure of a lumbar spine?

3. What is the adult exposure of a head CT?

4. What is the adult exposure of a abdominal CT?

CT Radiation Exposure

1. Chest X-ray is 0.02 mSv.

2. Lumbar spine is 1.3 mSv or 65 times a chest X-ray.

3. Head CT is 2.0 mSv or 100 times that of a chest X-ray.

4. Abdominal CT is 10 mSv or 500 times that of a chest X-ray.

References

McNitt-Gray MF: AAPM/RSNA Physics Tutorial for Residents: topics in CT: radiation dose in CT. *Radiographics* 22:1541–1553, 2002.

Brenner D, Elliston C, Hall E, et al.: Estimated risks of radiation-induced fatal cancer from pediatric CT. *Am J Roentgenol* 176(2): 289–296, 2001.

Comment

A current hot topic in radiology relates to computed tomography pediatric radiation exposure. Utilization has dramatically increased in CT over the past 5 years and continues to do so at an ever-increasing rate. This, along with a steadily growing stream of technologic advancements including helical and multidetector CT, has increased the number and scope of applications in pediatric imaging. The radiation impact of CT has recently been addressed by a number of authors who cite the importance of reducing exposure to the pediatric population. It has been estimated that pediatric head and abdominal CT in 1 year would be responsible for 480 deaths per year in the pediatric population. While the number of pediatric scans represents 4%, mortality is disproportionately estimated at 20% of all (adult and pediatric) CT-related cancer deaths.

The increased risks of CT in pediatric patients are twofold. Firstly, the smaller size of patients relative to adults creates a geometry that imparts increased exposure to the patient. Imagine a projectional PA radiograph of the chest. Radiation exposure is highest at the back skin surface as that is the closest to the radiation source. As the beam traverses the body it is attenuated by electrons subjecting the anterior skin surface the lowest exposure. In CT the X-ray source rotates around the patient creating concentric rings of differing exposure, higher in the superficial tissue and lower in the deep tissues. In children, however, smaller size leads to reduced attenuation and uniform high exposure. A simpler way of understanding it is the more intuitive grilling analogy. If you make a small hamburger it is likely to cook quickly and uniformly. Alternatively, big thick hamburgers will cook on the outside while remaining pink and cool on the inside.

The second component in increasing CT risk relates to the patient's age. Radiation risks are always higher in younger patients as they undergo a greater number of cell divisions in a lifetime each with an additive risk of mutation and resulting malignancy.

Studies indicate that children receive two to six times the necessary dose for diagnostic quality images. There are many strategies to reducing dose. Numerous studies suggest that dose may be reduced without loss of diagnostic quality. Reducing the mAS will lower exposure as fewer photons bombard the patient. The downside is decreasing signal to noise. kVp may be raised; however, this will lower contrast. The pitch refers to the distance the table moves during one rotation of the gantry. Lowered pitch will lower radiation, much like walking quickly over hot coals is preferred over a slow stroll. The price paid for increasing pitch is increased effective slice thickness with associated increased volume averaging. One caveat: a number of today's multidetector scanners will automatically increase mAS with an increase in pitch; consult your vendor. Increasing slice thickness will lower radiation exposure but increase volume averaging as well.

New strategies are currently being built into today's scanners to modulate current in real time, allowing for the optimization of diagnostic image as a function of dose.

Notes

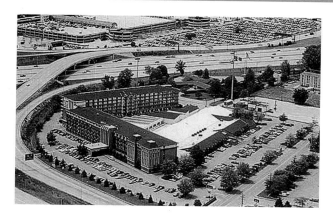

1. What is the correct pronounciation of centimeter?
2. What is the distinction between significance and substantial?
3. What is the local pronunciation of Louisville, Kentucky?
4. How long did it take to write this book?

Executive West

1. Centimeter is pronounced SEN-ti-meter, **NOT** SAHN-ti-meter.

2. Substantial refers to quantity, while significant implies that one phenomenon implies another.

3. LOO-uh-vul

4. Six years, four cities, four jobs, three girlfriends (RJW), a fortune in long distance charges and air fares (JGB), four publishers, and one patient series editor.

Comment

Let's face it, chances are you are not in one of those Fiji lagoon huts leisurely flipping through this book in hopes of gleaning some radiology knowledge. You are, however, frantically banging through case book after case book in anticipation of the American Society for Irritable Bowel Syndrome conference held annually in Louisville, Kentucky at the posh Executive West, resort of choice for the radiology academic elite. It's most likely February, March, or even May and you're feeling the pressure of boards approaching. Much stress, anxiety, and attention is paid to the boards during training, some deserved and some not. The best overall strategy is start early, real early. First year would be ideal but as you read this first year was probably 2.5 years ago. Here are some of the strategies that have worked in the past.

Firstly, take care of housekeeping. As soon as you find out your date, book a flight to Louisville. As UPS is the only carrier that is hubbed in Louisville you may be looking at a connection unless you are willing to crate up and send yourself United Parcel. Make sure your flight is no more than one connection as multiple segments only increase your chances of missing your plane, a serious setback. Book a room close by; there are several options in the area.

The exam is like every other test you've taken over the last 10 years. It has to be studied for specifically. Don't believe anyone who says the key to the boards is sitting at the alternator/PACS workstation and reading cases. Not true, unless you routinely see thanatophoric dwarfs, pyknodysostosis, or Canavan disease. Having said that, there are a substantial number of board cases devoted to everyday management issues. The boards are not all about the esoteric. Remember the rationale for the exam: to make sure that the radiologists that enter practice are not a danger to patients, themselves, and the field.

Case books and board reviews are your main tools. Book your attendings early, you never know when schedules may conflict. Remember that this is their personal time and reviews are out of the goodness of their heart. Try to choose attendings that are either board examiners or have had recent experience with the boards. A well-meaning attending with a bunch of "interesting cases" may be a waste of precious time. In preparation, steer clear from lengthy didactic texts unless you want to delve deeper into a specific area in which you feel weak. And start early. Begin getting it together a month or so after the writtens; it will lower your overall stress level and allow your years of hard work to shine through.

Ten sections, 10 rooms, 10 examiners. Be courteous and quiet. Let them know you understand the weight of the examination. A flippant attitude may put your examiner off and tarnish your performance. Alternatively, a competitive and defensive posture may produce the same undesirable effect. The overwhelming majority of examiners are there to facilitate your passing. Let them help you—these guys want you to pass. If you sense they are pushing you in one direction then play along, don't fight them, you will lose. Be careful not to say too much. The conventional wisdom dictates that you give a few reasonable differentials in cases that call for them. Don't give differentials for aunt Minnies. Examiners are looking for a sense of how you might interpret films once you are in practice. If you don't know what you are looking at, take a deep breath and think again, you've probably seen it. Alternatively, you may begin verbalizing a coherent thought process so they know at least you are thinking. Don't let a single case rattle you, you can easily recover.

After the morning and afternoon sessions the group gets together and decides who passes, conditions, and fails. The decision will probably be made before your plane touches down at your home airport. You'll spend about 5 hours after the exam second guessing yourself. Don't be discouraged, you will have done better than you thought. The next step is the waiting. Mail service in the same city can be variable. The ABR doesn't mail the passes out early followed by failures and conditions so be patient despite the rising anxiety. When you do receive the letter, treat yourself to opening it in a memorable location as it will undoubtedly be emblazoned in your memory for a very long time.

Good luck.